Surgical Complications

Guest Editor

CHRISTOPHER A. ADIN, DVM

VETERINARY CLINICS OF NORTH AMERICA: SMALL ANIMAL PRACTICE

www.vetsmall.theclinics.com

September 2011 • Volume 41 • Number 5

SAUNDERS an imprint of ELSEVIER, Inc.

W.B. SAUNDERS COMPANY
A Division of Elsevier Inc.

1600 John F. Kennedy Blvd. • Suite 1800 • Philadelphia, PA 19103-2899

http://www.vetsmall.theclinics.com

VETERINARY CLINICS OF NORTH AMERICA: SMALL ANIMAL PRACTICE Volume 41, Number 5
September 2011 ISSN 0195-5616, ISBN-13: 978-1-4557-1042-3

Editor: John Vassallo; j.vassallo@elsevier.com
Developmental Editor: Donald Mumford

Veterinary Clinics of North America: Small Animal Practice (ISSN 0195-5616) is published bimonthly (For Post Office use only: volume 41 issue 5 of 6) by Elsevier Inc., 360 Park Avenue South, New York, NY 10010-1710. Months of issue are January, March, May, July, September, and November. Business and Editorial Offices: 1600 John F. Kennedy Blvd., Ste. 1800, Philadelphia, PA 19103-2899. Customer Service Office: 3251 Riverport Lane, Maryland Heights, MO 63043. Periodicals postage paid at New York, NY and additional mailing offices. Subscription prices are $262.00 per year (domestic individuals), $427.00 per year (domestic institutions), $128.00 per year (domestic students/residents), $347.00 per year (Canadian individuals), $525.00 per year (Canadian institutions), $385.00 per year (international individuals), $525.00 per year (international institutions), and $186.00 per year (international and Canadian students/residents). To receive student/resident rate, orders must be accompanied by name of affiliated institution, date of term, and the signature of program/residency coordinator on institution letterhead. Orders will be billed at individual rate until proof of status is received. Foreign air speed delivery is included in all *Clinics* subscription prices. All prices are subject to change without notice. **POSTMASTER:** Send address changes to *Veterinary Clinics of North America: Small Animal Practice,* Elsevier Health Sciences Division, Subscription Customer Service, 3251 Riverport Lane, Maryland Heights, MO 63043. Customer Service (orders, claims, online, change of address): Elsevier Periodicals Customer Service, Elsevier Health Sciences Division, Subscription Customer Service, 3251 Riverport Lane, Maryland Heights, MO 63043. Tel: 1-800-654-2452 (U.S. and Canada); 314-447-8871 (outside U.S. andCanada). Fax: 314-447-8029. E-mail: journalscustomerservice-usa@elsevier.com (for print support); journalsonlinesupport-usa@elsevier.com (for online support).

Reprints. For copies of 100 or more of articles in this publication, please contact the Commercial Reprints Department, Elsevier Inc., 360 Park Avenue South, New York, NY 10010-1710. Tel.: 212-633-3812; Fax: 212-462-1935; E-mail: reprints@elsevier.com.

Veterinary Clinics of North America: Small Animal Practice is also published in Japanese by Inter Zoo Publishing Co., Ltd., Aoyama Crystal-Bldg 5F, 3-5-12 Kitaaoyama, Minato-ku, Tokyo 107-0061, Japan.

Veterinary Clinics of North America: Small Animal Practice is covered in *Current Contents/Agriculture, Biology and Environmental Sciences, Science Citation Index, ASCA, MEDLINE/PubMed (Index Medicus), Excerpta Medica,* and *BIOSIS*.

Printed in the United States of America.

Contributors

GUEST EDITOR

CHRISTOPHER A. ADIN, DVM
Diplomate, American College of Veterinary Surgeons; Associate Professor, Small Animal Surgery, Department of Veterinary Clinical Sciences, College of Veterinary Medicine, The Ohio State University, Columbus, Ohio

AUTHORS

CHRISTOPHER A. ADIN, DVM
Diplomate, American College of Veterinary Surgeons; Associate Professor, Small Animal Surgery, Department of Veterinary Clinical Sciences, College of Veterinary Medicine, The Ohio State University, Columbus, Ohio

PIERRE AMSELLEM, Docteur Vétérinaire, MS
Diplomate, American College of Veterinary Surgeons, Wey Referrals, Woking, United Kingdom

DENNIS J. CHEW, DVM
Diplomate, American College of Veterinary Internal Medicine (Internal Medicine); Professor, Department of Veterinary Clinical Sciences, College of Veterinary Medicine, The Ohio State University, Columbus, Ohio

JOAO FELIPE DE BRITO GALVAO, MV, MS
Currently, Diplomate, American College of Veterinary Internal Medicine (Internal Medicine); Internist, Arboretum View Animal Hospital, Downers Grove, Illinois; Formerly, Resident, Small Animal Internal Medicine, The Ohio State University, Columbus, Ohio

GARY W. ELLISON, DVM, MS
Diplomate, American College of Veterinary Surgeons; Professor and Service Chief, Small Animal Surgery, Department of Small Animal Clinical Sciences, College of Veterinary Medicine, University of Florida, Gainesville, Florida

LAUREN R. MAY, VMD
Diplomate, American College of Veterinary Surgeons; Veterinary Specialists of Rochester, Rochester, New York

PHILIPP D. MAYHEW, BVM&S, MRCVS
Diplomate, American College of Veterinary Surgeons; Assistant Professor of Small Animal Surgery, School of Veterinary Medicine, Department of Surgical and Radiological Sciences, University of California-Davis, Davis, California

MARY A. MCLOUGHLIN, DVM, MS
Diplomate, American College of Veterinary Surgeons; Associate Professor, Department of Veterinary Clinical Sciences, College of Veterinary Medicine, The Ohio State University, Columbus, Ohio

STEPHEN J. MEHLER, DVM
Diplomate, American College of Veterinary Surgeons; Veterinary Specialists of Rochester, Rochester, New York

ANDREW MERCURIO, DVM, MS
Department of Small Animal Surgery, The Ohio State University Veterinary Medical Center, Columbus, Ohio

LAURA L. NELSON, DVM, MS
Diplomate, American College of Veterinary Surgeons; Assistant Professor, Department of Small Animal Clinical Sciences, Michigan State University College of Veterinary Medicine, East Lansing, Michigan

BRIAN A. SCANSEN, DVM, MS
Diplomate, American College of Veterinary Internal Medicine (Cardiology); Assistant Professor of Cardiology and Interventional Medicine, Department of Veterinary Clinical Sciences, College of Veterinary Medicine, The Ohio State University, Columbus, Ohio

DANIEL D. SMEAK, DVM
Diplomate, American College of Veterinary Surgeons; Chief of Surgery, Department of Veterinary Clinical Sciences, Colorado State University, College of Veterinary Medicine and Biomedical Sciences, Veterinary Teaching Hospital, Fort Collins, Colorado

Contents

> Metabolic complications of endocrine surgery occur commonly and precautions should be taken to avoid potentially life-threatening situations and to lessen expense associated with a more extended hospital stay. Common complications of endocrine surgery as well as prevention strategies will be reviewed for pancreatic, parathyroid, and adrenal surgery.

> Due to the negative effects of urine on wound healing, the high rate of complications associated with surgical incisions in the ureter and a desire to avoid large open approaches to the abdomen, there is a strong trend in human medicine toward the use of endoscopic methods in the treatment of upper urinary tract disease. However, the small size of urogenital structures in companion animals has prevented the widespread application of endoscopy of the upper urinary tract and surgery continues to be the mainstay of treatment. Through careful decision making, veterinary surgeons now use microsurgical technique and interventional radiology to provide a high success rate. The current review will discuss complications pertaining to surgery of the kidney and ureter in companion animals, using experimental and clinical data to guide the detection and avoidance of these complications.

> Surgical procedures of the lower urinary tract are commonly performed in small animal practice. Cystotomy for removal of uroliths and urethrostomy diverting urine outflow due to urethral obstruction are the most commonly performed surgical procedures of the bladder and urethra respectively. Surgical procedures of the lower urinary tract are typically associated with few complications, including leakage of urine, loss of luminal diameter (stricture or stenosis), urine outflow obstruction, tissue devitalization, denervation, urinary incontinence, urinary tract infection, and death. Complications can result from inappropriate or inadequate diagnosis, localization, and surgical planning; failure to respect regional anatomy, and other causes.

The small animal surgeon creates wounds in the gastrointestinal (GI) tract for biopsy, for foreign body or neoplasm removal, or to relieve obstruction. Unlike a skin wound, dehiscence of a wound of the GI tract often leads to generalized bacterial peritonitis and potentially death. Technical failures and factors that negatively affect GI healing are of great clinical significance. Surgery of the GI tract must be considered clean-contaminated at best; as one progresses aborally down the GI tract, the bacterial population increases. Intraoperative spillage, wound dehiscence, or perforations that occur in the lower small intestine or colon tend to be associated with a relatively higher mortality rate.

The most common hepatic procedures performed in companion animals are liver biopsies and partial or complete liver lobectomies. Although these procedures are relatively simple to perform in healthy animals, surgery in clinical patients with liver disease is often complicated by the presence of significant systemic illness or by the technical challenges associated with removing massive hepatic tumors. An in-depth understanding of the possible complications that can occur with hepatic surgery helps to provide the best possible outcome for the patient by allowing the surgeon to not only take precautions to try to prevent complications but allows one to monitor for them postoperatively and treat them early if noted.

Surgery of the biliary tract is demanding and is associated with several potentially life-threatening complications. Veterinarians face challenges in obtaining accurate diagnosis of biliary disease, surgical decision-making, surgical hemostasis and bile peritonitis. Intensive perioperative monitoring is required to achieve early recognition of common postoperative complications. Proper treatment and ideally, avoidance of surgical complications can be achieved by gaining a clear understanding physiology, anatomy, and the indications for hepatobiliary surgery.

Surgery of the upper airway is performed in dogs for the correction of brachycephalic airway syndrome and laryngeal paralysis and for temporary or permanent tracheostomy. Although technically simple to perform, upper airway surgeries can lead to the development of significant postoperative complications. This article reviews complications associated with common surgical conditions of the upper airway. It involves a discussion of brachycephalic airway syndrome and associated respiratory and gastrointestinal complications. It also covers laryngeal paralysis with a focus on unilateral arytenoid lateralization and the complication of aspiration pneumonia. The condition of acquired laryngeal webbing/stenosis and potential treatment options is also discussed. Finally, tracheostomies and associated complications in dogs and cats are reviewed.

Total ear canal ablation combined with bulla osteotomy is a salvage procedure recommended primarily for end-stage inflammatory ear canal disease but also for neoplasia and severe traumatic injuries. Due to the complexity of the procedure and the poor exposure associated with the surgical approach, there is significant risk for a variety of complications. This review discusses intraoperative, early postoperative, and late postoperative complications reported in large retrospective studies, the causes for these complications, and recommendations about how to prevent them.

Factors that affect wound healing include the general health of the patient, nutritional status, and wound factors. Treatments such as corticosteroids, chemotherapy, or radiation are also common causes of delayed healing. Multimodal cancer treatment has become more common and the veterinary surgeon may be required to perform reconstructive procedures on an animal that has received or will receive chemotherapy and/or radiation treatments. Complications of reconstructive cutaneous procedures include seroma, hematoma formation, infection, wound dehiscence, distal tip necrosis of skin flaps, paresthesia, and free skin graft failure. Procedures such as maxillectomy or hemipelvectomy also have complications. Knowledge of common complications can facilitate client education and even allow the surgeon to avoid these complications.

Minimally invasive surgery (MIS) has become increasingly popular in recent years for diagnosis and treatment of an ever-expanding list of disease processes in small animal patients. Reports in the veterinary literature have documented a large number of MIS alternatives to traditional open surgery albeit mostly in small cohorts of patients. Advantages of MIS have been documented by many investigators and include significant decreases in postoperative pain, length of hospital stay, and analgesic requirements, as well as other types of morbidity, with some procedures now being performed on an outpatient basis. However, MIS procedures are not without surgical morbidity and in some cases may be associated with higher levels or different types of complications compared to open surgery.

Complications following elective spay or neuter procedures are particularly feared by new graduates. However, even the most experienced surgeons may encounter surgical or postoperative complications. At best, complications associated with elective procedures can harm the doctor-client relationship. At worst, these can present legal and financial problems. Veterinary surgeons should be aware of the potential complications associated with elective sterilization, these should be communicated to the client, and there should be a clear plan for action when a complication occurs. This article reviews the reported complications encountered in elective sterilization surgery in companion animals, with a special focus on early detection and prevention.

Surgical site infections (SSIs) are a significant source of morbidity, mortality, and cost associated with small animal surgery. The most well-established strategies to reduce the impact of SSI are preventive, focusing on bolstering host immunity while decreasing wound contamination during surgery. When SSI is identified, the use of consistent definitions and culture-based therapy help to facilitate surveillance and appropriate management. Debridement and open wound management of infected wounds are important for successful treatment.

THE CLINICS ARE NOW AVAILABLE ONLINE!

Access your subscription at:
www.theclinics.com

Preface

Surgical Complications

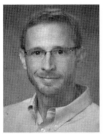

Christopher A. Adin, DVM
Guest Editor

"Although today we are spared the horror of operations without anesthesia and the misery of mortality from uncontrolled hospital gangrene, we still find there are other problems that we have to face with steadfastness, self-control and intensity of purpose if we are to achieve that very great contentment and happiness in successful treatment of our patients . . .. I remember at an early stage of our development of the surgery of mitral valve stenosis, about 1948 or 1949, we had four successive deaths in one ward. Despair stalked before us and everyone's morale was low. I recall saying to my team that we could only do one of two things, give up or go on; that it was impossible to give up as we were certainly in the right; the only thing therefore, that we should do was go on. This we did and had 30 consecutive successful cases. Tenacity of purpose must be accompanied by serenity of purpose and a surgeon requires this serenity in addition to technical dexterity."

— *Sir Russel Brock, MS, FRCS (Eng), FRACS (Hon.), FACS (Hon.), from "Philosophy of Surgery," an address given upon his receipt of the Gairdner Foundation International Award in 1961 and published in the Canad Med Assoc J 1962;86:370-2.*

This quotation, from a pioneer in open heart surgery, reflects an ongoing trend in veterinary surgery. As we continue to achieve technological advancements in both diagnosis and treatment of surgical disease, surgeons will continually be challenged with new and more complicated procedures that will, initially, have a steep learning curve. As an introduction to this excellent series of articles concerning surgical complications in veterinary surgery, I think that it is appropriate to point out that, although complications must give us pause and compel us to improve, they must not be allowed to create a feeling of self-doubt that prevents us from achieving our ultimate goal: successful care for our patients. I would like to thank the authors for

Vet Clin Small Anim 41 (2011) xi–xii
doi:10.1016/j.cvsm.2011.07.002   **vetsmall.theclinics.com**
0195-5616/11/$ – see front matter © 2011 Elsevier Inc. All rights reserved.

their own "tenacity of purpose" in continuing to improve our approach to veterinary surgery.

Christopher A. Adin, DVM
Department of Veterinary Clinical Sciences
College of Veterinary Medicine
The Ohio State University
610 Vernon Tharp Street
Columbus, OH 43210, USA

E-mail address:
Christopher.Adin@cvm.osu.edu

Metabolic Complications of Endocrine Surgery in Companion Animals

Joao Felipe de Brito Galvao, MV, MS*
Dennis J. Chew, DVM

KEYWORDS

- Hyperparathyroidism • Insulinoma • Adrenalectomy
- Hypercalcemia • Thromboembolism • Hypertension

Metabolic complications of endocrine surgery occur commonly and precautions should be taken to avoid potentially life-threatening situations and to lessen expense associated with a more extended hospital stay. Common complications of endocrine surgery as well as prevention strategies will be reviewed for pancreatic, parathyroid, and adrenal surgery.

PANCREATIC SURGERY

Pancreatic surgery is indicated as the primary means of therapy for canine insulinoma. Unfortunately, surgical manipulation of the pancreas can result in a variety of complications, including vomiting, refractory pancreatitis, pancreatic exocrine insufficiency, and diabetes mellitus. The prevalence and consequences of metastasis, benefits and goals of surgery, and possible complications and mortality should be discussed with clients before surgery.

Approximately 45% (129 of 285) of dogs with insulinoma were reported to have metastasis detected at the time of surgery.[1–8] Additionally, 11.5% (7 of 61) of dogs had multiple pancreatic nodules.[2,6] Whenever possible, partial pancreatectomy is recommended to achieve maximal local disease control in dogs with insulinoma. The only study that reported data on nodulectomy for insulinoma described a median survival time (345 days in 10 dogs)[2] that was shorter than the reported median survival times in dogs undergoing partial pancreatectomy (534 days in 60 dogs).[2,6,7] The goals of surgery are to achieve a definitive diagnosis of insulinoma and to potentially increase the overall median survival time by decreasing gross disease. Combining the

The authors have nothing to disclose.
Small Animal Internal Medicine, The Ohio State University, 601 Vernon Tharp Street, Columbus, OH 43210, USA
* Corresponding author. Arboretum View Animal Hospital, 2551 Warrenville Road, Downers Grove, IL 60515.
E-mail address: jfgalvao@me.com

Vet Clin Small Anim 41 (2011) 847–868
doi:10.1016/j.cvsm.2011.05.012
0195-5616/11/$ – see front matter © 2011 Elsevier Inc. All rights reserved.

results of previous retrospective studies, the median survival time for medical management as the only treatment was 124 days (22 dogs),[6,7] and for surgical intervention with or without medical management, 436 days (102 dogs).[2,6,7] These results support the need for surgical intervention whenever possible.

Insulinomas are considered malignant in dogs. Location of the tumors is variable, with tumors located near the accessory pancreatic duct and biliary duct being considered less amenable to resection. Ideally, dogs with nonresectable tumors would not undergo surgery because fasting or manipulation of the pancreas can lead to refractory hypoglycemia and pancreatitis after surgery. Unfortunately, it can be extremely challenging to classify tumors as resectable or nonresectable based on standard methods of preoperative staging and surgical exploration is typically required.

Preoperative Considerations

The patient should not be fasted for longer than 8 to 10 hours, to minimize the risk for hypoglycemic seizures. Clinical signs should be closely monitored to avoid the development of seizures. Ideally, dextrose supplementation should be avoided unless the dog has clinical signs compatible with hypoglycemia (eg, tachycardia, muscle tremors, weakness, seizures). The use of anesthetic premedications that alter glycemic control such as dexmedetomidine is controversial. Alpha-2 agonists may exacerbate hyperglycemia due to decreased insulin secretion occasionally seen immediately after partial pancreatectomy.

Intraoperative Considerations

Inability to achieve complete resection of the primary tumor and the presence of gross metastasis at the time of surgery are important markers of postoperative complications and should be considered. Dogs with gross metastasis at the time of surgery or those with non-resected primary tumors are more prone to persistent hypoglycemia after surgery, which may be exacerbated by pancreatitis or stimulation of the neoplastic islet cells during surgical manipulation. Moreover, even though partial pancreatectomy may offer better disease control, this technique may be associated with a higher morbidity, especially when en bloc resection is performed at the central portion of the pancreas, necessitating biliary and intestinal reconstruction. These consequences should be addressed a priori when weighing the cost-benefit ratio for surgical intervention. Many surgeons will perform aggressive resection with partial pancreatectomy in dogs that have peripheral lesions near the tip of the left or right pancreatic lobes. In dogs with central lesions, nodulectomy can be considered in an attempt to minimize surgically induced morbidity while still achieving some degree of cytoreduction.

Postoperative Considerations

Postoperative complications of pancreatectomy include persistent hypoglycemia, seizures, pancreatitis, and transient hyperglycemia. These complications are discussed in detail next.

Hypoglycemia is the most common postoperative complication following insulinoma surgery (**Table 1**). Based on the compilation of data available from previously published retrospective case series on insulinomas, hypoglycemia is estimated to occur in one third of dogs undergoing surgery and one third of those may die from complications associated with hypoglycemia.[1,2,4–7] Glycemic control after surgery is usually accomplished in a stepwise approach (**Table 2**). First, supplementation of 2.5% dextrose in intravenous fluids is routinely performed until the dog has recovered from surgery and is eating. More dextrose is added only if the patient develops clinical

Table 1
Postoperative complications in canine insulinoma with compiled prevalence and mortality available

Complications	Prevalence (affected, total)	Mortality (affected, total)
Hypoglycemia	35.5% (72, 203)[1,2,4–7,11]	12.8% (5, 39)[1,7]
Pancreatitis	18.1% (26, 144)[2,5–7,11]	3.5% (4, 113)[2,6,7,11]
Hyperglycemia	16.6% (33, 171)[1,2,4–7]	
Delayed wound healing	12.9% (4, 31)[5]	
Death	9.7% (3, 31)[5]	9.7% (3, 31)[5]
Ventricular arrhythmias	6.5% (2, 31)[5]	
Hemorrhage	6.5% (2, 31)[5]	
Seizures	5.1% (3, 59)[2,5]	1.7% (1, 59)[2,5]
Duodenal necrosis	3.6% (1, 28)[2]	3.6% (1, 28)[2]
Sepsis	3.0% (2, 66)[6,11]	3.0% (2, 66)[6,11]
Cardiac arrest	3.0% (3, 100)[1,2,11]	3.0% (3, 100)[1,2,11]

signs compatible with hypoglycemia (ie, tremors, significant lethargy, seizures). It is not recommended to oversupplement patients with dextrose as the neoplastic beta cells are usually responsive to serum glucose and a rebound effect can be seen.[9] If dextrose supplementation (2.5%–5%) is not effective in controlling clinical signs, glucagon as a constant rate infusion (5–40 ng/kg/min IV diluted in saline) can also be used.[10] Glucagon has been reported to be effective as a sole therapy, although the authors prefer to use it in conjunction with dextrose in animals that are refractory to dextrose alone.[10] If these treatments fail to prevent clinical signs of hypoglycemia, glucocorticosteroids or diazoxide should be considered. Glucocorticosteroids (dexamethasone 0.3 mg/kg/d IV) should be used with caution due to the potential for negative effects on wound healing in the surgical patient. Diazoxide is a nondiuretic benzothiadiazide that increases blood glucose by blocking insulin release, stimulating epinephrine release, and inhibiting cellular glucose uptake.[10] Diazoxide (6.6–40 mg/kg/d divided doses) may be used on a long-term basis, and though it is considered to be moderately effective (up to 70%) in controlling hypoglycemia, it is not commonly used because of the high cost of this drug[2,11,12] (see **Table 2**). The most common side effects of this drug are gastrointestinal. As a last resort, octreotide, a somatostatin analog, can be administered at 10 to 50 μg (alternatively 2–4 μg/kg) SC q 8–12 h.[13] This drug has been successful in humans to decrease hypoglycemia and is used before tumor resection. In humans, it has been thought to decrease the potential for pancreatitis.[14] Unfortunately, this drug has shown disappointing results in controlling hypoglycemia in dogs.[13] If the previously described therapy fails or if the dog develops refractory seizures, we recommend anesthetizing the dog with propofol or pentobarbital for 4 to 12 hours while continuing the therapy just described (see **Table 2**).

Seizures are typically a direct continuation of progressive hypoglycemic signs. It is important to be aggressive in the control of seizures to prevent permanent brain injury. Most seizures are directly related to current hypoglycemia, but seizures may persist even after the correction of hypoglycemia due to the presence of underlying brain damage (neuroglycopenia leading to superficial neuronal necrosis). Increased intracranial pressure and cerebral edema may develop as consequences of hypoglycemia, even after hypoglycemia has resolved.[15,16] To our knowledge, there are no

Table 2
Treatments for hypoglycemia and postoperative seizures in dogs with insulinoma

Treatment	Doses	Possible Side Effects
Dextrose (maintenance)	2.5%–5% in IV fluids	Higher doses may lead to rebound hypoglycemia
Dextrose (crisis)	25% dextrose 1 mL/kg IV	May lead to rebound hypoglycemia
Prednisone	0.5–1 mg/kg/d PO	May lead to delayed healing when used postoperatively
Dexamethasone	0.2–0.3 mg/kg/d IV	May lead to delayed healing when used postoperatively
Diazoxide	6–40 mg/kg/d (divided, start at lower doses)	Gastrointestinal side effects
Glucagon	5–40 ng/kg/min IV diluted in saline	
Octeotride	10–50 μg SC q 8–12 h	
Propofol	Initial: 3–6 mg/kg IV CRI: 0.1–0.6 mg/kg/min IV	
Pentobarbital	3–15 mg/kg IV to create heavy sedation, then repeat every 4–8 h as needed	
Mannitol	0.5–1.5 g/kg over 10–20 min q 6–8 h IV	
Diazepam, midazolam	0.5–1.0 mg/kg IV 1.0–2.0 mg/kg per rectum CRI: 0.1–1.0 mg/kg/h	
Phenobarbital	Loading dose: 16–20 mg/kg/d (divided) Maintenance dose: 1–5 mg/kg q 12 h PO	
Levetiracetam (Keppra)	20 mg/kg PO q 8–12 h	

studies regarding the efficacy of osmotic diuretic (ie, mannitol) to decrease intracranial pressure and aid in the control of seizures in these animals (**Table 2**). The use of anticonvulsants may also be beneficial if the dog has developed a seizure focus. Dogs that develop refractory seizures following restoration of normoglycemia have a very poor prognosis. Postoperative seizures have been reported to occur in approximately 5% of dogs, resulting in 2% mortality (**Table 1**).[2,5]

Pancreatitis is the second most common postoperative complication reported in dogs that undergo insulinoma resection. Pancreatitis is estimated to occur in almost 20% of dogs that undergo surgery, resulting in 3.5% mortality (**Table 1**). Some degree of pancreatic trauma is unavoidable during pancreatic surgery. We recommend administering intravenous fluids preoperatively and postoperatively with 2.5% to 5% dextrose at a rate of 60 to 110 mL/kg/d (1–2 times maintenance to maintain perfusion and reduce risk of pancreatitis). Historically, a prolonged period of fasting was recommended in dogs with acute pancreatitis. Currently, it is recommended that feeding is continued postoperatively in small, frequent meals as soon as animals are able to eat. A low-fat, low-simple-carbohydrate, high-fiber diet (eg, Hills W/D, Purina OM) is preferred to prevent pancreatitis and insulin surge postoperatively. Frequent meals are important for maintaining euglycemia as dogs with insulinoma will invariably develop hypoglycemia after prolonged fast due to the low likelihood of achieving complete excision of this tumor.[17] Despite all precautions, a portion of dogs are expected to develop acute pancreatitis after surgery, resulting in prolonged hospitalization and a need for intensive care. As a result, clients should be counseled about this risk before surgery is pursued.

Postoperative hyperglycemia is thought to be due to atrophy of and lack of insulin production by the remaining islet cells in the pancreas (**Table 1**).[1,2,4-7] Temporary hyperglycemia has been reported to occur in 28% of dogs in the first 2 to 3 days after insulinoma resection; however, only 7% required insulin therapy.[2] Glucose-containing fluids should be discontinued in dogs that develop hyperglycemia. As long as the hyperglycemia is mild (<350 mg/dL), we recommend waiting 2 to 3 days after discontinuation of dextrose supplementation before instituting insulin treatment, in the hope that spontaneous resolution of surgically induced pancreatitis will occur. In dogs that require insulin therapy, the lower end of the dose range is selected initially, using 0.25 U/kg of NPH insulin SC bid. Insulin therapy is usually required for less than a month in the majority of cases so the clinician should anticipate that hypoglycemia will occur as the transient diabetes mellitus resolves. Owners should be instructed to monitor urine glucose and clinical signs of hypoglycemia at home to identify when insulin is no longer necessary (persistently negative urine glucose likely indicates resolution of diabetes mellitus). Those dogs undergoing the most aggressive tumor debulking and loss of pancreatic mass are most likely to have postoperative hyperglycemia due to loss of beta cell mass and subsequent development of diabetes mellitus.

Other, much less common complications of insulinoma resection include cardiac arrest and sepsis (**Table 1**), which are likely to be secondary results of severe, acute pancreatitis rather than direct results of surgical procedures in these animals.

PARATHYROID SURGERY

Primary hyperparathyroidism (PHPT) is the third most common cause of ionized hypercalcemia in dogs, ranking behind cancer and renal failure as the first and second most common causes, respectively.[18] Dogs with cancer or renal failure are generally sick when they present for evaluation and hypercalcemia is discovered. However, dogs with PHPT are generally healthy with no or mild clinical signs usually characterized by polyuria, polydipsia, lethargy, occasional gastrointestinal signs, dysuria, and mild anorexia.[19-23] It is important for surgeons to be able to distinguish the physiologic causes and implications of hypercalcemia prior to considering therapeutic parathyroidectomy.

Preoperative Considerations

Chronic kidney disease
Chronic hypercalcemia from PHPT leads to chronic kidney disease (CKD) characterized by nephrocalcinosis and azotemia in some dogs, which has been used as an argument for early treatment of PHPT.[21] Calcium-containing uroliths can occur in the kidney or ureter, which can contribute to CKD and can also cause urinary obstruction leading to azotemia.[22] One study of dogs that underwent parathyoidectomy to treat PHPT reported that 41% (7 of 17) of dogs developed CKD postoperatively and that this was more likely to occur in dogs with higher preoperative total calcium (mean 16 mg/dL, range 14.4–23.2 mg/dL for dogs that did develop azotemic CKD; mean 13.2 mg/dL, range 12–16.8 mg/dL for dogs did not develop CKD).[21] Compiled data from previous reports suggested a lower prevalence of postoperative renal disease (**Table 3**).[21,22] Interestingly, one report that compared dogs with PHPT to a control population found that mean kidney values (ie, blood urea nitrogen [BUN] and creatinine) were actually lower in dogs with PHPT compared to control animals preoperatively.[22] Hypercalcemic dogs often have lower urine specific gravity (USG) (<1.030) due to acquired nephrogenic diabetes insipidus caused by the effects of hypercalcemia in the

Table 3		
Postoperative complications of parathyroidectomy		
Postoperative Complications and Consequences of Primary Hyperparathyroidism	**Prevalence (affected, total)**	**Mortality (affected, total)**
Hypocalcemia	40.5% (34, 84)[21,24,27]	5.3% (1, 19)[24]
Tetany	10.5% (2, 19)[24]	
Urolithiasis	29.8% (75, 252)[21,22,24,25]	
Urinary tract infection	29.0% (67, 231)[22,24]	
Renal failure	13.0% (27, 207)[21,22]	10.5% (2, 19)[21]
Hypercalcemia	4.3% (2, 47)[27]	

collecting tubule.[23] Serum biochemistry panels that are collected preoperatively can reveal prerenal azotemia that is associated with dehydration. USG of less than 1.030 is often encountered due to the diuretic effects of the hypercalcemia, so it is easy to conclude that any azotemia that is discovered is from intrinsic renal disease, when in reality it might be prerenal. Since most of these dogs are older, there is increased chance of CKD not associated with hypercalcemia; therefore, it is important to fully examine the kidneys using ultrasound imaging, urine protein-to-creatine ratios, and blood pressure measurement during the presurgical workup. Since calcium-containing urinary stones are common in dogs with PHPT, preoperative screening for bladder stones is indicated, so that they can be removed during the same anesthetic procedure. Some clinicians recommend parathyroidectomy early during the course of PHPT to lessen the chances of encountering postoperative hypocalcemia. Others have recommended surgical intervention only to treat clinical signs commonly associated with hypercalcemia, most commonly to ameliorate polyuria and polydipsia.[22]

Adenoma versus hyperplasia

In the vast majority of dogs with PHPT, hypercalcemia is due to uniglandular disease caused by an adenoma (84.9%).[21,22,24–27] However, some dogs may be affected with hyperplasia, multiglandular disease (12.4%),[21,22,24–27] or carcinoma (5.4%) (**Table 4**).[21,24,25,27] It is important to consider the possibility of multiglandular disease during diagnostic evaluation of PHPT (**Fig. 1**), because dogs may remain hypercalcemic after surgery due to multiglandular disease or hyperplastic ectopic parathyroid tissue that is not addressed during initial surgery. Ultrasonographic evaluation is an important step to surgical planning; however, this imaging modality has been reported to either overestimate (2 of 12) or underestimate (5 of 17) the number of affected glands in dogs.[26] Adenomatous hyperplasia or secondary HPT is

Table 4	
Histologic and morphologic characteristics of primary hyperparathyroidism in dogs	
Histologic Diagnosis	**Prevalence (dogs affected, total)**
Adenoma	84.9% (247, 291)[21,22,24–27]
Hyperplasia	12.4% (36, 291)[21,22,24–27]
Carcinoma	5.4% (8, 149)[21,24,25,27]

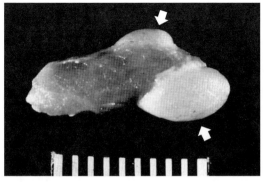

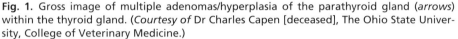

Fig. 1. Gross image of multiple adenomas/hyperplasia of the parathyroid gland (*arrows*) within the thyroid gland. (*Courtesy of* Dr Charles Capen [deceased], The Ohio State University, College of Veterinary Medicine.)

considered when glands measure less than 4 mm, while adenomas or carcinomas measure more than 4 mm.[28] Whenever the parathyroid glands are undetected by ultrasound or measure less than 4 mm or when multiple glands are visible but not clearly enlarged (ie, 2–4 mm in diameter), the surgeon needs to consider the pros and cons of surgical intervention. Even though ultrasound is not perfect in estimating the extent of PTH disease, it is commonly available and more reliable than other techniques, including scintigraphy.[29,30] A rapid PTH assay has been developed to assist surgeons in achieving complete excision of abnormal parathyroid tissue in dogs.[26] Based on this assay, the surgery is considered successful when PTH values drop greater than 50% compared to preoperative values. In the future, this assay may assist surgeons in decision making, especially when dealing with multiglandular disease. In general, it is recommended to explore the parathyroid glands and remove all grossly abnormal tissue. It is more common to have bilateral disease than multiple ipsilateral nodules when dealing with multiglandular disease.[27] If all glands appear to be affected, the surgeon will be required to decide whether to remove all parathyroid gland tissue and risk iatrogenic hypocalcemia, or to leave one gland and risk persistent hypercalcemia due to incomplete resection. Rarely, some dogs will remain hypercalcemic even after removal of all obvious parathyroid gland tissue. This is thought to occur because of the presence of ectopic parathyroid tissue in the mediastinum or in other areas of the neck. Identification of ectopic parathyroid tissue can be exceedingly difficult as it can be located anywhere from the mediastinum to the higher cervical regions. Nuclear scintigraphy has been used to locate ectopic parathyroid gland tissue in humans with PHPT but has only 25% sensitivity in dogs.[30] In the future, other imaging techniques using fluorescent methods at the time of surgery may facilitate identification of parathyroid tissue.[31] The clear disadvantage of fluorescent techniques is that they help to identify parathyroid tissue only within the surgical field.

Pretreatment with calcitriol (prevent hypocalcemia)
Hypocalcemia is the most common and clinically relevant postoperative complication encountered in dogs undergoing correction of PHPT, affecting approximately 40% of dogs undergoing parathyroidectomy (see **Table 3**). Although rarely life threatening, the costs of prolonged calcium monitoring and intravenous calcium therapy can often equal or exceed the costs of surgery. It has been reported that dogs with a higher

magnitude of preoperative hypercalcemia are more likely to develop postoperative hypocalcemia, presumptively based on atrophy of remaining parathyroid glands.[21,24] In two separate studies, mean preoperative total calcium was 13.7 mg/dL[24] and 13.6 mg/dL[21] in dogs that did not develop hypocalcemia, whereas total calcium in dogs that did develop postoperative hypocalcemia was 15.4 mg/dL[24] and 16.8 mg/dL,[21] respectively. Eleven of 12 dogs that developed hypocalcemia had not received prophylactic treatment (eg, calcium salts, active vitamin D) preoperative.[24] These findings have led to recommendations of treating dogs orally with active vitamin D metabolites and calcium salts preoperatively to prevent hypocalcemia. Active vitamin D metabolites increase enterocyte absorption of calcium from the intestinal lumen, "priming the pump" so that sufficient calcium can be available to enter the circulation after the sudden withdrawal of PTH. Calcitriol is the preferred therapy based on its activity, short time to achieve biological effect (1–4 days), short circulating half-life, and quicker resolution of hypercalcemia should overdose occur, compared to cholecalciferol or ergocalciferol treatments. Although the efficacy of this protocol has not been rigorously studied, we currently recommend starting calcitriol 3 to 5 days before surgery at a dose of 10 to 20 ng/kg PO, q 12 h for 2 to 3 days, then decreasing the dose to 5 ng/kg PO q 12 h until surgery. Postoperative calcitriol therapy is described later in this chapter (see Management of Hypocalcemia under Postoperative Considerations). Hypercalcemia can develop in association with preoperative or postoperative administration of calcitriol therapy, although this effect should resolve after discontinuation of calcitriol.

Pretreatment with bisphosphonate (prevent "hungry bone syndrome")

The preoperative use of bisphosphonates has been advocated in humans to prevent post-op hypocalcemia.[32–35] Hypocalcemia after parathyroidectomy is related to the sudden decrease in PTH release and subsequent attenuation of its effect on bone turnover. Bisphosphonates inhibit osteoclast-mediated bone resorption, decreasing calcium uptake by bone that occurs in the absence of PTH.[34] Administration of bisphosphonates may lead to inhibition of bone formation/mineralization and prevention of hungry bone syndrome (HBS).[33] However, the use of bisphosphonates can also prolong remodeling and mineralization that occurs post-op. HBS is defined by a postoperative calcium level of less than 8.5 mg/dL in humans.[36] Pretreatment with bisphosphonates significantly decreased the likelihood of HBS in one study of humans.[36] However, unlike what was previously thought, the level of hypercalcemia did not predict which human patients would develop HBS. Preoperative treatment with bisphosphonates intravenously or orally has not been evaluated in dogs with PHPT. Intravenous bisphosphonates are sometimes given to dogs to lessen the degree of preoperative hypercalcemia; usually pamidronate is chosen as a more cost-effective treatment over the more potent zolendronate. The effects of this treatment on the development of postoperative hypocalcemia have not been studied in dogs. We have observed that some dogs develop hypocalcemia after surgery despite adequate pretreatment with calcitriol, raising the suspicion of HBS. Although we are tempted to speculate that dogs with severely elevated levels of circulating calcium are at increased risk for HBS, this does not appear to be the case in humans.[36] Because dogs are often more hypercalcemic by the time of surgery compared to humans, this potential risk factor warrants further study. Diagnosis of postoperative HBS would be based on detection of an elevated level of PTH in dogs with persistent hypocalcemia, while PTH would be low if hypocalcemia is due to hypoparathyroidism; combinations of both could be present early on as hypocalcemia develops. Serial measurements of PTH during the evolution of hypocalcemia will provide pivotal information on this pathophysiology. Further development and evaluation of protocols using bisphosphonates for the effective and safe control of preoperative hypercalcemia and postoperative hypocalcemia in dogs are needed.

Urolithiasis and Urinary Tract Infections

Urine culture and imaging of the urinary system are recommended in all dogs with suspected PHPT, as these animals are predisposed to urinary tract infections (UTI) and urolithiasis.[21,22,24,25] A compilation of data previously published revealed that approximately 29.8% and 29.0% of dogs have UTI and urolithiasis, respectively.[21,22,24,25] Surgical intervention to remove bladder stones may be performed at the same time as parathyroidectomy.

Postoperative Considerations

Measurement of postoperative circulating calcium is needed to determine the trend and magnitude of any developing hypocalcemia. It is best to intervene with supplemental calcium treatments before there are overt signs of hypocalcemia (ie, tremors, seizures). Ideally, use of ionized calcium measurements is preferred over the use of total serum calcium monitoring. Measurement of total serum calcium can be used when measurement of ionized calcium concentrations is not readily available, especially for the detection of trends. We recommend monitoring ionized calcium every 12 hours postoperatively for the first 2 days, then once daily until the fifth day. Dogs are hospitalized during this entire period for 24-hour monitoring, allowing immediate therapy for any signs of hypocalcemia. Dogs with higher preoperative calcium or those that developed postoperative hypocalcemia are monitored the longest (up to the fifth or sixth day). This is based on the fact that hypercalcemia typically resolves within 1 to 6 days (mean of 1.6 ± 1.1 days).[27] Sixty-three percent of dogs had the largest drop in their calcium concentration during the first 24 hours postoperatively, while in 30% of dogs, this occurred by 72 hours.[24]

Persistent or recurrent hypercalcemia

Dogs remaining hypercalcemic for 7 to 10 days after surgery are likely to remain hypercalcemic. This complications is thought to be uncommon and has been described in approximately 6% of dogs in a previous study.[27] Recurrent hypercalcemia is thought to occur in 7%[21] to 17%[26] of cases and can occur months to years after the initial surgery. In these cases, we recommend repeating PTH measurements and parathyroid ultrasound to rule out multiglandular disease. If there is still inappropriate PTH concentration in the face of ionized hypercalcemia, it is recommended to consider surgical reexploration. Parathyroid ultrasound may help determine if other glands are affected. However, occasionally the ultrasound is unremarkable in the presence of inappropriately high concentrations of circulating PTH. This can happen in cases of multiglandular disease or when there is ectopic hyperplastic parathyroid tissue. In dogs with multiglandular disease, we consider removing all parathyroid glands and instituting therapy to prevent hypocalcemia. As an alternative therapy for dogs with persistant hypercalcemia due to suspected ectopic parathyroid tissue, we have used alendronate (1–4 mg/kg PO twice weekly) to control hypercalcemia. One dog recently managed with this protocol developed sudden hypocalcemia almost 1 year after initiation of therapy. We speculate this may have been caused by parathyroid tissue necrosis following infarction, as has been reported to spontaneously occur rarely with parathyroid gland adenoma in the dog.[37] This dog went on to require lifelong calcitriol and calcium supplementation.

Management of hypocalcemia: acute and subacute/chronic

Acute Intravenous calcium salts may occasionally be necessary following parathyroidectomy, even in dogs pretreated with calcitriol. At any time the dog becomes clinical for hypocalcemia, calcium gluconate 10% solution IV (9.3 mg of Ca/mL) is given slowly to effect (0.5–1.5 mL/kg; 50–150 mg/kg), then maintained at 5 to 15 mg/kg/h (0.05–0.15 mL/kg/h). It is important to remember not to mix calcium solution with bicarbonate-containing fluids as precipitation may occur. The heart rate should be serially determined during the infusion of IV calcium salts. If the heart rate decreases markedly or if absolute bradycardia develops, stop the infusion and then restart at a slower rate. Progressive shortening of the QT interval on the ECG should prompt a slower rate of calcium salt infusion. After stabilization with IV calcium gluconate, the oral dose of calcitriol is increased from 5 ng/kg q 12 h to 10 to 20 ng/kg q 12 h if the dog becomes acutely hypocalcemic postoperatively even when not showing clinical signs of hypocalcemia. Oral calcium carbonate (50 mg/kg/d of elemental calcium) is usually added if not previously being administered.

Subacute/chronic Though subcutaneous protocols for injection of calcium gluconate have been described, they should not be used. Potential side effects of subcutaneous calcium gluconate administration include calcinosis cutis, severe pain, inflammation, sterile abscess formation, and necrosis. We have observed severe reactions that have actually resulted in euthanasia of several dogs, so we strongly recommend against the subcutaneous administration of calcium salts, even when diluted.[38,39] Oral calcium carbonate (25–50 mg/kg/d PO of elemental calcium) is generally given in addition to oral calcitriol to help support the level of circulating calcium because it is less expensive than calcitriol and can facilitate non–vitamin D–dependent intestinal absorption of calcium. It is possible that concurrent administration of vitamin D metabolites would predispose to soft tissue mineralization associated with subcutaneous fluids that contain calcium salts, so 0.9% NaCl is recommended as a safe alternative in dogs that require supplemental fluid therapy.The calcitriol dose is discontinued or markedly reduced if dog remains hypercalcemic by the end of the second day after surgery. If the dog is normocalcemic while receiving twice-daily calcitriol, this dose remains the same for 1 week postoperatively. Ionized calcium levels are rechecked weekly and the calcitriol doses are decreased in half at each recheck (ie, 2.5 ng/kg/d, 2.5 ng/kg every other day, discontinued) as long as the animal remains either hypercalcemic or normocalcemic. Caution is taken while tapering the calcitriol dose because the biologic effects of this drug can last up to 1 week, though it is typically shorter. Owners are instructed to monitor for signs of hypocalcemia during the tapering period.

ADRENAL SURGERY

Adrenal masses are often diagnosed incidentally. In one study of 50 dogs with pheochromocytomas, approximately half of the adrenal masses identified were found incidentally.[40] Another study, where most dogs had cortical carcinoma, only 10% of the masses were incidental.[41] Adrenal masses can be secretory or nonsecretory and are commonly caused by hyperplasia, adrenocortical carcinoma, adrenocortical adenoma, or pheochromocytoma. According to the Veterinary Medical Database (1985–1996), cortical adenomas are more than 2 times (41%) as common as pheochromocytomas (15%) or cortical carcinomas (14%).[42] In this study, only 3% of dogs had metastatic lesions. However, the pooled results of previous studies indicate that metastasis is present in approximately one third of dogs with pheochromocytomas or adrenal cortical neoplasia (**Tables 5** and **6**). Incidental adrenal masses are

Table 5
Complications associated with pheochromocytomas

Complications	Prevalence (dogs affected, total)	Mortality (dogs affected, total)
Locally invasive	55.1% (70, 127)[40,47,63,80]	
Tumor thrombi	34.5% (20, 58)[41,47,61]	30.0% (3, 10) for thrombi and 25.0% (6, 24) for no thrombi[61]
Metastasis	36.8% (43, 117)[40,49,80]	5.9% (1, 17)[80]
Death	29.5% (51, 173)[40,41,49,61,63,80]	29.5% (51, 173)[40,41,49,61,63,80]
Hypertension	36.7% (40, 109)[40,41,49,63,80]	
Hypotension	41.6% (37, 89)[41,63,80]	16.7% (1, 6)[80]
Tachycardia	66.7% (4, 6)[80]	
Arrhythmias	29.8% (14, 47)[63,80]	
Hemorrhage	15.1% (13, 86)[41,63]	
Cardiac arrest	32.0% (8, 25)[47,49]	32.0% (8, 25)[47,49]
Thromboembolism	17.6% (3, 17)[49]	

Includes data from a study containing both pheochromocytomas and adrenocortical tumors.[41,44]

often called "adrenal incidentalomas" and pose a treatment dilemma in that clinicians must decide whether to pursue surgical interventions in an animal with no clinical signs related to the adrenal enlargement.[42] Adrenalectomy is the treatment of choice if an adrenal mass is malignant and has not metastasized, but adrenalectomy may not be indicated if the mass is benign, small, and hormonally inactive and has not invaded

Table 6
Complications and characteristics associated with adrenocortical neoplasia

Complications	Prevalence (dogs affected, total)
Carcinoma	65.8% (52, 79)[41,46,77]
Adenoma	34.2% (27, 79)[41,46,77]
Metastasis (carcinoma only)	29.0% (20, 69)[44,46,77]
Caval invasion	32.9% (27, 82)[44,46,61]
Euthanasia during surgery	12.7% (9, 71)[44,46,77]
Perioperative mortality (carcinoma only)	25.4% (18, 71)[44,61,77]
Cardiac arrest	20.0% (3, 15)[44,77]
Renal failure	10.4% (8, 77)[41,44,46,77]
Pneumonia	13.3% (2, 15)[44,77]
Pancreatitis	10.0% (7, 70)[41,44,46]
Addison's	16.1% (10, 62)[41,46]
Other	10.3% (3, 29)[44,46]
Perioperative mortality (adenoma only)	36.4% (4, 11)[77]
Pulmonary thromboembolism	18.2% (2, 11)[77]
Pancreatitis	9.1% (1, 11)[77]
Gastroenteritis	9.1% (1, 11)[77]

Includes data from a study containing both pheochromocytomas and adrenocortical tumors.[41,44]

surrounding structures. Guidelines to suggest malignancy include mass size, invasion of the mass into surrounding tissues and blood vessels, and identification of additional mass lesions with abdominal ultrasound and thoracic radiographs. The bigger the mass, the more likely it is that it is malignant and that metastasis has occurred, regardless of findings on abdominal ultrasound and thoracic radiographs. These issues are specifically important because understanding of the adrenal pathology affects decision making, treatment considerations both preoperative and postoperative. These factors will ultimately affect treatment success. This section will focus on complications associated with resection of cortisol-secreting adrenal tumors and pheochromocytomas.

Adrenal-dependent hyperadrenocorticism

In approximately 10% to 20% of dogs with hyperadrenocorticism, cortisol excess is related to a primary tumor in the zona faciculata of the adrenal cortex.[43,44] These tumors occur most commonly in one gland leading to atrophy of the contralateral adrenal gland. However, bilateral cortisol-secreting tumors have been described.[45,46] It is important to differentiate bilateral adrenocortical tumors from bilateral hyperplasia secondary to pituitary-dependent hyperadrenocorticism.

Pheochromocytoma

Pheochromocytomas are catecholamine-producing tumors derived from chromaffin cells of the adrenal medulla.[40,47–49] Primary actions of catecholamines include response to acute stress and regulation of intermediary metabolism, especially in response to hypoglycemia.[50,51]

Preoperative Considerations

Perioperative treatment and expected complications are highly dependent on the particular type of adrenal tumor that is being approached, and it is therefore recommended that specific diagnostic tests are used in an attempt to differentiate whether an adrenal mass is likely to be a pheochromocytoma, an adrenocortical carcinoma, or a nonsecretory benign mass. Generally, arterial blood pressure, fundic exam, fine-needle aspirate of the adrenal mass (if possible), urinalysis, complete blood count, chemistry profile, urine cortisol-to-creatinine ratio (3-day pooled sample collected at home), and abdominal ultrasound are recommended after detection of an adrenal mass. Depending on these findings and clinical signs, further endocrine diagnostic tests are recommended to support the diagnosis, as discussed in the following sections on each adrenal tumor type.[52–55]

While abdominal ultrasound imaging does not offer a definitive method to differentiate between various types of adrenal tumors, this test can provide a significant amount of information. Bulbous enlargement of the cranial or caudal pole of the adrenal gland is common in dogs with normal adrenal glands and can often be misinterpreted as an adrenal mass.[56] Diagnosis of an adrenal mass is made when maximum width of the adrenal gland exceeds 1.5 cm, the gland loses its typical "peanut" shape (left adrenal) or "V" shape (right adrenal), and the gland is asymmetric in shape and size when compared with the contralateral adrenal gland.[51,57,58] It has been previously shown that adrenal masses with a thickness greater then 2 cm tend to be malignant, while all masses greater than 4 cm are malignant.[57] Pheochromocytomas and adrenocortical tumors (ie, carcinomas) tend to appear more as rounded masses, whereas hyperplasia and adenomas have a more nodular appearance.[57] If the maximal width of the smaller adrenal gland (when asymmetric) is less than 5 mm, this is consistent with pituitary independent hyperadrenocorticism.[59] It is important to note that bilateral adrenal

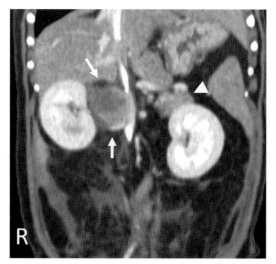

Fig. 2. Abdominal computed tomography scan with contrast (reconstructed sagittal view) of right adrenal mass (*arrows*) with normal sized left adrenal gland (*arrowhead*). This mass is a pheochromocyotoma causing extramural compression of the caudal vena cava. (*Courtesy of Dr Bridget Urie and the Radiology Department, The Ohio State University, College of Veterinary Medicine.*)

neoplasia is rarely diagnosed. When present, it hinders the ability to diagnose pituitary-dependent hyperadrenocorticism based on lack of atrophy of the contralateral gland.[44] Adrenal asymmetry may represent a functional neoplasm; however, other differentials include hypertrophy of normal tissue, granuloma, cyst, hemorrhage, or an inflammatory nodule.[51] Mineralization is not pathognomonic for malignancy as only 57% (4 of 7) of dogs with mineralized masses had adenocarcinoma.[57] Even though thrombus formation may be seen in benign lesions, local vascular invasion appears to be a feature of malignancy.[57] Because of the risk of intraoperative hemorrhage, blood is submitted for cross-matching in anticipation of a blood transfusion during or after surgery. If surgery is planned, computed tomography (CT)[60] or magnetic resonance imaging (MRI) is recommended to more accurately assess the size of the adrenal mass, its location relative to the aorta, presence and size of any tumor thrombi, and evidence of infiltration of the mass into the kidney and body wall (**Fig. 2**). Cross-sectional imaging is especially important if a caval thrombus was detected during abdominal ultrasound, to evaluate the cranial extent of the thrombus prior to attempted resection.

Adrenal-dependent hyperadrenocorticism
The right adrenal gland is covered by the caudal extension of the right lateral liver lobe; access to the region can be further complicated by hepatomegaly that accompanies hyperadrenocorticism.[51] The mass may compress or invade adjacent blood vessels and organs; these findings are suggestive of carcinoma.[61]

The low-dose dexamethasone suppression test (LDDST) is used to establish a diagnosis of hyperadrenocorticism. We tend to perform an ACTH stimulation test only if we believe the dog may have pituitary-dependent hyperadrenocorticism, as this test does not have good sensitivity (33%[46]–60%[62]) for diagnosing cortisol-secreting adrenocortical neoplasia. Determination of a single baseline plasma

ACTH concentration may aid in distinguishing dogs with adrenal-dependent hyperadrenocorticism from those with pituitary-dependent hyperadrenocorticism.[43,63] Dogs with a functional adrenal tumor are likely to have low or undetectable levels of ACTH.[64] We recommend submitting a plasma sample from a control dog whenever using this assay because ACTH is very labile and easily degraded during manipulation and transport.[64]

Potential postoperative complications in dogs with adrenocortical tumors include cortisol-induced immunosuppression, impaired wound healing, systemic hypertension, hypercoagulation, development of hypoadrenocorticism, and pancreatitis (see **Table 6** for pooled data).[51] Treatment with trilostane (Vetoryl; Dechra Veterinary Products, 1–3 mg/kg q 12 h initially) for 3 to 4 weeks before surgery can reverse metabolic derangements of hyperadrenocorticism and potentially minimize many of the complications associated with surgical removal of a cortisol-secreting adrenal tumor.[65] Goals of therapy are post-ACTH serum cortisol concentration between 2 and 5 μg/dL (collected at 4–6 hours post dosing) and improvement of clinical signs. The dosage of trilostane is increased if these goals have not been attained at the 10- to 14-day recheck. Surgery is recommended 1 to 2 weeks later.

Proposed causes of hypertension in hyperadrenocorticism include activation of the renin-angiotensin system, increased vascular responsiveness to catecholamines, as well as decreased concentrations of vasodilator prostaglandins.[66] Initial treatment may include use of angiotensin-converting enzyme inhibitors to reduce peripheral vasoconstriction and aldosterone secretion and are typically effective to control hypertension associated with hyperadrenocorticism.

Pheochromocytoma

In dogs with pheochromocytoma, high levels of circulating catecholamines pose a significant risk for cardiovascular arrest, hypertension, hypotension, and arrhythmias. These complications are typically associated with surgical intervention due to massive catecholamine release during manipulation of the tumor.

Clinical signs, when present, develop as a result of the space-occupying nature of the tumor and its metastatic lesions or, more commonly, as a result of excessive secretion of catecholamines. The most common clinical signs of pheochromocytomas are generalized weakness and episodic collapse, which have been associated with poorer outcome.[40,63] Abnormalities identified during physical examination may include excessive panting, tachypnea, tachycardia, weakness, and muscle wasting. Excess catecholamine secretion may also cause severe systemic hypertension, resulting in retinal hemorrhage or detachment. There are no consistent abnormalities identified in routine blood and urine tests that would raise suspicion for pheochromocytoma.[40,63] Atrophy of the contralateral adrenal gland does not occur with pheochromocytoma and atrophy of the adrenal cortex is not always apparent ultrasonographically.[57] Supportive evidence for preoperative diagnosis of pheochromocytoma can be obtained by measurement of urine catecholamines. Samples collected at home are recommended to avoid stress-associated catecholamine secretion.[52] Normetadrenaline-to-creatinine ratio or normetanephrine in the urine has high sensitivity for diagnosing pheochromocytomas when very elevated.[53,54] It is important to note that illness has a significant impact on urine catecholamines.[55] Unfortunately, there is no established protocol for diagnosing pheochromocytomas in veterinary patients and the previously mentioned tests are not readily available to veterinary clinicians.

Arrhythmias and Hypertension

Electrocardiograpic monitoring is recommended preoperatively, intraoperatively, and postoperatively due to a risk of ventricular arrhythmias in dogs with pheochromocytoma. Chronic catecholamine exposure in dogs can also cause generalized vasoconstriction. Upon removal of a pheochromocytoma, an acute decline in circulating catecholamine levels can result in decreased vascular tone and a precipitous drop in vascular resistance. In addition, anesthetic induction and intraoperative tumor manipulation are often associated with surges in blood catecholamine concentrations that can produce episodes of intraoperative hypertension, ventricular tachycardia, arrhythmias, and even cardiac arrest.[63] In one study, preoperative administration of a noncompetitive alpha-adrenergic receptor blocker (phenoxybenzamine) reduced perioperative mortality from 48% to 13% in dogs with pheochromocytoma.[63] If pheochromocytoma is suspected, phenoxybenzamine therapy is initiated 2 to 3 weeks before surgery at a dosage of 0.5 mg/kg q 12 h. Because of the infrequency of clinical signs in affected dogs, it is difficult to make dosage adjustments based on improvement in clinical signs and blood pressure. However, some clinicians propose that this initial dosage is often ineffective in preventing severe intraoperative hypertension, especially because there was no difference in blood pressure when phenoxybenzamine was or was not used.[63] Therefore, it has been recommended to gradually increase the phenoxybenzamine dosage every few days until clinical signs of hypotension (eg, lethargy, weakness, syncope), adverse drug reactions (eg, vomiting), or maximum dosage of 2.5 mg/kg q 12 h is attained.[51,61] Surgery is recommended 1 to 2 weeks later, and the drug is continued until the time of surgery.[51] Phenoxybenzamine is very expensive, which impairs its widespread use. Prazosin has been recommended as an alternative treatment in human beings with pheochromocytoma. In humans, prazosin had similar effects to phenoxybenzamine in patients with essential hypertension.[67] In this same study, heart rate was slightly higher in patients receiving prazosin and prazosin appeared to be a more effective antihypertensive than phenoxybenzamine.[67] Another study indicated that prazosin lowered arterial blood pressure by reducing total peripheral resistance. No difference in the operative and postoperative blood pressure as well as plasma volume control was seen in humans with pheochromocytomas undergoing preoperative preparation with either prazosin or phenoxybenzamine.[68] A study in beagles aiming to evaluate urodynamic and hemodynamic effects of prazosin and phenoxybenzamine showed a significant drop in blood pressure after administration of intravenous prazosin but not phenoxybenzamine or placebo.[69] These results indicate the need to evaluate prazosin in a clinical setting as a pretreatment in canine cases of pheochromocytomas.[67,69–71]

If severe persistent tachycardia is identified, beta-adrenergic antagonist therapy (eg, propranolol [0.2–1.0 mg/kg PO q 8 h] or atenolol [0.2–1.0 mg/kg PO q 12–24 h]) may be utilized during the preoperative period.[51] Arrhythmias and hypertension may still occur despite prior treatment with alpha-adrenergic blocking drugs; close monitoring of the dog during the perioperative period is critical for a successful outcome following adrenalectomy.

Anesthetic drugs that are arrhythmogenic, exert anticholinergic effects on alpha receptors, or potentiate the effects of catecholamines should be avoided when possible (eg, thiobarbiturates, halothane). Anesthetic induction is a period of high risk for development of arrhythmias or severe hypertension; consequently, serial electrocardiography and blood pressure should be monitored before and after inducing anesthesia. Severe sinus tachycardia may be treated with intravenous propranolol (0.3–1 mg/kg), as needed. Esmolol, a short-acting beta-1 antagonist, provides a more specific chronotropic effect.[61] Pathologic ventricular arrhythmias (rate > 180 bpm, polymorphic complexes, or R-on-T phenomenon) are treated with intravenous boluses of lidocaine (2–4 mg/kg IV). Anesthetists should also be prepared to treat intraoperative episodes of arterial hypertension. Administration of a short-acting alpha antagonist (phentolamine, 0.1 mg/kg loading dose, then 1–2 μg/kg/min) can be effective, although random surges of catecholamines can overcome this competitive inhibitor and a direct vasodilator (nitroprusside, 0.1–0.8 μg/kg/min) may be required.[61]

Risks of Surgery

Hemorrhage

The anatomy of the adrenal glands in relationship to that of the great vessels creates significant risk of hemorrhage during surgery in this region. The left adrenal gland is adjacent to the left side of the abdominal aorta medially, and its caudal aspect borders the left renal artery. The right adrenal is located ventral to the 13th thoracic vertebra and is adhered to the right side of the vena cava.[72] The right adrenal vein empties directly into the vena cava, while the left adrenal vein empties into the left renal vein.[72] Arterial supply to the adrenal glands consists of 20 to 30 small branches arising from the phrenicoabdominal, renal, and cranial abdominal arteries and directly from the adjacent aorta.[72] The likelihood of intraoperative complications is dependent upon the size of the adrenal mass and invasion of the adjacent vena cava or kidney.

Caval invasion (tumor, thrombi)

Caval thrombi are reported in both adrenocortical tumors and pheochromocytomas (**Tables 5** and **6**). Although caval invasion is more commonly associated with right-sided adrenal masses, it was also noted in 20% of dogs with left-sided tumors in one series.[61] Tumor thrombi were not associated with poorer outcome as previously thought.[61] Some surgeons advocate use of intraoperative hypothermia in all dogs that are undergoing adrenalectomy, in preparation for temporary occlusion of the caudal vena cava during tumor resection.[41,61] Surface cooling is applied to achieve an esophageal temperature of 32°C (89.6°F) before vascular occlusion. Experimental studies in normal dogs indicate that acute, permanent occlusion of the suprarenal vena cava will lead to unacceptable hemodynamic consequences, causing a 60% decrease in cardiac output, temporary or permanent renal dysfunction, and even death.[73,74] In an attempt to avoid these complications, one group has investigated the use of gradual occlusion of the caudal vena cava by applying an inflatable silicone hydraulic occluder in dogs.[75] In this study, gradual occlusion of the suprarenal vena cava was achieved in normal dogs without hemodynamic compromise, although some evidence of renal injury was detected. The technique has not been described in dogs with naturally occurring adrenal tumors. Interestingly, a recent case report described the successful application of acute suprarenal caval resection in a Cairn terrier with extensive tumor thrombus, suggesting that chronic partial obstruction may lead to development of collateral circulation in some dogs with malignant adrenal masses that will allow aggressive resection of the vena cava without the morbidity seen in normal dogs.[76]

Thromboembolism

Dogs with adrenal-dependent hyperadrenocorticism are often hypercoagulable and prone to thromboembolic events. Perioperative pulmonary thromboembolism is a common complication associated with removal of a cortisol-secreting adrenal tumor in dogs.[41,46,61,77] When it occurs, thromboembolism is typically noted within the first 72 hours after surgery and is associated with a high mortality rate. There are no controlled studies in dogs with adrenal-dependent hyperadrenocorticism reporting decreased incidence of postoperative thromboembolism with perioperative anticoagulation.[61] In an effort to minimize thromboembolism, we routinely initiate anticoagulant therapy during and after surgery. Heparinized plasma (35 U/kg of heparin added to 10 mL/kg of canine plasma) is administered intravenously during surgery as a source of antithrombin III, which can help prevent thromboembolism.[51] After surgery, subcutaneous heparin (35 U/kg) is administered 2 additional times at 8-hour intervals and then at tapered doses for an additional 2 to 3 days (eg, day 2: 25 U/kg/injection q 8 h SC; day 3: 15 U/kg/injection q 8 h SC). It may be beneficial for dogs to go for frequent short walks within hours of surgery to promote blood flow and minimize clot formation; therefore, anesthetic drugs and pain medications should be administered at dosages that allow the dog to be ambulatory within 4 hours of surgery.[51] Anecdotally, despite use of perioperative anticoagulants, thromboembolism remains a common perioperative complication.

Postoperative Considerations

Pheochromocytoma
Perioperative or postoperative hormonal and anticoagulant therapies are not indicated for animals with pheochromocytoma; however, blood pressure and cardiac rhythm should be monitored closely for 24 hours following surgery. Fluid balance is carefully monitored because rapid resolution of peripheral vasoconstriction can occur after tumor removal, causing a state of relative hypovolemia.

Adrenal-dependent hyperadrenocorticism
Thromboembolism Clinical signs of thromboembolism are nonspecific and highly variable, depending on the amount of physiological impairment.[78] We believe pulmonary thromboembolism (PTE) is the most common form of thromboembolic events where the most common signs are dyspnea, tachypnea, and lethargy. Less common signs of PTE include coughing, hemoptysis, cyanosis, syncope, collapse, and sudden death. Clinical signs of right heart failure (eg, jugular distention, ascites) or poor contractility (poor pulses, prolonged capillary refill time, pallor) may develop. Changes in serum biochemistry are nonspecific, and routine coagulation profiles (prothrombin time and partial thromboplastin time) are typically normal. On auscultation, harsh lung sounds or crackles may be heard, and the heart may have a louder or split second heart sound. Sounds may be muffled if pleural effusion is present. Typical blood gas changes include hypoxemia, hypocapnea, and an increased alveolar-arterial gradient on room air; however, Pao_2 and $Paco_2$ may be normal. Depending on the severity of the ventilation-perfusion mismatch, some (but not all) affected animals will have poor response to oxygen therapy. Thoracic radiographs may be normal; however, pulmonary alveolar or alveolar interstitial infiltrates are most commonly seen. Selective pulmonary angiography is the gold standard for diagnosis; however, it requires general anesthesia and is therefore risky for unstable patients; CT and MRI have the same disadvantage. In the end, PTE is often a diagnosis of exclusion.[78] Treatments include supportive and anticoagulant (eg, unfractionated heparin) therapies. Oxygen is provided, and some patients may require mechanical ventilation. Fluids are administered judiciously to support pressures while preventing right ventricular overload. Theophylline may be beneficial by increasing bronchodilation, pulmonary vasodilation, and diaphragmatic contractility and reducing respiratory muscle fatigue. Administration of sildenafil, which causes selective pulmonary arterial

vasodilation, is considered if pulmonary hypertension is documented.[78] The least invasive way to diagnose pulmonary hypertension is by echocardiography.

Hypoadrenocorticism Glucocorticoids are not indicated before surgery; however, once the tumor is removed, dexamethasone (0.05– 0.1 mg/kg IV total dose) should be given. A tapering dose (0.03–0.07 mg/kg IV q 24 h) is given until oral prednisone can be given. Oral prednisone (0.2–0.5 mg/kg q 24 h) is given initially and gradually decreased to 0.1 to 0.2 mg/kg q 24 h and administered over 3 to 4 months.[61]Development of mild hyponatremia and hypokalemia is common within 72 hours of adrenalectomy and usually resolves in a day or two with exogenous glucocorticoids. Mineralocorticoid therapy is instituted if serum sodium concentration decreases to less than 135 mEq/L or if serum potassium concentration increases to greater than 6.5 mEq/L.[45] An injection of desoxycorticosterone pivalate (DOCP; Percorten-V; Novartis Pharmaceuticals) is recommended, with measurement of serum electrolytes performed 25 days after the injection.[79] If the dog is healthy and serum electrolytes are normal on day 25, the dog should be reevaluated 7 to 10 days later. If serum electrolytes are still normal, DOCP treatment is not needed. If hyponatremia or hyperkalemia is identified on day 25, another injection of DOCP should be administered, but the dosage reduced 50% (1.1 mg/kg SC), and serum electrolytes evaluated 25 days later. In dogs that have undergone bilateral adrenalectomy, prednisone and DOCP supplementation must be continued indefinitely.

Summary

Adrenalectomy for the treatment of malignant adrenal neoplasia is associated with significant risk in dogs, with reported perioperative mortality rates of 19% to 60% in dogs with adrenocortical neoplasms and 18% to 47% in dogs with pheochromocytoma.[41,44,46,49,77,80] Postoperative complications include dyspnea, thromboembolism, acute pancreatitis, oliguric renal failure, hypoadrenocorticism, and hemoperitoneum.[41,44,46,61,77] Interestingly, the best success rates (19% and 22% overall mortality)[41,49,61] were reported in the most recent case series, suggesting that improvements in preoperative management and anesthetic techniques have had a positive effect on outcome, a theory that is supported by a recent study on the effects of preoperative alpha blockade in dogs with pheochromocytoma.[63] In addition, recent data have contradicted the assumption that tumor invasion into the vena cava is associated with increased operative mortality, indicating that, with proper case selection and surgical experience, these cases can be managed successfully.[61]

REFERENCES

1. Kruth SA, Feldman EC, Kennedy PC. Insulin-secreting islet cell tumors: establishing a diagnosis and the clinical course for 25 dogs. J Am Vet Med Assoc 1982;181(1): 54–8.

2. Mehlhaff CJ, Peterson ME, Patnaik AK, et al. Insulin-producing islet cell neoplasms: surgical considerations and general: management in 35 dogs. J Am Anim Hosp Assoc 1985;21(5):607–12.

3. Braund KG, Steiss JE, Amling KA, et al. Insulinoma and subclinical peripheral neuropathy in two dogs. J Vet Intern Med 1987;1(2):86–90.

4. Caywood DD, Klausner JS, Oleary TP, et al. Pancreatic insulin-secreting neoplasms: clinical, diagnostic, and prognostic features in 73 dogs. J Am Anim Hosp Assoc 1988;24(5):577–84.

5. Trifonidou MA, Kirpensteijn J, Robben JH. A retrospective evaluation of 51 dogs with insulinoma. Vet Q 1998;20(Suppl 1):S114–5.

6. Tobin RL, Nelson RW, Lucroy MD, et al. Outcome of surgical versus medical treatment of dogs with beta cell neoplasia: 39 cases (1990–1997). J Am Vet Med Assoc 1999;215(2):226–30.

7. Polton GA, White RN, Brearley MJ, et al. Improved survival in a retrospective cohort of 28 dogs with insulinoma. J Small Anim Pract 2007;48(3):151–6.

8. Madarame H, Kayanuma H, Shida T, et al. Retrospective study of canine insulinomas: eight cases (2005-2008). J Vet Med Sci 2009;71(7):905–11.

9. Feldman EC, Nelson RW. Canine and feline endocrinology and reproduction. 3rd edition. St Louis: WB Saunders; 2004.

10. Fischer JR, Smith SA, Harkin KR. Glucagon constant-rate infusion: a novel strategy for the management of hyperinsulinemic-hypoglycemic crisis in the dog. J Am Anim Hosp Assoc 2000;36(1):27–32.

11. Leifer CE, Peterson ME, Matus RE. Insulin-secreting tumor: diagnosis and medical and surgical management in 55 dogs. J Am Vet Med Assoc 1986;188(1):60–4.

12. Parker AJ, Musselman EM, O'Brien D. Diazoxide treatment of canine insulinoma. Vet Rec 1981;109(9):178–9.

13. Simpson KW, Stepien RL, Elwood CM, et al. Evaluation of the long-acting somatostatin analogue octreotide in the management of insulinoma in three dogs. J Small Anim Pract 1995;36(4):161–5.

14. McKay CJ, Imrie CW, Baxter JN. Somatostatin and somatostatin analogues: are they indicated in the management of acute pancreatitis? Gut 1993;34(11):1622–6.

15. Shimada A, Morita T, Ikeda N, et al. Hypoglycaemic brain lesions in a dog with insulinoma. J Comp Pathol 2000;122(1):67–71.

16. Auer RN, Wieloch T, Olsson Y, et al. The distribution of hypoglycemic brain damage. Acta Neuropathol 1984;64(3):177–91.

17. Kar P, Price P, Sawers S, Bhattacharya S, et al. Insulinomas may present with normoglycemia after prolonged fasting but glucose-stimulated hypoglycemia. J Clin Endocrinol Metab 2006;91(12):4733–6.

18. Messinger JS, Windham WR, Ward CR. Ionized hypercalcemia in dogs: a retrospective study of 109 cases (1998–2003). J Vet Intern Med 2009;23(3):514–9.

19. Feldman EC. Disorders of the parathyroid glands. In: Ettinger SJ, Feldman EC, editors. Textbook of veterinary internal medicine: diseases of the dog and the cat, vol 2. 7th edition. St Louis: Elsevier Saunders; 2010. p. 1722–50.

20. Schenck PA, Chew DJ, Nagode LA, et al. Disorders of calcium: hypercalcemia and hypocalcemia. In: DiBartola SP, editor. Fluid, electrolyte, and acid-base disorders in small animal practice. 3rd edition. St Louis/London: Saunders Elsevier; 2006. p. 122–93.

21. Gear RN, Neiger R, Skelly BJ, et al. Primary hyperparathyroidism in 29 dogs: diagnosis, treatment, outcome and associated renal failure. J Small Anim Pract 2005;46(1):10–6.

22. Feldman EC, Hoar B, Pollard R, et al. Pretreatment clinical and laboratory findings in dogs with primary hyperparathyroidism: 210 cases (1987–2004). J Am Vet Med Assoc 2005;227(5):756-1.

23. Feldman EC, Nelson RW. Hypercalcemia and primary hyperparathyroidism. In: Feldman EC, Nelson RW, editors. Canine and feline endocrinology and reproduction. 3rd edition. St Louis: WB Saunders; 2004. p. 660–715.

24. Berger B, Feldman EC. Primary hyperparathyroidism in dogs: 21 cases (1976–1986). J Am Vet Med Assoc 1987;191(3):350–6.

25. DeVries SE, Feldman EC, Nelson RW, et al. Primary parathyroid gland hyperplasia in dogs: six cases (1982–1991). J Am Vet Med Assoc 1993;202(7):1132–6.

26. Ham K, Greenfield CL, Barger A, et al. Validation of a rapid parathyroid hormone assay and intraoperative measurement of parathyroid hormone in dogs with benign naturally occurring primary hyperparathyroidism. Vet Surg 2009;38(1):122–32.

27. Rasor L, Pollard R, Feldman EC. Retrospective evaluation of three treatment methods for primary hyperparathyroidism in dogs. J Am Anim Hosp Assoc 2007;43(2):70–7.

28. Wisner ER, Penninck D, Biller DS, et al. High-resolution parathyroid sonography. Vet Radiol Ultrasound 1997;38(6):462–6.

29. Matwichuk CL, Taylor SM, Wilkinson AA, et al. Use of technetium Tc 99m sestamibi for detection of a parathyroid adenoma in a dog with primary hyperparathyroidism. J Am Vet Med Assoc 1996;209(10):1733–6.

30. Matwichuk CL, Taylor SM, Daniel GB, et al. Double-phase parathyroid scintigraphy in dogs using technetium-99m-sestamibi. Vet Radiol Ultrasound 2000;41(5):461–9.

31. Prosst RL, Weiss J, Hupp L, et al. Fluorescence-guided minimally invasive parathyroidectomy: clinical experience with a novel intraoperative detection technique for parathyroid glands. World J Surg 2010;34(9):2217–22.

32. Davenport A, Stearns MP. Administration of pamidronate helps prevent immediate postparathyroidectomy hungry bone syndrome. Nephrology (Carlton) 2007;12(4): 386–90.

33. Gurevich Y, Poretsky L. Possible prevention of hungry bone syndrome following parathyroidectomy by preoperative use of pamidronate. Otolaryngol Head Neck Surg 2008;138(3):403–4.

34. Lee IT, Sheu WH, Tu ST, et al. Bisphosphonate pretreatment attenuates hungry bone syndrome postoperatively in subjects with primary hyperparathyroidism. J Bone Miner Metab 2006;24(3):255–8.

35. Rathi MS, Ajjan R, Orme SM. A case of parathyroid carcinoma with severe hungry bone syndrome and review of literature. Exp Clin Endocrinol Diab 2008;116(8): 487–90.

36. Brasier AR, Nussbaum SR. Hungry bone syndrome: clinical and biochemical predictors of its occurrence after parathyroid surgery. Am J Med 1988;84(4):654–60.

37. Rosol TJ, Chew DJ, Capen CC. Acute hypocalcemia associated with infarction of parathyroid gland adenomas in two dogs. J Am Vet Med Assoc 1988;192(2):212–4.

38. Ruopp J. Primary hypoparathyroidism in a cat complicated by suspect iatrogenic calcinosis cutis. J Am Anim Hosp Assoc 2001;37(4):370–3.

39. Schaer M, Ginn PE, Fox LE, et al. Severe calcinosis cutis associated with treatment of hypoparathyroidism in a dog. J Am Anim Hosp Assoc 2001;37(4):364–9.

40. Gilson SD, Withrow SJ, Wheeler SL, et al. Pheochromocytoma in 50 dogs. J Vet Intern Med 1994;8(3):228–32.

41. Schwartz P, Kovak JR, Koprowski A, et al. Evaluation of prognostic factors in the surgical treatment of adrenal gland tumors in dogs: 41 cases (1999–2005). J Am Vet Med Assoc 2008;232(1):77–84.

42. Myers NC 3rd. Adrenal incidentalomas. Diagnostic workup of the incidentally discovered adrenal mass. Vet Clin North Am Small Anim Pract 1997;27(2):38–99.

43. Reusch CE, Feldman EC. Canine hyperadrenocorticism due to adrenocortical neoplasia. Pretreatment evaluation of 41 dogs. J Vet Intern Med 1991;5(1):3–10.

44. van Sluijs FJ, Sjollema BE, Voorhout G, et al. Results of adrenalectomy in 36 dogs with hyperadrenocorticism caused by adreno-cortical tumour. Vet Q 1995;17(3):113–6.

45. van Sluijs FJ, Sjollema BE. Adrenalectomy in 36 dogs and 2 cats with hyperadrenocorticism. Tijdschr Diergeneeskd 1992;117(Suppl 1):29S.

46. Anderson CR, Birchard SJ, Powers BE, et al. Surgical treatment of adrenocortical tumors: 21 cases (1990–1996). J Am Anim Hosp Assoc 2001;37(1):93–7.

47. Bouayad H, Feeney DA, Caywood DD, et al. Pheochromocytoma in dogs: 13 cases (1980–1985). J Am Vet Med Assoc 1987;191(12):1610–5.
48. Maher ER Jr. Pheochromocytoma in the dog and cat: diagnosis and management. Semin Vet Med Surg (Small Anim) 1994;9(3):158–66.
49. Barthez PY, Marks SL, Woo J, et al. Pheochromocytoma in dogs: 61 cases (1984–1995). J Vet Intern Med 1997;11(5):272–8.
50. Guyton AC, Hall JE. The autonomic nervous system and the adrenal medulla. In: Textbook of medical physiology. 11th edition. Philadelphia: Elsevier Saunders; 2006. p. 748–60.
51. Adin CA, Nelson RW. Adrenal Gland. In: Tobias KM, Johnston SA, eds. Veterinary Surgery: Small Animal: Elsevier Health Sciences; 2011:2688.
52. Kook PH, Boretti FS, Hersberger M, et al. Urinary catecholamine and metanephrine to creatinine ratios in healthy dogs at home and in a hospital environment and in 2 dogs with pheochromocytoma. J Vet Intern Med 2007;21(3):388–93.
53. Kook PH, Grest P, Quante S, et al. Urinary catecholamine and metadrenaline to creatinine ratios in dogs with a phaeochromocytoma. Vet Re 2010;166(6):169–74.
54. Quante S, Boretti FS, Kook PH, et al. Urinary catecholamine and metanephrine to creatinine ratios in dogs with hyperadrenocorticism or pheochromocytoma, and in healthy dogs. J Vet Intern Med 2010;24(5):1093–7.
55. Cameron KN, Monroe WE, Panciera DL, et al. The effects of illness on urinary catecholamines and their metabolites in dogs. J Vet Intern Med 2010;24(6):1329–36.
56. Douglass J, Berry C, James S. Ultrasonographic adrenal gland measurements in dogs without evidence of adrenal disease. Vet Radiol Ultrasound 1997;38(2):124.
57. Besso JG, Penninck DG, Gliatto JM. Retrospective ultrasonographic evaluation of adrenal lesions in 26 dogs. Vet Radiol Ultrasound 1997;38(6):448–55.
58. Grooters AM. Ultrasonographic parameters of normal canine adrenal glands: comparison to necropsy findings. Vet Radiol Ultrasound 1995;36(2):126.
59. Benchekroun G, de Fornel-Thibaud P, Rodriguez Pineiro MI, et al. Ultrasonography criteria for differentiating ACTH dependency from ACTH independency in 47 dogs with hyperadrenocorticism and equivocal adrenal asymmetry. J Vet Intern Med 2010;24(5):1077–85.
60. Rosenstein DS. Diagnostic imaging in canine pheochromocytoma. Vet Radiol Ultrasound 2000;41(6):499–506.
61. Kyles AE, Feldman EC, De Cock HE, et al. Surgical management of adrenal gland tumors with and without associated tumor thrombi in dogs: 40 cases (1994–2001). J Am Vet Med Assoc 2003;223(5):654–62.
62. Peterson ME, Gilbertson SR, Drucker WD. Plasma cortisol response to exogenous ACTH in 22 dogs with hyperadrenocorticism caused by adrenocortical neoplasia. J Am Vet Med Assoc 1982;180(5):542–4.
63. Herrera MA, Mehl ML, Kass PH, et al. Predictive factors and the effect of phenoxy-benzamine on outcome in dogs undergoing adrenalectomy for pheochromocytoma. J Vet Intern Med 2008;22(6):1333–9.
64. Gould SM, Baines EA, Mannion PA, et al. Use of endogenous ACTH concentration and adrenal ultrasonography to distinguish the cause of canine hyperadrenocorticism. J Small Anim Pract 2001;42(3):113–21.
65. Vaughan MA, Feldman EC, Hoar BR, et al. Evaluation of twice-daily, low-dose trilostane treatment administered orally in dogs with naturally occurring hyperadreno-corticism. J Am Vet Med Assoc 2008;232(9):1321–8.
66. Goy-Thollot I, Pechereau D, Keroack S, et al. Investigation of the role of aldosterone in hypertension associated with spontaneous pituitary-dependent hyperadrenocorti-cism in dogs. J Small Anim Pract 2002;43(11):489–92.

67. Mulvihill-Wilson J, Graham RM, Pettinger W, et al. Comparative effects of prazosin and phenoxybenzamine on arterial blood pressure, heart rate, and plasma catecholamines in essential hypertension. J Cardiovasc Pharmacol 1979;1(6 Suppl): S1–7.

68. Kocak S, Aydintug S, Canakci N. Alpha blockade in preoperative preparation of patients with pheochromocytomas. Int Surg 2002;87(3):191–4.

69. Fischer JR, Lane IF, Cribb AE. Urethral pressure profile and hemodynamic effects of phenoxybenzamine and prazosin in non-sedated male beagle dogs. Can J Vet Res 2003;67(1):30–8.

70. Mulvihill-Wilson J, Gaffney FA, Pettinger WA, et al. Hemodynamic and neuroendocrine responses to acute and chronic alpha-adrenergic blockade with prazosin and phenoxybenzamine. Circulation 1983;67(2):383–93.

71. Stanaszek WF, Kellerman D, Brogden RN, et al. Prazosin update: a review of its pharmacological properties and therapeutic use in hypertension and congestive heart failure. Drugs 1983;25(4):339–84.

72. Hullinger RL. The endocrine system. In: Miller ME, Evans HE, editors. Miller's anatomy of the dog. 3rd edition. Philadelphia: Saunders; 1993. p. 574–9.

73. Brenner DW, Brenner CJ, Scott J, et al. Suprarenal Greenfield filter placement to prevent pulmonary embolus in patients with vena caval tumor thrombi. J Urol 1992;147(1):19–23.

74. Peyton JW, Stewart JR, Greenfield LJ, et al. Hemodynamics and renal function following experimental suprarenal vena caval occlusion. Surg Gynecol Obstet 1982; 155(1):37–42.

75. Peacock JT, Fossum TW, Bahr AM, et al. Evaluation of gradual occlusion of the caudal vena cava in clinically normal dogs. Am J Vet Res 2003;64(11):1347–53.

76. Louvet A, Lazard P, Denis B. Phaeochromocytoma treated by en bloc resection including the suprarenal caudal vena cava in a dog. J Small Anim Pract 2005;46(12): 591–6.

77. Scavelli TD, Peterson ME, Matthiesen DT. Results of surgical treatment for hyperadrenocorticism caused by adrenocortical neoplasia in the dog: 25 cases (1980–1984). J Am Vet Med Assoc 1986;189(10):1360–4.

78. Goggs R, Benigni L, Fuentes VL, et al. Pulmonary thromboembolism. J Vet Emerg Crit Care (San Antonio) 2009;19(1):30–52.

79. Lynn RC, Feldman EC, Nelson RW. Efficacy of microcrystalline desoxycorticosterone pivalate for treatment of hypoadrenocorticism in dogs. DOCP Clinical Study Group. J Am Vet Med Assoc 1993;202(3):392–6.

80. Gilson SD, Withrow SJ, Orton EC. Surgical treatment of pheochromocytoma: technique, complications, and results in six dogs. Vet Surg 1994;23(3):195–200.

Complications of Upper Urinary Tract Surgery in Companion Animals

Christopher A. Adin, DVM*, Brian A. Scansen, DVM, MS

KEYWORDS

- Upper urinary tract • Ureters • Kidneys • Endoscopy
- Interventional radiology

SURGERY OF THE KIDNEY

Renal Biopsy

Renal biopsy is indicated for the diagnosis of primary or metastatic neoplasia of the kidney or for treatment planning in animals with protein-losing nephropathy secondary to glomerular disease. In guiding the location for biopsy, it is important to note that protein-losing diseases are typically characterized by glomerular lesions, which are located in the renal cortex. Medullary tissue is less useful for histopathologic interpretation and biopsy of this area increases the chance of injury to the renal pelvis and/or renal vascular pedicle. Therefore, the ideal renal biopsy contains only cortical tissue and has several (>5) glomeruli to allow adequate interpretation of morphology, but debate continues on the best method to obtain safe and interpretable biopsy samples. Wedge kidney biopsy may be obtained through an open abdominal approach to the kidney. The cortex is incised with a scalpel and the defect is then closed by placing sutures in the renal capsule, aiding in hemostasis by creating tamponade. Although wedge biopsy is highly successful in obtaining diagnostic samples of renal cortex, the requirement for animals to undergo general anesthesia and open abdominal surgery was a major deterrent to obtaining diagnostic biopsy samples. Percutaneous needle biopsy of the kidney has now been available for several decades and is one of the first examples of minimally invasive procedures used in veterinary medicine.[1] Original publications suggested that complications included hematuria (>80% of dogs), gross hematuria (10%), and hydronephrosis (only 3 of 82 dogs and 1 of 19 cats) due to temporary obstruction by a blood clot in the renal pelvis/ureter.[1] Although there was some concern regarding the ability to achieve diagnostic samples through use of this technique, more recent studies have confirmed that percutaneous needle biopsy was of diagnostic quality in 87% of dogs

Department of Veterinary Clinical Sciences, College of Veterinary Medicine, The Ohio State University, 601 Vernon Tharp Street, Columbus, OH 43210, USA
* Corresponding author.
E-mail address: adin.1@osu.edu

Vet Clin Small Anim 41 (2011) 869–888
doi:10.1016/j.cvsm.2011.05.015   vetsmall.theclinics.com
0195-5616/11/$ – see front matter © 2011 Elsevier Inc. All rights reserved.

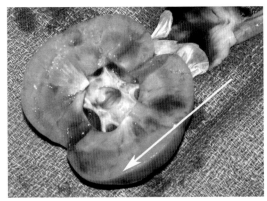

Fig. 1. This sagittal section of a kidney depicts the ideal course of a renal biopsy needle (*arrow*) placed longitudinally through the renal cortex to gain the maximal number of glomeruli for histologic interpretation, while avoiding injury to the deeper interarcuate vessels and renal pelvis.

and 86% of cats.[2] The complication rate was 13.4% in dogs and 18.5% in cats, with severe hemorrhage being the most common complication.

Avoidance

Factors that have been shown to increase the complication rate of percutaneous renal biopsy are body weight (<5 kg), species (cat>dog), and serum creatinine level greater than 5 mg/dL.[2] Quality of the biopsy sample was increased by general anesthesia, and chances of obtaining pure cortical samples were improved in surgically obtained biops samples.[2] Although a large clinical study[2] showed that percutaneous ultrasound-guided samples were equal in quality to those obtained using laparoscopy, an experimental study in dogs suggested that laparoscopic-guided needle biopsy increased the chances of a obtaining a diagnostic sample.[3] In summarizing these findings, it would be reasonable to consider using laparoscopic guidance to increase the chances of obtaining a diagnostic sample when obtaining renal biopsy specimens in animals cats or dogs less than 5 kg. Regardless of the technique used to access the kidney, proper insertion of the needle must be performed to maximize the chances of diagnostic biopsy while avoiding injury to the renal pelvis, ureter, and renal vasculature (**Fig. 1**).

Nephrotomy

Historically, access to the renal pelvis was performed using a technique termed "bisection nephrotomy." The kidney is freed from the retroperitoneal space and renal blood flow is temporarily occluded using digital compression of the entire pedicle or, preferably, with atraumatic vascular clamps placed on the renal artery. Access to the renal pelvis is obtained by making a sagittal incision in the renal capsule; then blunt dissection of the parenchyma is performed using the scalpel handle. After urolith removal, the renal parenchyma and capsule are apposed with large mattress sutures to aid in hemostasis. A landmark publication by Gahring in 1977 demonstrated that dogs undergo a 20% to 40% decrease in glomerular filtration rate (GFR) by 6 weeks after bisection nephrotomy using this technique.[4]

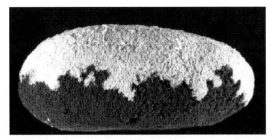

Fig. 2. This corrosion cast depicts the vascular distribution of the dorsal branch (*dark*) and ventral branch (*light*) of the renal artery. The intersegmental line is undulating and does not correspond with simple bisection nephrotomy. (*From* Stone EA, Robertson JL, Mecalf MR. The effect of nephrotomy on renal function and morphology in dogs. Vet Surg 2002;31:394; with permission.)

Advances in human surgery have occurred in this area, using knowledge of vascular anatomy. The human kidney is actually supplied by 2 branches of the renal artery (anterior and posterior). Vascular supply from each of these arteries can be mapped by performing intravenous administration of dyes during temporary occlusion of one branch of the renal artery, allowing visualization of the intersegmental line in the renal parenchyma (**Fig. 2**). Using this technique as a guide, the nephrotomy incision may be directed to avoid inadvertent trauma to intersegmental arteries and improving function after nephrotomy. A study by Stone and others[5] in 2002 sought to investigate the use of this technique in dogs and to compare postoperative GFR to dogs undergoing traditional bisection nephrotomy. Similar to humans, the canine renal artery forms 2 branches (termed dorsal and ventral renal arteries), allowing selective occlusion and evaluation of the segmental vasculature. Interestingly, Stone and colleagues' results showed that there were no significant differences in GFR measurements when dogs that underwent bisection nephrotomy were compared with those that underwent intersegmental nephrotomy. Even more notably, both groups actually had improved GFR in the first 4 weeks after surgery (176% of baseline). These results have directly contradicted earlier findings and have caused rethinking of how nephrotomy may be applied in surgical practice. Potential explanations for differences in results include the fact that Stone and colleagues' study used simple continuous closure of the renal capsule, avoiding large bites of renal parenchyma that were previously advocated. In addition, the more recent study used modern anesthetic inhalant drugs and preischemic administration of mannitol (as per standard of care), which may have decreased ischemic injury to the kidney during vascular occlusion. We must also keep in mind that both studies were performed in normal dogs and may not reflect the conditions in animals with compromised renal function at baseline. Although bisection nephrotomy was found to cause slightly more tissue trauma and renal hemorrhage, this study has maintained bisection as the more expedient and simple technique in dogs.[5]

In line with the trend of research, 2 additional recent studies[6,7] used a similar study design to evaluate the effects of bisection nephrotomy in normal cats. Both studies showed no significant changes in GFR compared with the contralateral kidney when using noninvasive means of assessing postoperative GFR, with one group following cats to 79 weeks of follow-up.[6] It is notable that 2 normal cats had documented ureteral obstruction following nephrotomy in one experimental study,[7] a problem that would not have been as easily handled in a cat with contralateral renal dysfunction.

URETERAL SURGERY
Inability to Localize the Lesion

Ureteral obstruction is a common indication for surgical intervention in small animals. Although ureteral obstruction in dogs and cats is most commonly associated with the presence of radiopaque ureteral calculi (eg, calcium oxalate), diagnosis and localization of these and other causes of obstruction can be challenging in companion animals and imaging findings could lead to surgical intervention on the wrong ureter in up to 5% of animals that receive ureteral surgery.[8-13] In a retrospective study of cats with suspected ureteral obstruction,[12] radiography was found to have 100% specificity in identifying radiopaque calculi (there are few false-positive results) but had a sensitivity of only 60% (not all obstructions are detected). Radiography can be limited in cases where an obstruction is caused by nonradiopaque lesions (eg, a stricture or mucus plug), when calculi are too small to be detected, or when superimposition of the colon and vertebral column obstructs detection or lateralization of ureteral lesions.[12] In contrast, ultrasound was found to have a very high sensitivity (100%) in detecting ureteral obstruction, due to the early onset of hydronephrosis and renal pelvic dilatation in most animals.[8] However, pelvic dilatation can occur secondary to pyelonephritis and other nonobstructive conditions, which decreased the specificity of this technique to 33% for correct detection of ureteral obstruction in cats.[8] Due to the complementary nature of these 2 techniques, the use of combined radiography and ultrasound was found to improve the sensitivity of detecting ureteral calculi in cats to 90% in a recent large retrospective study.[12]

Even when preoperative imaging is successful in locating the source of urinary obstruction, intraoperative migration of urinary calculi can occur during manipulation of the ureter, causing difficulty in locating and mobilizing small stones into the site of a ureterotomy incision. Although this complication can often cause delay in completing surgery, it has also been documented to cause a need for additional procedures, with proximal migration of a ureteral calculus causing a need for conversion to nephrotomy in 1 cat.[14]

Avoidance

Based on the information gleaned from previous studies,[12,14] it appears that the use of complementary abdominal radiographic and ultrasound imaging techniques is indicated to maximize correct diagnosis and localization of ureteral obstructions in small animals. Sensitivity of radiography in detecting small ureteral calculi may be improved by the use of techniques that empty or physically displace the colon when obtaining a lateral abdominal projection, preventing superimposition of fecal material over the distal ureter. When standard imaging techniques are inconclusive, use of antegrade pyelography, contrast computed tomography (CT), or retrograde ureteropyelography can improve identification and localization of ureteral obstruction in cats.[8,12,15] Antegrade pyelography facilitates identification of both radiopaque and nonradiopaque ureteral obstructive lesions by using percutaneous, ultrasonographic, and fluoroscopic-guided contrast injection into the renal pelvis. With this technique, a bolus of contrast material can be directly instilled into the renal pelvis and ureter, improving the detail that can be obtained compared with intravenous urography in animals with a poor GFR.[8] CT excretory urography carries similar advantages but also allows the use of cross-sectional imaging to prevent superimposition of structures that occurs in 2-dimensional radiographs. In addition, the noninvasive nature of CT eliminated the risk of iatrogenic renal or ureteral injury that has been described after antegrade pyelography.[8] Retrograde ureteropyelography can be performed in female

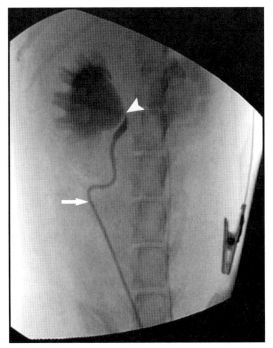

Fig. 3. An example of retrograde ureteropyelography in a dog. A ureteral catheter (*arrowhead*) is advanced into the right ureteral orifice via a guidewire and cystoscopic visualization. The iodinated contrast delineates the ureteral lumen, a ureteropelvic junction stenosis (*arrow*), and the hydronephrotic renal pelvis. Note that a ureteral stent has previously been placed in the left ureter and kidney.

cats and dogs as well as large breed male dogs (**Fig. 3**). Cystoscopy is used to visualized the ureteral orifice; then a hydrophilic guidewire (0.018-inch in a cat, 0.035-inch in a dog) is used to access the ureter over which a ureteral catheter (3Fr in a cat, 4Fr in a dog) is advanced to the distal ureter under fluoroscopic guidance.[15] The wire is then removed and contrast is injected through the catheter to visualize the ureter and renal pelvis. The benefits of this technique are that the minimally invasive approach is used, that maximal ureteral dilation can be achieved, and that the contrast is only infused into the ureter and pelvis, avoiding the potential for contrast-induced nephropathy. Drawbacks to retrograde ureteropyelography include the requirement for cystoscopic and fluoroscopic guidance and potential difficulty in accessing the ureteral orifice of cats and small dogs.

Correct intraoperative localization of ureteral calculi can be facilitated by a number of surgical techniques. First, the surgeon should be prepared to fully explore both the right and left ureters by visual examination and palpation to gain an appreciation of all potential lesions before executing a ureteral incision and removing any suspected calculi. Complete exploration of the right and left ureters requires a ventral midline abdominal approach in the dog and cat. After locating a suspected ureteral calculus or other obstructive lesion, the author will typically place a vessel loop proximal and distal to a suspected area of obstruction, partially occluding the ureter by traction so that ureteral calculi are prevented from retrograde migration into the proximal dilated ureter or renal pelvis during attempts to retrieve the stone. If proximal migration does occur, the author has had success in inserting a 20-gauge, spinal needle into the renal pelvis and gently flushing calculi out of a more distal ureterotomy incision with a 6-mL syringe. When the site of obstruction cannot be located by direct visual and digital examination of the ureters, a cytotomy incision can be made to access the ureteral papilla, allowing the surgeon to insert a piece of fine colored suture (5-0 monofilament polypropylene in a cat), a hydrophilic guidewire (0.018-inch-diameter in cat, 0.035-inch-diameter in a dog), or a small urinary catheter into either ureter. The suture, wire, or catheter is then advanced in a retrograde fashion until the site of obstruction is encountered, guiding the location of the ureterotomy incision.

Postoperative Urine Leakage

Urine leakage was the most commonly reported complication of upper urinary tract surgery in a series of 101 cats undergoing upper urinary tract surgery for urinary calculi.[14] Uroabdomen occurred in 16% (14 of 88) cats that survived surgery, representing more than half of the overall complications that occurred in this series.[14] Leakage occurred in 11 of 70 (16%) cats following ureterotomy and in 4 of 27 (15%) cats in which ureteroneocystostomy was performed, suggesting that there is no significant advantage in one technique over another.[14] Although urinary diversion has been advocated as a means of preventing urine leakage after ureteral surgery,[16] uroabdomen was actually more common in cats that received nephrostomy tubes (6 of 24 [25%]) compared with cats that did not (8 of 64 [12%]). Ironically, urine leakage was actually related to the nephrostomy tube insertion site in 6 of the 24 cats.[14] There are no large case series have presented comparative data on complications of ureteral surgery in dogs. The author's clinical experience is that surgical complications are similar in this species, although the larger luminal diameter of the canine ureter makes surgery of the canine ureter less technically demanding than in cats.

Diagnosis

Urine leakage typically occurs within the first 3 to 5 days after ureteral or renal surgery. Recognition of clinical signs is crucial for early detection of uroabdomen, prior to the development of severe metabolic derangements. Animals with uroabdomen develop noticeable abdominal discomfort secondary to a chemical peritonitis that is induced by exposure to urine. Abdominal distention, progressive bruising of the ventral abdomen, lethargy, and loss of appetite are all common sequelae. Although urine production may remain adequate due to function of the contralateral kidney and ureter, weight gain will be noted as fluid is retained in the peritoneal cavity. Patients should be monitored by daily abdominal palpation, body weight measurement, and serum creatinine/blood urea nitrogen (BUN) and electrolytes for the first 3 days after surgery. In animals with signs of uroabdomen, diagnosis is confirmed by abdominal ultrasound and abdominocentesis. In animals with active urine leakage, abdominal fluid creatinine and potassium concentrations will be far in excess of those in the serum.

Treatment

Urine leakage after upper urinary tract surgery is unlikely to resolve spontaneously and therapeutic intervention is indicated. To date, surgical revision has been the standard approach to failed ureterotomy or ureteroneocystostomy in companion animals, and in the author's experience, revision of leaking ureterotomy sites or uteroneocystostomy sites has had some success, without concurrent urinary stenting or ureteronephrectomy. In the previously described study of ureteral surgery in 101 cats, uroabdomen developed in 11 of 70 cats that had a ureterotomy, with a second surgery being performed in 9 of these cats.[14] Revision of ureterostomy closure was successful in 5 of 7 cats with leakage observed at that site. One cat was euthanized due to continued urine leakage at another site, while another underwent ureteronephrectomy and renal allograft transplantation. In cats that developed leakage from the kidney or renal pelvis secondary to nephrostomy tube placement or antegrade pyelography, resolution of urine leakage was not achieved with revision of primary closure. Overall mortality in cats that developed postoperative uroperitoneum was 27% (3 of 11), with another 3 cats being euthanized without additional surgery.[14] In the future, clinicians may consider performing temporary urinary diversion procedures (described later) at the time of the original surgery or as a means of draining urine from the operative site after leakage has been noted in the postoperative period.

Avoidance

The small size of the canine and feline ureter adds to the technical difficulty of obtaining an immediate, water-tight closure on incisions into this structure. Thus, most authors have advocated the use of surgical magnification to minimize the likelihood of urine leakage after ureteral surgery in companion animals. Magnifying loupes ($\times$3.5 magnification) provide sufficient visualization of the canine ureter to allow meticulous apposition of mucosa during closure,[16] but an operating microscope ($\times$8 to $\times$10 magnification) is recommended for ureteral surgery in cats.[7,14,17] Use of fine monofilament, absorbable suture on a small (vascular) taper point needle is recommended, with 6-0 suture being sufficient for most dogs and 8-0 to 9-0 suture being most appropriate in cats. There is an extremely limited selection of absorbable sutures in the 8-0 to 9-0 size range. Of these, only coated polyglactin 910 is available on a taper needle that is suited for ureteral repair. Full-thickness sutures should be placed in close apposition to achieve perfect mucosal apposition, using a simple continuous pattern to achieve a watertight seal where possible.[17]

Urinary diversion for 48 to 72 hours had been advocated to eliminate urine leakage after ureteral surgery, allowing urinary epithelium to migrate over any mucosal defects.[16] Historically, urinary diversion was performed by placement of a nephrostomy catheter,[18] as intraluminal stents that bridged the ureteral defect were thought to contribute to stricture formation at the operative site.[16] Over time, even nephrostomy tubes were abandoned as the high rate of tube dislodgement, occlusion, and urine leakage from the insertion site actually appeared to increase complication rate after surgery.[14] It is now known that intraluminal stenting has significant benefits in reducing postoperative complications with urine leakage after ureterotomy, and implantation of stents for 7 to 10 days has become the standard of care in human ureteral surgery.[19] Recent advances in veterinary interventional radiology have spurred a reconsideration of the use of both nephrostomy tubes and intraluminal stenting in canine and feline ureteral surgery. Original attempts at nephrostomy tube placement were hampered by a lack of available catheters designed for use in small animals. Red rubber feeding tubes were often inserted through the renal parenchyma and into the renal pelvis using a mosquito hemostat.[20] This technique created a large entry hole that was predisposed to urine leakage. In addition, tube dislodgement occurred frequently due to a lack of any mechanical interlock between the straight catheter and the renal pelvis. Modern pediatric nephrostomy catheters have solved these problems and are designed to be introduced percutaneously using the Seldinger technique (over a wire), preventing leakage from the insertion site in the kidney. In addition, modern nephrostomy catheters have a pigtail design that mechanically retains the device in the renal pelvis and prevents inadvertent dislodgement and have been used

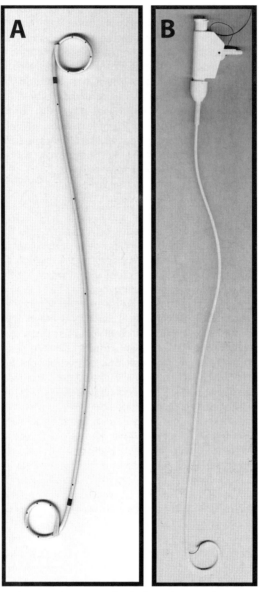

Fig. 4. A double-pigtail ureteral stent and a locking loop catheter used for percutaneous nephrostomy. Note, that the ureteral stent (*A*) has multiple side-holes to facilitate urine drainage, while the percutaneous nephrostomy catheter (*B*) contains a string which, when pulled taught, locks the pigtail loop in position and prevents migration of the nephrostomy tube from the renal pelvis. The stylet that straightens the catheter and facilitates advancement into the renal pelvis is not shown.

successfully in dogs and cats as a means of urine diversion.[15] Intraluminal ureteral stents that are anchored in both the bladder and renal pelvis are also available for use in cats and dogs (**Fig. 4**), allowing stenting of ureteral defects in association with surgical repair. While uroepithelium can migrate rapidly to cover small defects in the ureteral mucosa in 48 hours, the remainder of the repaired ureteral wall is composed of fibrous tissue[21] and large defects that are allowed to heal over a urinary stent will develop a significant decrease in lumen size, predisposing to ureteral obstruction. In addition, a recent experimental study in dogs showed that collagen deposition in the ureter is different than in other areas of the urinary tract, with ureteral anastomoses failing to reach full breaking strength at 6 weeks.[22] Unfortunately, prolonged retention of urinary stents has been shown to actually contribute to obstructive uropathy, even in normal unoperated ureters.[23] These findings suggested a possible explanation for the frequent problems of healing that are noted after ureteral surgery in both animals and human beings, reinforcing that urinary stenting alone is not a substitute for meticulous, tension-free repair of ureteral defects and that stenting itself can have detrimental effects. As a general recommendation, short-term ureteral stenting is indicated to reinforce ureteral anastomoses or ureterotomy closures in cases where there is significant concern regarding the likelihood of postoperative urine leakage.

Ureteral Obstruction

Ureteral surgery is one of the more challenging aspects of soft tissue surgery, particularly in cats, and has therefore been a focus of ongoing research. Clinical reports of renal pelvic dilatation and ureteral obstruction were common in cats that had undergone initial attempts at microscopic reimplantation of the ureter during renal transplantation.[24] A recent report of feline ureteral strictures in 10 cats described that previous ureteral surgery was the most common cause of stricture formation in that population.[25] Ureteral obstruction was also described as the second most common complication in cats treated for ureteral calculi, occurring in 5 of 101 (5%) cats undergoing ureterotomy (2 of 70 [2.9%]) or neoureterocystostomy (3 of 27 [11%]).[14] The authors acknowledged that they were likely to have underestimated the rate of postoperative obstruction in these animals, since prospective imaging was not performed unless clinical signs of complications were noted and contralateral renal function may have prevented development of azotemia. Although the risk of temporary ureteral obstruction was realized, the results of a landmark study by Barthez and others showed that persistent partial ureteral obstruction occurs for up to 1 to 2 weeks after ureteral implantation, even in normal dogs weighing 10 to 17 kg.[9] Despite these challenges, ureteral surgery is required with some frequency for treatment of ureteral calculi, ureteral ectopia, and to restore urinary tract patency in cases of vehicular or iatrogenic surgical trauma to the ureters.

Diagnosis

Detection of unilateral postoperative ureteral obstruction can be difficult when contralateral renal function is normal, since azotemia will not be detected on serum biochemical analyses. In addition, onset of obstruction can occur at a variety of time periods after surgery that correlate with the stages of wound healing, with obstruction in the early (1–7 days) postoperative period occurring secondary to inflammation,[9] while late obstructions (weeks to months after surgery) are more commonly due to stricture formation.[25] Unfortunately, early detection and intervention are essential as the degree of renal injury is directly proportional to the duration of urinary obstruction, with 30% of function lost at 1 week and nearly complete loss of function within 6 weeks.[26,27] In contrast to unilateral obstructive lesions, bilateral complete ureteral obstruction will cause a rapid onset of uremia, with death occurring in 3 to 6 days.[26] Scintigraphic assessement of renal function using technetium DTPA has been to shown to be a sensitive indicator of obstruction in an experimental canine model,[28] although this technique is not widely available in veterinary practice. Abdominal

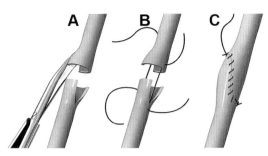

Fig. 5. (*A*) Ureteral anastomosis (ureterouretorostomy). The ends of the ureteral segments are spatulated by making a longitudinal incision to widen each ureteral orifice. (*B*) The anastomosis is performed using fine (5-0 to 9-0) synthetic absorbable suture material. Two sutures are placed at the points of each incision, 180° apart to align the anastomosis. (*C*) A continuous or interrupted suture pattern is used to complete the repair. (*From* McLoughlin MA, Bjorling D. Ureters. In: Slatter DH, editor. Textbook of small animal surgery. 3rd edition. Philadelphia: Saunders; 2003. p. 1625; with permission.)

ultrasonography provides a more readily accessible, noninvasive method to detect early signs of hydronephrosis or progressive ureteral dilation that are consistent with ureteral obstruction.[8,14,29] Early detection of unilateral ureteral obstructions requires a more proactive diagnostic approach and the author recommends serial ultrasound examinations at 2 days after ureteral surgery (prior to discharge), at the time of suture removal, and every 3 to 6 months following surgery. In this manner, serial measurements of the renal pelvis and ureteral lumen diameter can be performed and compared to baseline measurements obtained after surgery. Concurrently, animals can be monitored for recurrence or migration of ureteral/renal calculi. Definitive diagnosis of strictures or stenoses is typically achieved by percutaneous antegrade ureteropyelography or by surgical or endoscopic retrograde ureteropyelography.[25]

Treatment

Some animals with evidence of ureteral obstruction due to inflammation or crush injury will undergo spontaneous resolution of the obstruction without intervention.[9,10] The decision to intervene in an animal that is experiencing problems with postoperative ureteral obstruction is based on (1) evidence of progressive renal pelvic/ureteral dilatation on serial ultrasound examinations and/or (2) worsening postrenal azotemia. Therapy for postoperative ureteral obstruction involves reestablishing urine drainage through temporary urinary diversion procedures (nephrostomy tube or ureteral stent)[25] or by revision of the surgical site in the affected ureter(s). Goals of revision surgery would be to remove inflamed or fibrous tissue and to achieve a tension-free closure to avoid stricture formation at the operated site. Typically, the most efficient means of achieving these goals is to perform resection and anastomosis of the original ureterotomy/ureterostomy site, followed by primary closure. Lumen diameter is maximized by incising the ureter ends at an angle and is further increased by using a fine scissor to make an additional 3- to 4-m longitudinal incision in the ureter, spatulating the ends to increase luminal diameter at the site of anastomosis (**Fig. 5**).[26]

There is now early evidence that ureteral stenting can be used as an alternative means of treating postoperative ureteral strictures in cats.[25] Application of ureteral stents led to decreases in renal pelvic dilatation in 6 of 6 cats, with decreased azotemia in 5 of 6 cats.[25] In these cats, stent application was performed as a permanent treatment for ureteral stenosis,[25] while stent application in human beings is used only as a temporary means of establishing drainage as a result of to long-term complications of stent occlusion, migration, encrustation of the stent, and poor patient tolerance due to discomfort caused by the implant.[30–32] Treatment of ureteral strictures in human beings has now advanced to the use of balloon dilation catheters, a technique that has similar efficacy to open surgery.[19,30–32] Although not routine, balloon dilation of ureteral strictures has also been performed in veterinary patients by using small coronary balloon dilation catheters.[33]

Avoidance

A variety of factors contribute to the development of postoperative ureteral obstructions, including tissue ischemia that leads to stricture formation, postoperative inflammation, and surgeon error. Crush injuries typically produce temporary obstruction that can resolve spontaneously, while devascularization produced by stripping of the ureteral adventitia contributes to stricture formation.[34] As a result, it is crucial to preserve the longitudinal ureteral blood supply and to strip a minimal amount of adventitia at the site of ureteral anastomosis as the ureter is mobilized from the retroperitoneal space during surgical procedures. When handling the ureter and placing sutures, the surgeon should attempt to handle only the periureteral fat or adventitia, rather than grasping the mucosa of the ureter itself. A stay suture can be placed in the tip of the ureter during manipulation, to minimize crushing trauma caused by thumb forceps. Bleeding from the periureteral fat should be addressed with direct pressure or, when necessary, with stainless steel microclips rather than with electrocautery.

A series of recent studies have shown that adjustments in surgical technique can significantly reduce the likelihood of postoperative ureteral obstruction. For example, the original surgical procedure used for ureteral implantation in the cat involved a "drop-in" technique in which the ureter was pulled through a stab incision in the bladder wall, spatulated, and then attached to the bladder mucosa using a single suture. This technique led to high rates of obstruction due to granuloma formation at the implantation site.[24] After experience with microsurgery was improved, direct mucosal apposition was performed using 8-10 interrupted sutures to achieve direct apposition of bladder and ureteral mucosa in the cat.[35] This technique was used for many years until more recent studies showed that the intravesicular mucosal apposition technique led to significant increases in serum creatinine (mean of 9.4 mg/dL at 3 days after surgery), even in healthy cats undergoing experimental renal transplantation.[36] The mucosal apposition technique is performed through a ventral cystotomy with the bladder mucosa everted to maintain surgical exposure. Unfortunately, progressive edema of the bladder mucosa develops during the procedure, obscuring visualization and likely contributing to the noted incidence of postoperative ureteral obstruction. To address these challenges, veterinary surgeons have now adopted the use of extravesicular implantation techniques (also known as the modified Lich-Gregoir technique), in which the ureteral mucosa is sutured to the bladder mucosa through a small incision in the seromuscular layer of the bladder. Extravesicular neoureterocystostomy has been shown to improve outcome and decrease the rate of postoperative obstruction in experimental cats, and is now the procedure of choice for ureteral implantation in small animals.[36]

When tension is considered to be a contributor to postoperative ureteral stricture formation, or in cases of ureteral shortening due to resection of a stenosed or traumatized segment, alternatives to ureteral reimplantation in the bladder have also been raised. One option in animals with a shortened ureter is to shorten the distance between the bladder and kidney by performing renal descensus, dissecting the kidney from the retroperitoneal space and transposing it caudally, as far as the vessels allow, before pexying in a new location. Cystopexy to the dorsal body wall (psoas hitch) or kidney (nephrocystopexy) has also been described in cats as a means of relieving tension on ureteral anastomoses.[37] An alternative technique would be ureteroureteric anastomosis, as was described in a more recent report by Mehl and Kyles.[38] Due to the high incidence of postoperative ureteral obstruction documented in these experimental studies, the prophylactic use of temporary ureteral stents may need to be reconsidered in veterinary surgery.[15,25,33] It should be noted that the application of a ureteral stent may necessitate a second procedure to remove the stent via cystoscopy in the future. Interestingly, however, the reported complications of stent encrustment and diffuse ureteral obstruction, which dictate stent exchange or removal in human medicine within 3 to 12 months, have not been documented in any canine or feline patient, including indwelling durations of up to 4.5 years.[33]

Recurrence of urolithiasis

Recurrence of urolithiasis after surgical removal is common and was documented in 40% of cats (14 of 35) that underwent serial abdominal imaging after treatment for upper urinary calculi.[14] Thus, it is crucial that the surgeon takes responsibility for obtaining mineral analysis of all removed calculi and prescribing a follow-up regimen that is aimed toward preventing recurrence of urinary calculi. The vast majority of renal and ureteral calculi that are isolated from cats are composed of calcium oxalate (98%).[12] Interestingly, calcium oxalate urolithiasis has also been shown to recur in 25% of renal allografts after transplantation into cats with a history of previous stone disease.[39] Recurrence of calcium oxalate calculi in cats can be related to a number of risk factors, including diet (dry vs canned), environment (indoor or outdoor), and obesity.[40,41] In both cats and dogs, renal hypercalciuria is likely to be an important part of the underlying pathophysiology of oxalate disease. Other metabolic conditions such as canine primary hyperparathyroidism can occasionally cause primary urinary tract signs due to formation of calcium oxalate stones, reinforcing the importance of performing a complete biochemistry analysis on all animals prior to surgical intervention for urolithiasis. A small number of dogs will have ureteral or renal calculi that are composed primarily of struvite. In contrast to oxalate stones, which are commonly formed due to metabolic abnormalities, urease-producing bacteria are integral to the formation of struvite calculi in dogs.[42] Surgical factors that could contribute to postoperative calculus recurrence such as suture nidus due to intraluminal foreign material are discussed in the Complications of Lower Urinary Tract Surgery section of this text.

Diagnosis

Due to the high frequency of postoperative urolith recurrence in dogs and cats, serial imaging is recommended for the remainder of the pet's life. Since upper urinary tract calculi are nearly all composed of radiopaque calcium oxalate or struvite, abdominal radiography can be used as a readily accessible screening tool to locate and enumerate calculi throughout the urinary tract. Radiographs are recommended every 3 to 6 months, with additional ultrasound imaging in animals with evidence of decreased renal function secondary to post renal obstruction.

Avoidance

After ruling out metabolic conditions that cause hypercalcemia (hyperparathyroidism or malignancy) with serum biochemistry analyses, dietary therapy is the primary means of preventing calcium oxalate recurrence in dogs and cats. The primary goal of dietary therapy is to lower the concentration of calcium and oxalates in the urine, thereby decreasing the likelihood of calculus formation. Diets that are low in calcium have been shown to decrease calciuria in both dogs and cats with a history of calcium oxalate urolithiasis.[40,43] Increasing water intake through the use of canned diets is also recommended, encouraging calciuresis.[40,43] Potassium citrate may be added as a urine alkalinizer (50 mg/kg twice daily) to maintain urine pH at a range of 7.0 to 7.5.[42] In general, use of a canned prescription diet that is formulated for animals with calcium oxalate is a safe and convenient method for most owners,[40,43] provided that they are aware that this is the only food that is to be given to the animal, since treats and other supplements can contain large quantities of calcium or oxalate. It is important to note that dissolution of calcium oxalate calculi is not possible and that dietary modification can only be directed toward prevention of calculi, rather than being used as a primary means of therapy.

Prevention of recurrent struvite urolithiasis is directed primarily at effective treatment of the urinary tract infection based on bacterial culture and antimicrobial sensitivity testing. Culture of the calculus itself is more likely to yield positive results compared to urine culture.[42] Urine culture is often altered by preoperative administration of antimicrobial drugs, and in dogs with confirmed struvite urolithiasis, empirical therapy should be initiated with a broad-spectrum antibiotic that is effective against *Staphylococcus intermedius*, *Escherichia coli*, and *Proteus* sp. Follow-up evaluation should include recheck urine culture prior to cessation of antimicrobials and should be rechecked at 3-month intervals for life. Dietary dissolution of struvite stones can be accomplished in isolated cases using a prescription diet that is low in protein and ash content, although poor compliance due to low palatability of protein-restricted diets can be a problem in achieving successful dissolution.[42]

Therapy

Recurrent urinary calculi in dogs and cats are treated using the same guidelines that applied at the time of the original diagnosis. Fluid diuresis and analgesics may be used to treat initial azotemia and to encourage passage of ureteral calculi into the lower urinary tract.[14] If azotemia persists or there is evidence of progressive renal pelvic dilation on serial ultrasound imaging, then surgical intervention should be considered.

INTERVENTIONAL RADIOLOGY OF THE UPPER URINARY TRACT

The development of interventional radiology in veterinary medicine[44] has provided some novel techniques to deal with disease of the upper urinary tract in dogs and cats. In recent years, descriptive reports have focused on ureteral stenting,[15,25] percutaneous nephrostomy drainage,[15,44] and extracorporeal shockwave lithotripsy (ESWL).[33,45] These techniques will be briefly reviewed here, with the intent to introduce these techniques as a complement to traditional surgical approaches. Given the paucity of reports in veterinary medicine of these techniques, there are no direct comparisons evaluating the efficacy of surgery versus interventional radiology for treatment of upper urinary tract disease in animals. However, it is the author's opinion that an understanding of these techniques will help surgeons and internists widen the arsenal of available treatment strategies to manage animals with upper urinary tract disease and, in so doing, reduce or better manage complications of upper urinary tract surgery.

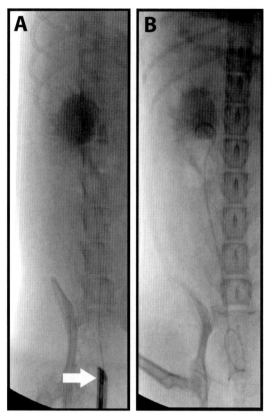

Fig. 6. Retrograde ureteral stent placement in a dog. (*A*) Cystoscope can be seen within the bladder (*arrow*) and a guidewire has been advanced into the right ureteral orifice and curled in the right renal pelvis. (*B*) Stent is advanced over the wire and the cranial loop resides in the renal pelvis, while the caudal loop is within the bladder.

Ureteral Stenting

Surgical ureteral (or ureteric) stenting was proposed in the early twentieth century as an aid to ureterotomy healing, and a temporary indwelling splint (termed an intubated ureterotomy) was performed in a human as early as 1915.[46] Minimally invasive placement of a ureteral stent, comparable to current technique, was first reported in a human in 1967.[47] Minimally invasive ureteral stenting in clinical veterinary patients was first reported in 2005,[48] with subsequent reports showing good success in both dogs and cats.[15,33,44,48] Current ureteral stents are made of polyurethane (prior materials included silicone and polyethylene; novel materials are under development) and have a double-pigtail design, meaning a straight shaft with a loop on each end that serve to hold the stent in the renal pelvis and the bladder (**Fig. 6**). Numerous sizes are available of variable diameter and length. In general, 3Fr to 3.7Fr diameter stents are suitable for very small dogs, 4Fr to 4.7Fr stents for small to medium-size dogs, and 6Fr stents for large dogs or those with severely dilated ureters. A novel feline stent has been developed and recently entered the market, available in a diameter of 2.5Fr with lengths of 12 cm, 14 cm, and 16 cm. Additionally, this stent comes from the manufacturer in polyurethane of variable stiffness: a soft stent (55 durometer) or a stiff stent (65 durometer). Indications for each will be discussed briefly later. The length of stent required can be estimated from abdominal films (measured from the renal pelvis to the urinary bladder) or intraoperatively with a sterile ruler. In general, erring toward a slightly longer stent is preferable to undersizing the stent as extra stent length can be extended into the bladder.

Ureteral stenting is useful as a means of urinary diversion after renal and/or ureteral surgery. Additionally, ureteral stenting may be considered as a primary therapy for obstructive ureterolithiasis or ureteral strictures in certain cases.[25] After placement of a ureteral stent, particularly current multifenestrated designs, the urine will flow through the stent lumen from pelvis to bladder but also around the stent. Furthermore, studies demonstrate that the ureter dilates passively around a stent within days to weeks, which further enhances urine drainage and stone passage.[49] Indeed, new experimental stent designs have no true lumen but alleviate obstruction solely through passive ureteral dilation around the stent and by straightening the pathway from renal pelvis to bladder.[50] In the setting of ureteral surgery, indications for ureteral stenting may then include animals with multiple sites of obstruction (whether stone, debris, or stricture) for which multiple ureterotomies would be required; ureteral strictures for which a high rate of surgical complication may be expected; to facilitate healing and prevent stricture formation in the setting of pyelotomy, ureteropyeloplasty, or ureterneocystostomy; for alleviation of external ureteral compression; or for facilitation of stone passage as in the setting of ESWL. The author believes ureteral stenting should be considered for nearly all cases of feline ureteral intervention, given the potential complications associated with ureteral surgery in cats. In addition, ureteral stents placed in cats are seldom, if ever, removed given the potential for recurrent urolithiasis and because placement of feline ureteral stents nearly always requires celiotomy. In dogs, the author primarily uses ureteral stents to facilitate healing after complex ureteral surgery (eg, ureteropyeloplasty), for ureteral stricture treatment, or to palliate malignant ureteral obstruction. Others perform ureteral stenting routinely for nephrolithiasis and ureterolithiasis in dogs.[44,48]

Briefly, the placement of a ureteral stent requires fluoroscopic and/or cystoscopic guidance and can be performed from an antegrade or retrograde approach. In the antegrade approach, access to the renal pelvis is obtained either percutaneously or directly if performed during an open surgical procedure. In the dog, an 18-gauge over-the-needle catheter or renal access needle is used; in the cat, a 22-gauge over-the-needle catheter is preferred. A hydrophilic guidewire (0.035-inch for a dog, 0.018-inch for a cat) is then directed through the catheter and down the ureter under fluoroscopic guidance (or direct visualization) and curled into the bladder. If performed percutaneously, this wire is then directed out the urethra and a vascular sheath (typically a 7Fr, 70-cm sheath) is advanced over the wire, up the urethra, and into the distal ureter. A second hydrophilic wire is advanced through this sheath and curled in the renal pelvis, and the stent is then delivered retrograde over a wire, advancing the cranial pigtail into the renal pelvis and positioning the caudal pigtail in the bladder (**Fig. 7**). If a ureterotomy or pyelotomy has been performed, the wire can be directed into the bladder through this incision and the stent delivered under direct visualization. The retrograde approach involves cystoscopic access or visualization of the ureteral orifices through a cystotomy/urethrotomy incision. In both techniques, a hydrophilic guidewire is advanced into the ureteral orifice, over which a ureteral catheter is placed. The wire is removed and contrast medium is injected to fluoroscopically visualize the ureter and renal pelvis. The wire is then replaced and advanced fluoroscopically until it has curled in the renal pelvis. The stent may then be advanced over the wire; once the cranial pigtail is within the renal pelvis, the wire is

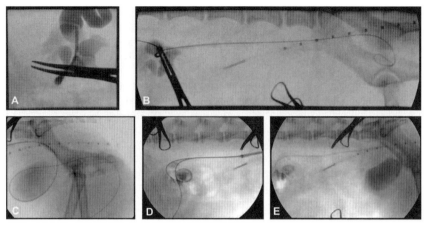

Fig. 7. Antegrade ureteral stent placement in a dog with malignant ureteral obstruction secondary to transitional cell carcinoma of the bladder. (*A*) Percutaneous renal access is obtained and iodinated contrast given to show the ureteral course. (*B*) Guidewire is then advanced down the ureter and to the level of the ureterovesicular junction. (*C*) Guidewire is manipulated through the obstruction, into the bladder, and out the urethra. (*D*) Long sheath is then advanced retrograde over-the-wire, up the urethra, and into the mid-ureter where a second guidewire is advanced into the renal pelvis. Over the second wire, the ureteral stent is advanced and cranial loop allowed to curl in the renal pelvis, while the caudal loop is brought back into the bladder facilitating drainage of the obstructed kidney (*E*).

removed and stent's curl is allowed to form. The caudal pigtail is then pushed with a radiopaque pusher (included with most stent systems) under fluoroscopic and cystoscopic guidance in the setting of a minimally invasive approach or directly positioned within the bladder if performed via cystotomy (see **Fig. 6**). In the cat, percutaneous or cystoscopic (only possible in female cats) approaches are quite challenging and an open abdominal procedure is the author's preferred technique for ureteral stenting. Usually, a retrograde approach via the ureteral orifice is attempted first, though conversion to an antegrade approach is occasionally required. Keeping the ureter as straight as possible via cranial retraction of the kidney is critical to successful stent advancement. Additionally, it should be noted that proximal or mid-ureteral obstructions are more difficult to stent as much of the ureter is not distended. The author prefers to attempt placement of the soft feline stent first as there is anecdotal evidence that this stent is better tolerated by cats, though in difficult cases the stiff feline stent may be required as this provides greater pushability through a nondistended feline ureter.

Complications of ureteral stenting in veterinary patients are not well-reported. While there is evidence that implantation of a ureteral stent induces some degree of mucosal edema and erosion in normal canine ureters,[21] clinically significant ureteral damage from stenting has not been documented in clinical feline or canine cases. Mild dysuria or hematuria is occasionally seen in the first week after ureteral stent placement in dogs and cats. This is typically self-limiting, though urine culture should be evaluated to rule out concurrent urinary tract infection. The author has seen 1 dog develop pyelonephritis and progressive hydronephrosis in the setting of a ureteral stent that had been implanted 3 months previously, which also argues for careful monitoring of urinary tract infection in animals with these implants.

Percutaneous Nephrostomy

As noted previously in this article, the use of nephrostomy tubes has fallen out of favor in veterinary medicine due to a high risk of dislodgement and complications.[14] However, newer designs optimized for percutaneous placement may prove useful as a means of emergent stabilization in the cat or dog with ureteral obstruction or as a means of urinary diversion postoperatively. In contrast to the red rubber catheters used in the past,[20] newer nephrostomy tubes are of a locking-loop design (see **Fig. 4**). These drainage catheters can be straightened with a stylet, advanced over a wire into the renal pelvis, and then a loop is formed that is "locked" in placed with a string knotted to the base of the catheter. The string retains the tip of the catheter in a tight loop, helping to prevent catheter migration (see **Fig. 4**). While no direct comparison to prior designs has been performed in veterinary medicine, it is the author's clinical impression that this design provides a more robust placement, though dislodgement is still possible and normal measures to prevent traction on the catheter should be used.

The technique of percutaneous nephrostomy tube placement requires that the animal be under general anesthesia, typically in lateral recumbency with the affected kidney elevated. Ultrasound is used to localize a direct path to the renal pelvis, free of other abdominal structures. A renal access needle or sufficiently long over-the-needle catheter is directed into the renal pelvis under ultrasonographic guidance with placement confirmed by aspiration of urine. Contrast (typically a 50:50 mixture of saline and iodinated contrast material) is injected to visualize the renal pelvis and proximal ureter fluoroscopically and a guidewire (0.035-inch for most drainage catheters, 0.018-inch is required for some 5Fr catheters) is advanced until it curls in the renal pelvis or is directed down the ureter. The drainage catheter is then advanced over the wire using the included stylet; a 1- to 2-mm stab incision can be made in the skin at the wire's entry site to facilitate advancement of the catheter. Using fluoroscopy, the catheter is advanced into the renal pelvis at which time the stylet is removed and the wire is slowly retracted to allow the loop to form within the pelvis. It should be noted that moderate to severe hydronephrosis should be present prior to attempting this technique as the loop requires a pelvis size of 8 mm to 10 mm to adequately form its shape. Once the loop has formed and the wire is removed, the suture is pulled taught to "lock the loop" and this tension is fixed by a screw or clasp mechanism on most catheters. Adhesive tape can also be applied over the suture to further prevent it from releasing and allowing the loop to deform. Additionally, the catheter should be sutured to the body wall via butterfly tape and/or a series of criss-crossing suture knots to prevent premature dislodgement. As with gastrotomy tubes, the nephrostomy tube should be kept in place for 2 to 4 weeks prior to removal to allow the tract to mature; alternatively, the site can be closed surgically if withdrawal of the catheter is necessary.

Extracorporeal Shockwave Lithotripsy

The use of ESWL has been described as a successful treatment of nephroliths and ureteroliths in the dog as well as of ureteroliths in the cat.[45] This noninvasive modality may be considered as a means to reduce complications of upper urinary tract surgery because it may prevent open surgery by fragmenting uroliths of the upper urinary tract and allowing their passage with time. ESWL has not adopted widespread application in veterinary medicine because the equipment is expensive, not all animals respond completely to the treatment (85% reported as successful in dogs), and complications may occur in about 10% of patients, with ureteral fragment obstruction being the most common complication seen.[45] The issue of ureteral obstruction after ESWL by the passage of fragments may be reduced by placing a ureteral stent (as described earlier) immediately prior to the treatment; however, a recent study in human patients suggests there is little benefit to ureteral stenting prior to ESWL.[51] Further investigation and refinement of ESWL in small animal patients may be warranted as a means to reduce the need for open surgical techniques.

SUMMARY

Surgery of the kidney and ureter is performed in dogs and cats for the treatment of urolithiasis, traumatic injuries, and congenital anomalies and, rarely, for resection of primary or metastatic neoplasia. Unfortunately, the healing characteristics of the ureter and the small size of the urogenital structures in companion animals have created a variety of challenges in surgical management of these conditions. Complications of upper urinary tract surgery are frequently life threatening, leading to the development of uroperitoneum or acute renal failure due to post renal obstructive uropathy. Increasing expertise in microsurgery and interventional radiology has improved the care of veterinary patients with upper urinary tract disease over the past 2 decades. Simultaneous with this increase in available skills have been a number of technological advances that have yielded vast improvements in clinical imaging, suture materials, and urinary stents. This review will discuss complications associated with upper urinary tract surgery in the dogs and cat, presenting the epidemiology, treatment, and, in particular, methods for avoiding these complications. Knowledge of the history and epidemiology of surgical complications is an important first step in improving success rates as we move forward in providing advanced care for animals with upper urinary tract disease.

REFERENCES

1. Jeraj K, Osborne CA, Stevens JB. Evaluation of renal biopsy in 197 dogs and cats. J Am Vet Med Assoc 1982;181:367–9.
2. Vaden SL, Levine JF, Lees GE, et al. Renal biopsy: a retrospective study of methods and complications in 283 dogs and 65 cats. J Vet Intern Med 2005;19:794–801.
3. Rawlings CA, Diamond H, Howerth EW, et al. Diagnostic quality of percutaneous kidney biopsy specimens obtained with laparoscopy versus ultrasound guidance in dogs. J Am Vet Med Assoc 2003;223:317–21.
4. Gahring DR, Crowe DT Jr, Powers TE, et al. Comparative renal function studies of nephrotomy closure with and without sutures in dogs. J Am Vet Med Assoc 1977; 171:537–41.
5. Stone EA, Robertson JL, Mecalf MR. The effect of nephrotomy on renal function and morphology in dogs. Vet Surg 2002;31:391–7.
6. Bolliger C, Walshaw R, Kruger JM, et al. Evaluation of the effects of nephrotomy on renal function in clinically normal cats. Am J Vet Res 2005;66:1400–7.
7. King MD, Waldron DR, Barber DL, et al. Effect of nephrotomy on renal function and morphology in normal cats. Vet Surg 2006;35:749–58.
8. Adin CA, Herrgesell EJ, Nyland TG, et al. Antegrade pyelography for suspected ureteral obstruction in cats: 11 cases (1995–2001). J Am Vet Med Assoc 2003;222: 1576–81.
9. Barthez PY, Smeak DD, Wisner ER, et al. Ureteral obstruction after ureteroneocystostomy in dogs assessed by technetium Tc 99m diethylenetriamine pentaacetic acid (DTPA) scintigraphy. Vet Surg 2000;29:499–506.
10. Chambers JN, Selcer BA, Barsanti JA. Recovery from severe hydroureter and hydronephrosis after ureteral anastomosis in a dog. J Am Vet Med Assoc 1987;191: 1589–92.

11. Kyles AE, Stone EA, Gookin J, et al. Diagnosis and surgical management of obstructive ureteral calculi in cats: 11 cases (1993–1996). J Am Vet Med Assoc 1998;213:1150–6.
12. Kyles AE, Hardie EM, Wooden BG, et al. Clinical, clinicopathologic, radiographic, and ultrasonographic abnormalities in cats with ureteral calculi: 163 cases (1984–2002). J Am Vet Med Assoc 2005;226:932–6.
13. Ross SJ, Osborne CA, Lulich JP, et al. Canine and feline nephrolithiasis. epidemiology, detection, and management. Vet Clin North Am Small Anim Pract 1999;29: 23150, xiii–xiv.
14. Kyles AE, Hardie EM, Wooden BG, et al. Management and outcome of cats with ureteral calculi: 153 cases (1984–2002). J Am Vet Med Assoc 2005;226:937–44.
15. Berent AC: Urological interventional techniques in the feline patient. In: August JR, editor. Consultations in feline internal medicine. 6th edition. Philadelphia: Saunders Elsevier; 2010. p. 516–30.
16. Lanz OI, Waldron DR. Renal and ureteral surgery in dogs. Clin Tech Small Anim Pract 2000;15:1–10.
17. Hardie EM, Kyles AE. Management of ureteral obstruction. Vet Clin North Am Small Anim Pract 2004;34:989–1010.
18. Nwadike BS, Wilson LP, Stone EA. Use of bilateral temporary nephrostomy catheters for emergency treatment of bilateral ureter transection in a cat. J Am Vet Med Assoc 2000;217:1862–5.
19. Auge BK, Sarvis JA, L'esperance JO, et al. Practice patterns of ureteral stenting after routine ureteroscopic stone surgery: a survey of practicing urologists. J Endourol 2007;21:1287–91.
20. Fossum TW. Surgery of the kidney and ureter. In: Fossum TW, editor. Small animal surgery. 3rd edition. St Louis (MO): Mosby; 2007. p. 635–62.
21. Marx M, Bettmann MA, Bridge S, et al. The effects of various indwelling ureteral catheter materials on the normal canine ureter. J Urol 1988;139:180–5.
22. Bhatnagar BN, Chansouria JP. Healing process in the ureter: an experimental study in dogs. J Wound Care 2004;13:97–100.
23. Galal H, Lazica A, Lampel A, et al. Management of ureteral strictures by different modalities and effect of stents on upper tract drainage. J Endourol 1993;7:411–7.
24. Kochin EJ, Gregory CR, Wisner E, et al. Evaluation of a method of ureteroneocystostomy in cats. J Am Vet Med Assoc 1993;202:257–60.
25. Zaid MS, Berent AC, Weisse C, et al. Feline ureteral strictures: 10 cases (2007–2009). J Vet Intern Med 2011;25:222–9.
26. McLoughlin MA, Bjorling D. Ureters. In: Slatter DH, editor. Textbook of small animal surgery. 3rd edition. Philadelphia: Saunders; 2003. p. 1619–28.
27. Kerr WS Jr. Effects of complete ureteral obstruction in dogs on kidney function. Am J Physiol 1956;184:521–6.
28. Barthez PY, Smeak DD, Wisner ER, et al. Effect of partial ureteral obstruction on results of renal scintigraphy in dogs. Am J Vet Res 1999;60:1383–9.
29. Lamb CR. Ultrasonography of the ureters. Vet Clin North Am Small Anim Pract 1998;28:823–48.
30. Soria F, Rioja LA, Blas M, et al. Evaluation of the duration of ureteral stenting following endopyelotomy: animal study. Int J Urol 2006;13:1333–8.
31. Ravery V, de la Taille A, Hoffmann P, et al. Balloon catheter dilatation in the treatment of ureteral and ureteroenteric stricture. J Endourol 1998;12:335–40.
32. Soria F, Sun F, Sanchez FM, et al. Treatment of experimental ureteral strictures by endourological ureterotomy and implantation of stents in the porcine animal model. Res Vet Sci 2004;76:69–75.

33. Berent AC. Veterinary endourology: reverse translational medicine from human to veterinary medicine. In: Proceedings of the 2010 ACVIM Forum. Anaheim; 2010.

34. Brodsky SL, Zimskind PD, Dure-Smith P, et al. Effects of crush and devascularizing injuries to the proximal ureter. an experimental study. Invest Urol 1977;14:361–5.

35. Gregory CR, Lirtzman RA, Kochin EJ, et al. A mucosal apposition technique for ureteroneocystostomy after renal transplantation in cats. Vet Surg 1996;25:13–7.

36. Mehl ML, Kyles AE, Pollard R, et al. Comparison of 3 techniques for ureteroneocystostomy in cats. Vet Surg 2005;34:114–9.

37. Kyles AE, Stone EA, Gookin J, et al. Diagnosis and surgical management of obstructive ureteral calculi in cats: 11 cases (1993–1996). J Am Vet Med Assoc 1998;213:1150–6.

38. Mehl ML, Kyles AE. Ureteroureterostomy after proximal ureteric injury during an ovariohysterectomy in a dog. Vet Rec 2003;153:469–70.

39. Aronson LR, Kyles AE, Preston A, et al. Renal transplantation in cats with calcium oxalate urolithiasis: 19 cases (1997–2004). J Am Vet Med Assoc 2006;228:743–9.

40. Lulich JP, Osborne CA, Lekcharoensuk C, et al. Effects of diet on urine composition of cats with calcium oxalate urolithiasis. J Am Anim Hosp Assoc 2004;40:185–91.

41. Thumchai R, Lulich J, Osborne CA, et al. Epizootiologic evaluation of urolithiasis in cats: 3,498 cases (1982–1992). J Am Vet Med Assoc 1996;208:547–51.

42. Ling GV. Urinary stone disease. In: Lower urinary tract diseases of dogs and cats. St Louis, MO: Mosby; 1995. p. 147–78.

43. Stevenson AE, Blackburn JM, Markwell PJ, et al. Nutrient intake and urine composition in calcium oxalate stone-forming dogs: comparison with healthy dogs and impact of dietary modification. Vet Ther 2004;5:218–31.

44. Weisse CW, Berent AC, Todd KL, et al. Potential applications of interventional radiology in veterinary medicine. J Am Vet Med Assoc 2008;233:1564–74.

45. Lulich JP, Adams LG, Grant D, et al. Changing paradigms in the treatment of uroliths by lithotripsy. Vet Clin North Am Small Anim Pract 2009;39:143–60.

46. Davis DM, Strong GH, Drake WM. Intubated ureterotomy: experimental work and clinical results. J Urol 1948;59:851–62.

47. Zimskind PD, Fetter TR, Wilkerson JL. Clinical use of long-term indwelling silicone rubber ureteral splints inserted cystoscopically. J Urol 1967;97:840–4.

48. Adams LG. Ureteroscopy and ureteral stents. In: Proceedings of the 2005 ACVIM Forum. Baltimore; 2005.

49. Lennon GM. Double pigtail ureteric stent versus percutaneous nephrostomy: effects on stone transit and ureteric motility. Eur Urol 1997;31:24–9.

50. Soria F, Delgado MI, Rioja LÁ, et al. Ureteral double-J wire stent effectiveness after endopyelotomy: an animal model study. Urol Int 2010;85:314–9.

51. Ather MH, Shrestha B, Mehmood A. Does ureteral stenting prior to shock wave lithotripsy influence the need for intervention in steinstrasse and related complications? Urol Int 2009;83:222–5.

Complications of Lower Urinary Tract Surgery in Small Animals

Mary A. McLoughlin, DVM, MS

KEYWORDS
- Surgery • Lower urinary tract • Small animal practice
- Cystotomy • Urethrostomy

Surgical procedures of the lower urinary tract are commonly performed in small animal practice. Cystotomy for removal of uroliths and urethrostomy to divert urine outflow due to urethral obstruction are the most commonly performed surgical procedures of the bladder and urethra, respectively. Surgical procedures of the lower urinary tract are typically associated with few complications, which may include leakage of urine, loss of luminal diameter (stricture or stenosis), urine outflow obstruction, tissue devitalization, denervation, urinary incontinence, urinary tract infection, and death. Complications can result from inappropriate or inadequate diagnosis, localization, and surgical planning; failure to respect regional anatomy, including nerve and vascular structures; hemorrhage; and failure to remove uroliths or provide adequate medical stabilization of azotemic patients with metabolic and/or hemodynamic alterations.[1]

ANATOMICAL CONSIDERATIONS

The veterinary surgeon must be knowledgeable of the regional anatomy and use this information to successfully manage patients requiring surgery of the lower urinary tract or when dealing with complications that develop after surgical procedures. The urinary bladder is a compound, musculomembranous reservoir within the ventral aspect of the peritoneal cavity cranial to the pubis. The triangle-shaped lateral ligaments formed by reflections of the peritoneum loosely suspend the bladder from a dorsolateral position. Within each lateral ligament lie the ureter, ureteral and urinary bladder vascular supply, and innervation to the bladder and vesicourethral junction. The size, shape, and position of the urinary bladder change dependent on the volume of urine contained within its lumen.[2] The urinary bladder is regionally divided into apex, body, trigone, and bladder neck (vesicourethral junction). Ureters enter the bladder wall from the dorsolateral surface as they exit the peritoneal reflections of the

Department of Veterinary Clinical Sciences, The Ohio State University, 601 Vernon L. Tharp Street, Columbus, OH 43210, USA
E-mail address: mcloughlin.1@osu.edu

Vet Clin Small Anim 41 (2011) 889–913
doi:10.1016/j.cvsm.2011.07.001
0195-5616/11/$ – see front matter Published by Elsevier Inc.

vetsmall.theclinics.com

lateral ligaments. Each ureter traverses the bladder wall to open within the lumen, forming a C-shaped orifice along the right and left apical border of the trigone. Vascular supply to the urinary bladder and vesicourethral junction is supplied from both the cranial and caudal vesicular arteries traversing within the lateral ligaments. Innervation of the bladder and vesicourethral junction is supplied from the pelvic, hypogastric, and sympathetic nerve fibers controlling the complex integrated process of micturition. Iatrogenic or traumatic injuries to either one or both lateral ligaments including inadvertent ligation, transection, or malpositioning of the bladder (torsion) can result in compromise of vascular and nerve supply to the bladder, which then compromises function and its integrity.[3,4]

The urethra is also a compound tubular organ arising from the bladder neck and extending to the external urethral orifice. The urethra is anatomically quite variable between genders and species in small animal patients. In both dogs and cats, the female urethra is relatively short and distensible, ranging in length from approximately 5 to 12 cm in dogs and from 4 to 7 cm in cats.[2] The female urethra is tethered dorsally and laterally as it passes through the pelvic canal to the perineum. A peritoneal reflection forming the vesicogenital pouch exists between the dorsal aspect of the urethra and the ventral aspect of the vagina, tethering these structures together. Both vascular and nerve supplies to the female urethra are located along the dorsal and lateral surface. Vascular supply arises from the vaginal artery and both external and internal pudendal arteries.[2] Motor innervation travels with the vascular supply arising from the pudendal nerve. The hypogastric and pelvic nerves are responsible for autonomic control.[2,5,6]

The canine male urethra is more complex, ranging in length from 10 to 35 cm depending on body size. The male urethra is divisible into 3 distinct portions: prostatic, membranous (pelvic), and cavernous or penile urethra.[2] The membranous portion of the male urethra from the caudal edge of the prostate gland to the glands of the penis is anatomically most similar to the female urethra, permitting some degree of luminal distention. This portion of the urethra is palpable both rectally and externally in the perineal region. The penile urethra is the least mobile and distensible of the 3 regions. The penile urethra is surrounded by the cavernous components of the penis (corpus spongiosum, corpus cavernosum, and bulbus glandis) and the os penis bone. The urethra is positioned ventral to the U-shaped os penis bone within the distal aspect of the penis. Vascular supply to the male urethra is complicated by blood flow to the cavernous tissues of the penis. Vascular supply to the prostatic urethra arises directly from the prostatic artery, whereas the membranous urethra receives blood supply from the urethral arteries that are branches of the internal pudendal and prostatic artery. Blood supply to the penile urethra and corpus spongiosum arises from the artery of the urethral bulb.

HEALING OF THE LOWER URINARY TRACT

Specialized uroepithelium lining the bladder, ureters, and urethra has tremendous regenerative capacity. Epithelialization of mucosal defects occurs via rapid migration of a single or double layer of marginal epithelial cells.[1,7] Mitosis of both surrounding and migrating epithelial cells is recognized within 1 day of mucosal injury. Reepithelialization of the entire bladder occurs within 30 days from uroepithelial cells of the ureteral orifices or proximal urethra.[7] This process involves greater mitotic division of cells than is typically seen in restoration of other epithelium-lined surfaces.[3] Both urinary bladder and urethra are compound organs due to their distinct tissue layers, including mucosa, submucosa, muscularis, and serosa. The submucosa is the surgical holding layer of both the bladder and urethra. Microscopic examination of healing bladder incisions shows typical scar formation without evidence of smooth muscle regeneration within the wound. Wound healing of the bladder wall occurs via synthesis, deposition, and remodeling of collagen to form a scar.[8,9] The urinary bladder is unique in respect to other tissues and organs because of its capacity to regain 100% of its presurgical strength within 14 to 21 days after wounding or incision. Other hollow organs may never achieve more than 65% to 70% of their presurgical strength, even months after surgery or traumatic injury.[8-10]

URINARY TRACT SUTURE

There are many choices of appropriate suture material for use in lower urinary tract surgery. It has long been recommended to avoid the use of both nonabsorbable and multifilament suture materials exposed within the lumen of the lower urinary tract because of the potential for nidus formation, infection, as well as adhesion of urinary metabolites and debris-forming concretions or calculi.[11,12] Ideal suture material should maintain its strength until wound repair is satisfactory and then undergo total absorption.[12] The rate of collagen synthesis within bladder wounds reaches a peak within 5 days of wounding and returns to that of unwounded tissue by 70 days.[12] The potential for rapid and complete healing of wounds or incisions of the lower urinary tract permits a wide range of suture materials to be consider for use. Characteristics of suture materials to consider include ease of handling, knot security, tissue reaction while undergoing complete absorption, and the mode and rate of suture degradation when exposed to acidic, alkaline, or infected urine.[11-14]

Recommendations for suture usage in lower urinary tract surgery have focused on a group of absorbable synthetic monofilament suture materials including polydioxanone (Ethicon Inc, Somerville, NJ, USA), polyglyconate (Covidien, Mansfield, MA, USA), Glycomer 631 (Covidien, Mansfield, MA, USA), and poliglecaprone 25 (Ethicon Inc). Although synthetic absorbable sutures are more expensive than chromic gut, their improved handling and prolonged strength retention makes these sutures more desirable than historical choices of natural products. While the predictable degradation of synthetic materials is desirable, several of the commonly used monofilament absorbable sutures require 3 to 6 months for complete degradation and the presence of suture materials within the urinary tract for periods of time up to 6 months may not be desirable. The presence of exposed suture material within tissues or lumen of the lower urinary tract can act as a foreign body and become a nidus for infection and stone formation. The exact mechanism by which foreign materials induce stone formation is unknown.[12] Experimental studies have demonstrated that multiple factors can have a direct impact on precipitation of solutes from the urine leading to calculus formation. These factors include presence of urine within the bladder, urine volume and concentration, frequency of urination, type of suture material exposed, presence of urinary tract infection, specific bacterial pathogen, alkaline urine pH, and species.[12,13]

PROCEDURES AND COMPLICATIONS OF LOWER URINARY TRACT SURGERY
Cystotomy Incision and Closure

Cystotomy is one of the most commonly performed surgical procedures in small animal practice. Surgical incisions into the bladder can be performed along the ventral, dorsal, or apical surface. Ventral midline incision into the bladder has been recommended to avoid transection or ligation of vital structures within the lateral ligaments.[15] This approach permits optimal visualization of the luminal surface including the ureteral orifices. The risk of adhesions of the bladder to the ventral body wall after ventral midline cystotomy has been shown to be negligible.[15] Traditionally, bladder closure is performed using absorbable, synthetic monofilament suture material in 1 or 2 layers, which must include the submucosal layer. Choice of suture patterns and number of layers involved in cystotomy closure is determined based on thickness of the bladder wall and ability to create a watertight seal, preventing urine leakage. Single-layer appositional (simple continuous) or slightly inverting closure (Cushing) patterns are most commonly used when the bladder wall is thicker due to edema, inflammation, or disease. When suturing a completely normal bladder wall, a single-layer appositional or inverting pattern may be adequate.[16,17] Insufflating the bladder to mild distention with sterile saline using a syringe and 22-gauge needle is recommended to evaluate the cystotomy incision for leakage. If leakage of fluid along the incision line is noted, a second closure layer is indicated. An inverting interrupted or continuous seromuscular closure (Lembert) can be used to enhance the incision line. Reevaluation of the cystotomy incision with saline insufflation should be performed until all leakage has ceased.

Loss of Bladder Lumen

Compromise of the luminal diameter of the bladder is rarely of concern when repairing traumatic wounds or surgical incisions of the bladder. Partial cystectomy is performed to surgically remove tissues devitalized by traumatic injury, vascular compromise, severe inflammation, infection, tissue emphysema, or neoplasia. The bladder has been shown to have a tremendous regenerative capacity including cellular hypertrophy. Approximately 75% of the bladder can be excised if the trigonal region remains intact with the ureteral orifices and lateral ligament attachments with minimal clinical repercussions. Reestablishment of "reasonable" bladder capacity in the remaining pouchlike bladder has been recognized as quickly as 2 to 6 months.[4,8] Use of colonic or other intestinal seromuscular augmentation cystoplasty has been reported to rapidly expand the luminal volume of the bladder after an aggressive partial cystectomy.[4] Edges of the bladder remnant are sutured to the seromuscular surface of the colon or small intestine, providing a nonabsorbing, nonsecreting surface that expands the size of the bladder lumen. Presence of urine within the urinary bladder lumen has been shown to accelerate the process of luminal reepithialization.[1,7,12] Therefore, diversion of urine from the bladder to promote healing of surgically repaired wounds is not indicated in small animal patients.[8,12]

Urolithiasis

Removal of uroliths from the bladder and urethra is the most common indication for cystotomy thorough an open or minimally assisted approach in small animal patients.[16,18] Diagnostic imaging before and after treatment has been recommended to assess the completeness of urolith removal particularly when there are multiple uroliths or the number of uroliths removed is less than the number detected prior to treatment.[19] Plain abdominal radiographs are useful for identification of radiodense calculi such as struvite (ammonium magnesium phosphate) and calcium oxalate. However, contrast radiography is necessary to rule out the presence of radiolucent calculi including urate, cystine, silicate, and possible mixed-composition uroliths. Double contrast cystography has been shown to be more sensitive than plain radiography, pneumocystography, and ultrasonography for the detection and enumeration of canine urocystoliths.[19,20]

Failure to remove all uroliths from the bladder and urethra at the time of surgery can result in complications including partial or complete urinary outflow obstruction, urinary tract infection, hematuria, stranguria, and discomfort. At the time of cystotomy,

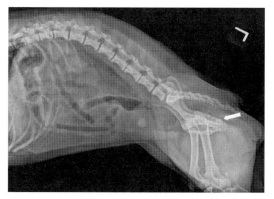

Fig. 1. Plain abdominal radiograph (lateral view) of 4-year-old female, spayed Pembroke Welsh corgi presented for depression, anorexia, and straining to urinate. Radiodense uroliths are observed within the bladder lumen. Arrow indicates additional urolith within the urethra that is causing lower urinary outflow obstruction.

varying sizes of hemostatic forceps or Ferguson gallstone scoops (Integra, Plainsboro, NJ, USA) can be used to remove uroliths from the bladder and urethra. Visual examination and manual palpation of the entire bladder lumen are necessary to ensure that all uroliths have been removed. Retrograde urethral catheterization and hydropulsion should be performed in all male patients (dogs and cats) to dislodge uroliths and crystalline material from the urethra into the bladder lumen for removal prior to bladder closure. Because the female urethra is shorter and more distensible, complete obstruction due to uroliths is uncommon. During the cystotomy procedure, a urethral catheter is passed antegrade from the bladder lumen into the urethra. The urethra is flushed with saline as the catheter is gently advanced until all crystalline material and stones are dislodged. Smaller uroliths and crystalline debris may be flushed from the distal urethra into the vestibule. Should a urolith become lodged within the distal aspect of the female urethra and cannot be displaced by gentle probing with blunt forceps or antegrade flushing, an epsiotomy approach providing exposure of the distal urethral orifice should be considered to dislodge and remove the obstructing urolith (**Fig. 1**). The bladder and abdominal incisions are routinely closed. Female patients are repositioned sternally in a reverse Trendelenburg position elevating the perineum and vulva for an episiotomy approach. The perineum and perivulvar region are clipped and aseptically prepared. Episiotomy provides direct visualization and surgical access to the external urethral orifice. An obstructive urolith lodged at the external urethral orifice can be gently manipulated into the vestibule or fragmented using hemostatic forceps or lithotripsy. Care is taken to avoid pushing the obstructive urolith back into the bladder lumen. If this complication occurs, retrieval of the urolith or its fragments is essential by cystotomy, transurethral cystoscopy and basket retrieval, lithotripsy with fragment retrieval, or urohydropulsion if stone fragments are small (<5 mm).[18,21,22]

Effectiveness of cystotomy for the complete removal of bladder and urethral calculi was recently reported in a study of 128 dogs.[19] Only 19 of 128 total dogs (15%) had appropriate imaging procedures performed after surgery. Uroliths were identified in 8 of these 19 dogs (42%) after cystotomy. This study highlights the importance of appropriate diagnostic imaging after cystotomy.[19,21,22]

Bladder Hematoma

An organized blood clot or hematoma compromising the bladder lumen is an uncommon occurrence in small animal patients. Excessive bleeding into the bladder lumen can occur after surgical incision through an inflamed or thickened bladder wall. Other causes of blood accumulation within the bladder lumen include upper urinary tract hemorrhage (idiopathic renal hematuria or neoplasia), coagulopathy, platelet dysfunction, trauma, neoplasia, drug therapy, or iatrogenic injury from invasive techniques including cystocentesis, transurethral catheterization, or uroendoscopy.[23] In most situations, hemorrhage into the bladder lumen results in gross hematuria and the presence of smaller clots that are expelled during voiding. Establishing diuresis and voiding after surgery is essential to eliminate accumulated blood. Failure to void in the face of persistent hemorrhage within the bladder lumen may contribute to hematoma formation. Bladder hematoma should be considered in patients presenting with clinical signs of gross hematuria, stranguria, or oliguria and presence of a palpably distended bladder. Luminal filling with a large organized hematoma can result in both upper and lower urinary outflow obstruction and uremia. Confirmation of an organized hematoma can be made with ultrasound or retrograde contrast cystography. In small animal patients, an obstructive hematoma is removed from the bladder lumen via cystotomy (**Fig. 2**). The luminal surface of the bladder is inspected for evidence of abnormalities and sites of persistent bleeding. If a specific site of bleeding is not located within the bladder lumen, catheterization of the ureteral orifices can be performed to rule out bleeding from either kidney. Bladder closure should include a simple continuous suture pattern in the mucosal layer to assist with hemostasis followed by routine closure including the submucosa and seromuscular layers. Establishing diuresis and bladder emptying after surgery through fluid therapy and frequent walking is critical to prevent recurrence. Transurethral catheter placement can be considered to monitor urine output and prevent accumulation of clotted blood and urine within the lumen.

Cystotomy Dehiscence/Leakage

Dehiscence of cystotomy incisions is an uncommon complication in small animal patients. The most likely cause of incisional dehiscence of the bladder is imperfect technical closure of the wound. Specific causes may be related to failure to incorporate the surgical holding layer (submucosa), inappropriate choice of suture material, suture failure/breakage, knot failure, or failure to check the incision for leakage at the time of surgery.[14,16,17] Careful handling of synthetic monofilament sutures is critical to avoid suture stress, fracture, and kinking. Care is taken to avoid grasping and damaging the structure of synthetic monofilament sutures with instruments such as needle holders, thumb forceps, and hemostatic forceps. Dehiscence or leakage of cystotomy closure generally occurs during the first 5 days after surgery.[12,13] Detection of urine within the abdominal cavity may take an additional 1 to 2 days after the onset of urine leakage.[24-27]

Uroabdomen

Accumulation of urine within the peritoneal cavity can occur from disruption or leakage of the upper or lower urinary tract. Leakage of urine from the upper urinary tract may accumulate within the retroperitoneal space if it is not disrupted or directly within the peritoneal cavity.[24] Leakage of urine from the bladder and proximal urethra tends to pool directly within the peritoneal cavity. Lower urinary tract urine leakage occurs as a complication of surgery, invasive techniques including transurethral

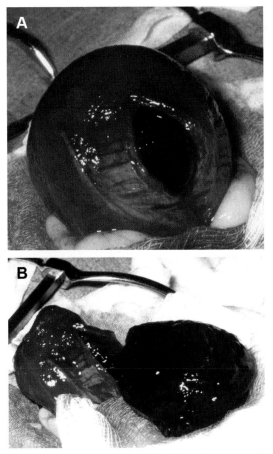

Fig. 2. (A) Intraoperative image of the urinary bladder of a 4-year-old neutered male cat presented for abdominal discomfort, palpable bladder distention, and inability to urinate following repeated catheterizations for lower urinary tract obstruction. An organized hematoma was completely filling the bladder lumen. (B) A ventral cystotomy incision was performed to remove the hematoma and flush the bladder lumen.

catheterization or uroendoscopy, overdistention of the bladder, overzealous attempts at manual expression of the bladder, as well as blunt or penetrating injury to the abdomen, pelvis, or perineum.[23–27]

Urine within the peritoneal cavity results in a delayed onset of clinical symptoms secondary to uremia and peritonitis.[24–27] Clinical signs are often vague and referable to diseases of a variety of organ systems. A history of recent abdominal surgery or invasive procedures may increase the clinician's index of suspicion of lower urinary tract leakage.[24] A detailed history is critical, characterizing the patient's attitude, appetite, and ability to urinate.[24] Normal voiding behavior is often reported in patients with confirmed leakage from the bladder or proximal urethra. Physical examination findings may be unremarkable. Abdominal tenderness or discomfort can be elicited in patients with a recent history of lower urinary tract surgical procedures and not necessarily referable to the presence of urine within the peritoneal cavity. It is critical to remember that the presence of a palpable urinary bladder and ability to void has no bearing on whether lower urinary tract leakage is ongoing. Detection of small or moderate amounts of abdominal fluid may be difficult to determine by abdominal palpation alone. Noninvasive sonographic evaluation of the abdominal cavity will greatly assist in determining the presence of free abdominal fluid, although further evaluation is indicated to determine the etiology. Rectal examination should also be performed to palpate and evaluate the pelvic canal, prostate (male patients), and urethra.[24] This examination cannot ensure the integrity of the bladder or urethra. Urethral catheterization should be carefully attempted. If resistance to the passage of a urethral catheter occurs, the procedure should be abandoned until further diagnostics are performed to evaluate lower urinary tract integrity. Forceful passage of a urethral catheter may cause additional damage to a disrupted urethra or bladder.[5,6,24,26]

Analysis of an abdominal fluid sample is essential to make the definitive diagnosis of uroabdomen.[24–27] Abdominal paracentesis is performed to obtain a diagnostic abdominal fluid sample. Ultrasound facilitates localization of fluid within the peritoneal cavity for abdominal paracentesis. This is especially helpful if there is only a small amount of fluid that may be localized into pockets surrounding abdominal viscera. Paracentesis is performed using a syringe and 22-gauge needle or 19-gauge butterfly catheter. Adherence to aseptic technique is critical to avoid introducing bacterial pathogens into the abdominal cavity. If an ultrasound unit is not available, abdominal paracentesis can still be performed. Fluid samples are readily retrieved from the peritoneal cavity of patients with moderate to large amounts of fluid. An area along the ventral midline from the umbilicus to the pubis is clipped and aseptically prepared. With the patient positioned in lateral recumbency, a needle or butterfly catheter is inserted into the abdominal cavity lateral to the ventral midline, 3 to 4 cm caudal to the umbilicus. This location should position the needle cranial to the bladder and caudal to falciform fat. Care is taken to avoid the spleen. If no fluid is retrieved, the needle can be aseptically repositioned.[24]

Definitive diagnosis of uroabdomen is made by comparison of the concentrations of urea nitrogen and creatinine in the peritoneal fluid to the concentrations of urea nitrogen and creatinine in the serum.[24–27] Leakage of urine into the peritoneal cavity results in the accumulation of fluid with an increased concentration of urea nitrogen and creatinine as well as nitrogenous waste products and electrolytes excreted in urine.[24,25] Urine in the peritoneal cavity typically incites only a mild chemical peritonitis due to its hyperosmolality. Following the accumulation of hyperosmolal urine within the peritoneal cavity, iso-osmolal fluid from the vascular and interstitial space moves into the peritoneal cavity to establish osmotic equilibrium.[24,25] Without aggressive supportive care, dehydration, hemoconcentration, and prerenal azotemia occur due to the third space loss of fluids.[25] The urea molecule is a relatively small molecule and will readily pass through the peritoneal membrane, reentering the vascular space along the concentration gradient. Therefore, an increase in the concentration of serum urea nitrogen occurs as a result of the urine accumulation within the peritoneal cavity.[24–27] However, the larger creatinine molecule does not effectively pass through the peritoneal membrane. Despite the concentration gradient between accumulated urine within the peritoneal cavity and the vascular circulation, creatinine is retained significantly longer within the peritoneal cavity. Therefore, the serum concentration of creatinine does not increase at as rapidly as the serum urea nitrogen in response to accumulated urine within the peritoneal cavity.[24,25] The definitive diagnosis of uroabdomen is made when the concentration of creatinine in the abdominal fluid sample exceeds that of the concentration measured in the serum.[24–27] Serial monitoring of serum concentrations of urea nitrogen, creatinine, and potassium in patients with suspected urinary tract leakage is not an efficient or definitive method of diagnosis. Increased concentrations of urea nitrogen, creatinine, and potassium can occur in small animal patients with primary renal failure, hypovolemic shock, severe dehydration, and urinary outflow obstruction.[24,26] Immediate surgical intervention is contraindicated in unstable small animal patients diagnosed with uroabdomen. Medical stabilization involving the treatment of dehydration, azotemia, and hyperkalemia will make the patient more metabolically and hemodynamically stable for general anesthesia and definitive surgical treatment.[24] Hyperkalemic patients can show bradycardia, small or absent P waves, prolongation of the P-R interval, widened QRS complexes, and spiked T waves. Potassium concentrations greater than 7.0 mEq/L may be associated with irregular idioventricular rhythms that can progress to atrial standstill.[24,26,27]

TREATMENT

Although repair of the site of urinary tract leakage is not considered a surgical emergency, immediate drainage of urine from the bladder and peritoneal cavity is required.[24–27] Stabilization of the patient with uroabdomen is a 2-fold process. First, correction of dehydration, azotemia, and electrolyte imbalances is accomplished with aggressive administration of appropriate fluid therapy. The use of isotonic fluids such as 0.9% saline solution is initiated. Normal saline solution will readily correct the hyponatremia, hypochloremia, and hyperkalemia associated with uroabdomen. Serum concentrations of potassium should be monitored as diuresis and drainage of urine from the abdominal cavity are established. Potassium supplementation will be indicated as the electrolyte imbalances are corrected. The rate of fluid administration should be calculated to correct dehydration over the first 4 to 6 hours and establish diuresis at 2 to 5 times maintenance rates.[24-26] Second, stabilization of the patient with uroabdomen relies on establishing a route of continuous drainage of urine from the peritoneal cavity. The specific site of urine leakage is unknown until contrast radiographic procedures are performed. Despite urine leakage into the peritoneal cavity or subcutaneous tissues, urine will continue to accumulate within the bladder lumen. Passage of a transurethral catheter into the bladder will assist in decompression of the bladder, reducing urinary leakage outside of the lower urinary tract. If the urethral catheter is inadvertently passed through a defect in the proximal urethra or bladder wall, this may aid in the drainage of urine from the peritoneal cavity. Most indwelling urethral catheters are constructed with a rounded closed end and 1 or 2 side ports for fluid drainage. Abdominal viscera or omentum can obstruct catheter drainage ports, preventing adequate fluid drainage from the peritoneal cavity. Commercially available percutaneous, trocar-mounted, multifenestrated abdominal/thoracic drainage catheters (SurgiVet, Waukesha, WI, USA) can be aseptically placed through the abdominal wall into the peritoneal cavity in patients using local anesthesia or light sedation. Multiple fenestrations along the catheter prevent complete obstruction and provide more effective drainage of fluid from the peritoneal cavity. If a commercially available catheter is not available, a balloon-tipped catheter (Bard Medical, Covington, GA, USA) can be fashioned to act as a sump drain providing temporary peritoneal drainage. The drainage end of the balloon-tipped catheter is passed through the lumen of an appropriate-size latex Penrose drain (Argyle Penrose Tubing; Covidien, Mansfield, MA, USA) with 4 to 6 fenestrations staggered along the distal third of the Penrose drain. The Penrose drain acts as a sheath, permitting fluid flow though the fenestrations to be drained by the side ports of the balloon-tipped catheter but protects the side ports of the internal catheter from becoming obstructed by abdominal structures. The Penrose drain is secured to the balloon-tipped catheter with

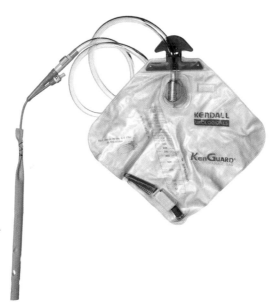

Fig. 3. Sump drain fashioned from balloon-tipped catheter and a fenestrated Penrose drain. The fenestrated Penrose drain is secured over the top of the balloon-tipped catheter with a 0 monofilament nonabsorbable suture using a finger trap. The sump drain is attached to a closed collection system.

a finger trap suture pattern using a 2-0 nonabsorbable monofilament suture (**Fig. 3**). The ventral abdomen is aseptically prepared from the umbilicus to the pubis. A local anesthetic is infused into the skin, subcutaneous tissues, and body wall at a site 2 to 3 cm caudal to the umbilicus on ventral midline. Light sedation or a short-acting anesthetic may be necessary to prevent patient discomfort. A small incision is made through the skin and body wall to insert the sump drainage catheter. The abdominal incision can be closed around the drain at the exit site. It is essential that a portion of the Penrose drain be exposed from the abdominal cavity to be assured that it will not become separated from the balloon-tipped catheter and displaced into the abdomen as a foreign body. The drainage system is secured to the skin with a finger trap suture pattern using a 2-0 nonabsorbable monofilament (**Fig. 4**). The balloon-tipped catheter is attached to a closed urine collection system to permit evaluation of volume and character of fluid drained from the peritoneal cavity.

Diagnostic Radiography

Diagnostic radiography is performed to localize the specific site of urine leakage. The location of site of leakage is determined prior to planning a definitive surgical correction. Radiographic evaluation of the lower urinary tract must always be performed in an orderly manner and based on medical parameters of the patient.[24,26] Survey radiographs of the abdominal cavity including the perineum and penile urethra are necessary but rarely diagnostic. Accumulation of fluid within the peritoneal cavity reduces serosal detail and inhibits visualization of abdominal structures. Changes in the appearance of the retroperitoneal space that include widening, increased density, and streaking are associated with fluid accumulation.[24,25] Contrast radiographic procedures are necessary to identify the specific site of lower urinary tract leakage.

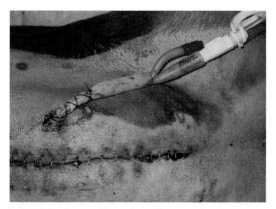

Fig. 4. Placement of abdominal sump drain into the peritoneal cavity. The sump drain exits the abdominal wall at a site separate from a celiotomy incision. The Penrose drain should be partially exposed from the peritoneal cavity to prevent dislodgment from the balloon-tipped catheter creating an abdominal foreign body. The drain is secured to the skin as it exits the abdomen with a finger trap suture.

Positive contrast studies of the lower urinary tract are considered to be a relatively fast and safe diagnostic tool that can be performed as patients undergo metabolic stabilization.[24]

Positive contrast retrograde cystourethrography is performed to evaluate the integrity of both the urethra and bladder.[24,26,27] This technique requires the passage of a balloon-tipped urethral catheter into the distal aspect of the urethra. Use of a balloon-tipped catheter prevents leakage of urine and contrast material around the catheter. A positive contrast agent is administered retrograde through the urinary catheter. Contrast material will enter the bladder if the urethra is not completely disrupted. Extravasation of contrast material from the urethra into the peritoneal cavity, retroperitoneal space, or subcutaneous tissues positively identifies a defect in urethral wall. The positive contrast cystogram is completed to evaluate the integrity of the bladder. Complete distention of the urinary bladder with contrast material is necessary to identify small tears in the bladder wall and determine bladder wall thickness, mucosal irregularities, and filling defects.[24,26] Once again, extravasation of contrast material into the peritoneal cavity or retroperitoneal space identifies a site of bladder wall disruption (**Fig. 5**). Successful management of small animal patients with complications of lower urinary tract leakage is based on severity of injury, location of leakage, as well as the condition of the patient at the time of diagnosis.

Bladder Leakage/Dehiscence

Conservative noninvasive management should first be attempted when leakage from a bladder wall incision is documented after surgery. Placement of a transurethral catheter into the bladder lumen will divert urine flow, minimizing or eliminating urine leakage into the peritoneal cavity. Maintaining the urinary bladder in a decompressed state for 24 to 48 hours may permit a site of incisional leakage to seal without surgical intervention. Retrograde cystography should be performed prior to removal of the urinary catheter to document that leakage is not persistent on expansion of the bladder. Persistent leakage of a cystotomy incision after attempts at noninvasive management will require celiotomy and surgical revision of the leaking incision site.

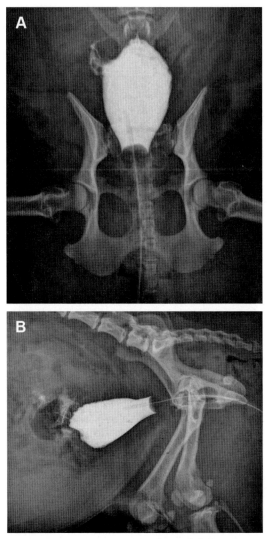

Fig. 5. Retrograde positive contrast cystogram (lateral [A] and ventrodorsal [B] views) demonstrating leakage from the bladder wall into the peritoneal cavity. Loss of detail within the abdominal cavity suggests the accumulation of fluid.

Urethral Leakage/Dehiscence

Surgically induced or traumatic wounds of the urethra heal rapidly by epithelial migration, fibrous protein synthesis, and scar contraction.[8] Surgical procedures are facilitated by the urethra's larger luminal diameter compared with the ureter(s). Placement of an intraluminal stent, such a urethral catheter, is used to maintain luminal diameter, direct epithelial migration, and channel urine flow. Intraluminal stents have been recommended for use in urethral reconstruction in small animal patients.[5,6,8,28] Size of a urethral stent should be the same as the maximum desired diameter of the urethra.[5,6] Although the fibrous protein synthesis of the submucosal

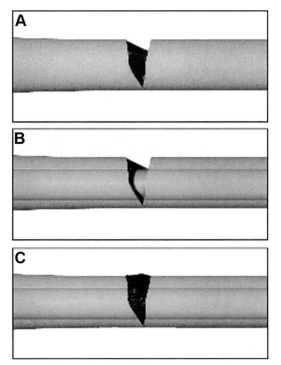

Fig. 6. Partial disruption of the urethral wall (*A*), placement of transurethral catheter stent filling the urethral lumen (*B*), and granulation tissue filling the disrupted area of the urethral wall (*C*). (*Courtesy of* The Ohio State University; with permission.)

layer of the urethra is not typically excessive, narrowing of the luminal diameter can occur after surgical repair or injury. If less than 80% of the circumferential diameter of the urethra is disrupted without substantial loss of tissue, the urethra will heal over a luminal stent without complete surgical reconstruction.[5,6,8,12,28] Lack of mucosal continuity results in granulation and fibrous tissue proliferation within the urethral defect (**Fig. 6**). Later, contraction of the fibrous component can lead to luminal narrowing or stricture.[5,6,8]

Clinical diagnosis of partial urethral disruption with urine leakage can be challenging. The anatomical location of urethral disruption and leakage determines the likely path of urine flow and accumulation. Urine leakage from the proximal urethra including the vesicourethral junction, prostatic urethra, and proximal third of the membranous urethra will generally accumulate within the peritoneal cavity resulting in uroabdomen. Retroperitoneal accumulation of urine from leakage of the membranous urethra is unlikely unless disruption of soft tissue structures within the pelvic canal occurs as a result of trauma or surgery. Urethral disruption and urine leakage from the pelvic, perineal, or ischial portions of the membranous urethra can result in urine accumulation within the retroperitoneal space (intrapelvic or perineal leakage) or subcutaneous tissues of the perineum, thighs, or inguinal region (**Fig. 7**). Extravasation of urine into the subcutaneous tissues results in edema, cellulitis, and bruising that can progress to tissue necrosis. Surgical debridement and open wound management may be necessary to treat devitalized tissues. Management of these wounds in the perineum or medial aspect of the thighs may require second-intention healing,

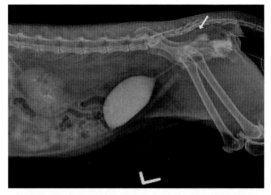

Fig. 7. Retrograde positive contrast urethrogram (lateral view) of a 2-year-old male neutered cat 2 days after perineal urethrostomy. The cat was depressed, anorexic, and azotemic and had a palpably distended urinary bladder. There was no visible swelling or bruising of the perineal region. Retrograde contrast injection demonstrated leakage of contrast between the skin and urethral stoma. Contrast was noted in the pelvic canal and retroperitoneal space as indicated by the arrow.

delayed closure, or the use of local axial pattern skin flaps such as the caudal superficial epigastric flap for wound closure. Conservative or temporary management of the urethral leakage is accomplished by placement of a transurethral catheter channeling urine from the site of leakage until diagnostic retrograde contrast radiography (urethrocystogram) is performed.[8,28–32]

Urine leakage following urethral surgery is uncommon if a transurethral stent is left in place to divert urine flow. If urine leakage is identified from a recent surgical site without a stent, gentle passage of an appropriate-size red rubber or balloon-tipped urethral catheter past the site of leakage into the bladder should be attempted. If attempts at retrograde catheter placement fail, passage of a small hydrophilic guide wire transurethrally into the bladder may facilitate passage of a smaller catheter over the guide wire past points of resistance from urethral swelling or partial disruption. Urethral stents should be maintained for a minimum of 5 to 14 days to ensure local reepithelialization at the site of urine leakage.[5,6,28–32] Evaluation of urethral healing with positive contrast radiography or uroendoscopy is recommended prior to removal of a urethral stent.

Complete Urethral Disruption/Transsection

Complete urethral transection results from trauma, penetrating wounds, or iatrogenic causes including inadvertent prostatectomy while performing cryptorchid castration, or urethral transection during complicated abdominal or perineal surgery. Urethral transection should be considered in patients that fail to urinate after an abdominal, pelvic, or perineal surgical procedures or trauma. Inability to pass a urethral catheter does not confirm the diagnosis of urethral transection but may raise the level of suspicion. Complete assessment of the patient is critical to determine if sites of urine accumulation outside of the lower urinary tract have occurred. Retrograde contrast radiography can confirm the diagnosis of complete urethral disruption and identify the site of injury. Placement of a cystostomy catheter across the abdominal wall directly into the bladder is indicated to temporarily divert urine flow away from the disrupted urethra, preventing urine accumulation within the peritoneal cavity or tissues.[5,6,33] Surgical management is indicated once the patient is stabilized. Surgical exploration

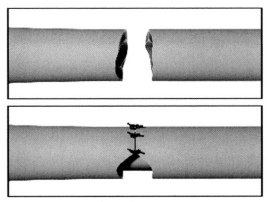

Fig. 8. Complete urethral transection (*above*) and partial urethral anastomosis with a transurethral catheter stent in place (*below*). Loss of tissue at the site of anastomosis will result in second-intention healing by epithelial migration filling the defect. (*Courtesy of* The Ohio State University; with permission.)

is necessary to expose, identify, and realign the ends of the transected urethra. A retrograde transurethral catheter stent is used to bridge the site of disruption.[5,6,31–33] The specific surgical approach is determined based on the location of the injury. A caudal abdominal celiotomy permits access to the proximal third of the membranous urethra in female patients while exposing only the preprostatic and prostatic urethra in male patients. Complete transection of the prostatic urethra is the most commonly reported site of transection injury due to iatrogenic inadvertent prostatectomy during cryptorchid castration in male dogs.[29,30] A ventral midline celiotomy extending to the pubis exposes the bladder and proximal urethra. A stay suture is placed through the bladder apex for manipulation during surgery. Retrograde advancement of a transurethral catheter will aid in identifying the distal transected end of the urethra. Once the tip of the urethral catheter is visualized, two 4-0 stay sutures are placed approximately 180° apart through the wall of the distal urethral segment. The tip of the urethral catheter is gently manipulated into the lumen of the proximal urethral segment and advanced into the bladder lumen. Stay sutures on the distal segment will assist bringing together the transected ends. [6,31,32] Devitalized tissues may need to be debrided at the site of injury, shortening the urethral length. Urethral anastomosis can be attempted if the transected ends of the urethra are brought together without tension. Urethral anastomosis is performed using a 4-0 or 5-0 synthetic absorbable monofilament suture in an interrupted pattern. Careful alignment of urethral mucosa and submucosa is critical.[32,33] Partial or complete suturing of the anastomosis can be performed based on tension and viability of the tissues along the transected ends of the urethra. Granulation tissue will fill any remaining defect provided the urethral mucosa is continuous over at least 20% of the closure (**Fig. 8**). A transurethral stent filling the luminal diameter is maintained for a period of 5 to 14 days as previously described. Prior to stent removal, evaluation of the surgical site for evidence of leakage or narrowing is performed using retrograde positive contrast radiography or uroendoscopy.

Transection of the intrapelvic membranous urethra in both male and female patients requires pelvic symphisotomy or pubic osteotomy to expose this portion of the urethra. The surgical approach for pubic symphyisotomy is made on ventral midline extending from the caudal aspect of the abdominal cavity over the pubis. In male dogs, scrotal testes are retracted from the field or closed castration is performed. The soft tissue structures along ventral midline of the pelvis are elevated to expose the pubic symphysis and medial aspect of each obturator foramen. After the caudal abdominal cavity is opened, the pubic symphysis is separated on midline using an osteotome and mallet or oscillating bone saw.[6] A self-retaining retractor is positioned to separate and retract the pubic bones, exposing the ventral aspect of the pelvic canal. Although the urethra is positioned ventrally, this procedure provides a limited amount of exposure. Alternatively, pubic osteotomy provides improved exposure within the pelvic canal for surgical procedures of the urethra and more dorsally located structures. This procedure requires 3 separate osteotomy sites: cranially through both pubic bones on the right and left sides and caudally across the symphysis into the medial aspect of each obturator foramen. The centrally located segment of pubis is elevated and removed for exposure.[6] Although the urethra is located ventrally within the pelvic canal, trauma or hemorrhage of surrounding tissues associated with the injury can make identification of the transected urethral ends very challenging. Retrograde passage of a transurethral catheter as previously described will facilitate identifying the distal end of the transected urethra. Avoid excessive soft tissue dissection in the region to minimize further injury to nerve and vascular structures or disruption of the pelvic diaphragm. A ventral cystotomy incision is made to permit antegrade passage of a urethral catheter, identifying the transected end of the proximal urethral segment. Once the urethra ends are identified and evaluated for viability and tension, partial or complete urethral anastomosis is performed over a transurethral catheter stent as previously described. If partial or complete urethral anastomosis is not possible due to loss of urethral length or excessive tension, second-intention healing of the urethra over a catheter stent can be attempted or permanent urinary diversion such as prepubic urethrostomy considered.[31–34] Urethral stricture has been shown to be a common complication after intrapelvic urethral alignment over a catheter stent when a sutured anastomosis is not performed.[31,32]

Replacement of the pubic bone is performed on completion of the surgical procedure by wiring together the pubic bones with appropriate-size orthopedic cerclage wire.[6] Predrilling holes for placement of cerclage wire on each side of the 3 osteotomy sites facilitates this process. Prolonged discomfort can be associated with healing of the pubic osteotomy sites.

Urethral Stricture

Stricture or stenosis of the urethral lumen can occur as a complication after surgical procedures including urethrotomy, urethrostomy, urethral anastomosis, or treatment of urethral disruption.[5,6,28–30] Intraluminal injury from iatrogenic causes such as catheter-induced trauma and uroendoscopy or chronically lodged urethral calculi can also narrow the lumen.[5,6,23] Urethral strictures are most often diagnosed due to clinical signs of partial or complete lower urinary tract obstruction including stranguria, pollakiuria, or inability to urinate. Confirmation of urethral narrowing is made with retrograde positive contrast radiography. Isolated, short urethral strictures can be treated by mechanical balloon dilation, intraluminal stent placement, or urethroplasty.[33,35–39] Location and length of a urethral stricture play a major role in determining the mode of treatment and potential for success. Patients with multiple sites of urethral stricture or a site of stricture longer than 2 to 3 cm carry a less favorable prognosis for surgical intervention.[5,6,33] If applicable based on location, permanent urinary diversion may be the best treatment option to avoid further complications.[34]

Areas of urethral stricture located within the pelvic canal or penis surrounded by cavernous tissues make direct surgical access extremely challenging. Balloon dilatation of an isolated short stricture using a small, high-pressure angioplasty balloon with fluoroscopic or cystoscopic guidance has been successfully reported.[35–37] After balloon dilation, an intraluminal stent is passed through the affected site and maintained. The size of the intraluminal stent should approximate the maximal luminal diameter achieved after the dilatation procedures. Intraluminal stents should remain in place for a minimum period of 5 to 14 days, allowing tissue inflammation to subside and promoting healing of the disrupted scar tissue around the stent at the site of stenosis. Repeated balloon dilation procedures at 3- to 21-day intervals may be necessary to achieve adequate urethral widening permitting unobstructed urination. If balloon dilation is unable to achieve or maintain adequate widening of the strictured area, consideration should be given to interventional placement of a covered self-expanding urethral stent (Infiniti Medical, Malibu, CA, USA) (**Fig. 9**). Urethral stenting has been successfully reported in both dogs and cats for malignant obstructions of the urethra.[38,39] Potential complications associated with placement of intraluminal urethral stents include granulation tissue ingrowth and resultant obstruction, urinary incontinence, stent displacement, or fracture.[38] If at all possible, surgical intervention of urethral strictures should be used only when medical management and noninvasive therapies have failed.

Strictures within the penile urethra in both dogs and cats are most commonly treated with permanent urinary diversion (urethrostomy) at a site proximal to the luminal obstruction.[34,40–42] Urethrostomy provides a new site of urinary outflow, avoiding the complexity and complications associated with primary surgical repair of regional stenosis involving the penile urethra. Hemorrhage from cavernous tissues can be difficult to control both during and after surgery. Prolonged bleeding from the surgical site can impact healing of the urethra and lead to excessive bruising or hematoma formation.[40–43]

Strictures or narrowing of the membranous urethra is frequently located within the pelvic canal. However, in male dogs, the membranous urethra extends over the ischium into the perineal region before it enters the cavernous tissue of the penis. The portion of membranous urethra housed within the pelvic canal can be challenging to approach surgically, requiring a pubic symphisotomy or pelvic ostotomy.[6]

Urethroplasty is a primary surgical intervention to widen or resect an area of urethral narrowing or stricture. Urethroplasty involves resection of a discreet area of urethra followed by end-to-end anastomosis or widening of a stricture area by augmentation, graft, or tissue advancement.[5,6,36,44] Loss of urethral length and ability to mobilize the transected ends of the urethra for anastomosis are significant limitations when considering the use of these procedures. Widening of an isolated segment of urethral narrowing can be attempted by performing longitudinal incision through the narrowed region of the urethra, exposing the lumen. Transverse closure of the urethrotomy incision is performed with an interrupted pattern using a 5-0 synthetic monofilament absorbable suture material to create a focal widening at the site of stricture (**Fig. 10**). Augmentation of proximal urethral strictures following inadvertent prostatectomy in male dogs using porcine intestinal submucosa or rectus abdominis muscle flaps has been successfully reported in dogs.[36,38]

COMPLICATIONS OF URETHROSTOMY

Urethrostomy is the permanent diversion of urine at a location proximal to a site of urethral obstruction or disease. Creation of a "new" permanent urethral orifice requires surgical exposure of the urethral lumen and primary closure of the luminal mucosa to the skin. Meticulous soft tissue handling technique and adherence to basic principles of urethrostomy are essential for a successful surgical outcome avoiding

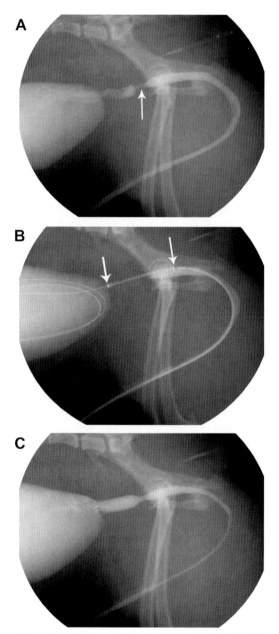

Fig. 9. Lateral radiographic views (*A–C*) of a 6-year-old mixed-breed male dog with a proximal urethral stricture following inadvertent prostatectomy during cryptorchid castration. Complete urethral anastomosis was performed at the time of urethral injury. Clinical symptoms of urinary outflow obstruction began to occur within 4 weeks of the injury. Positive contrast retrograde urethrogram identified the site of urethral stricture denoted by the arrow (*A*). A hydrophilic guide wire was passed transurethrally into the bladder lumen and a self-expanding urethral stent was positioned for deployment. The length of the self-expanding stent is denoted with arrows (*B*). A positive contrast urethrogram documented the luminal diameter of the urethra with the urethral stent in place. The hydrophilic guide wire has been removed (*C*). (*Courtesy of* Brian A. Scansen, DVM, Columbus, OH.)

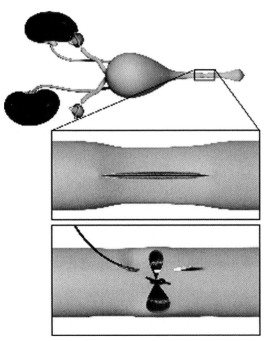

Fig. 10. Stricture of the membranous urethra. Urethroplasty is performed by making a longitudinal urethrotomy incision through the length of the narrowed urethra. Closure of the urethrotomy incision is performed in a transverse pattern using a 5-0 absorbable monofilament suture in an interrupted pattern to widen the urethra at the site of stricture. (*Courtesy of* The Ohio State University; with permission.)

complications.[5,34,40,41] A variety of complications have been reported after urethrostomy procedures including stricture, hemorrhage, dehiscence, subcutaneous leakage of urine, perineal hernia, urinary or fecal incontinence, rectal prolapse, and ascending urinary infection.[5,34,40,41,45–51] Due to anatomical differences between small animal species, recommended sites for urethrostomy differ between dogs and cats. Although specific complications vary with the anatomical location of the urethrostomy site, stricture, hemorrhage, dehiscence, and subcutaneous leakage of urine are common to all locations. Successful urethrostomy requires accurate apposition of urethral mucosa to the skin without tension to achieve primary healing of the permanent stoma without scar tissue formation or stricture.[5] In properly sutured wounds under minimal tension, the epidermal cells at the cut edge thicken, and basal cells of the skin margin become mobile and migrate across the wound gap. Within 48 hours these epidermal cells bridge the gap. Rapid contact inhibition of cells from apposed wound edges minimizes wound contraction and scarring.[5,51] Care must be taken to avoid excessive soft tissue dissection within the pelvic canal, preserving innervation to the bladder and urethra and avoiding urinary incontinence or disruption of the pelvic diaphragm and resultant perineal hernia.[45–48] Control of local hemorrhage is critical. Excessive bleeding from the urethrostomy site can lead to bruising, hematoma formation, and wound dehiscence.[5,40,43,45–47]

Patient management after any type of urethrostomy procedure is critical to outcome and long-term success. All urethrostomy patients should wear an Elizabethan collar until suture removal to prevent physical trauma and oral contamination of the stoma and surrounding tissues. The stoma should be kept free of excessive blood clots and scabs, which can be removed with the gentle application of warm compresses once or twice daily. Removal of all suture material at 10 to 14 days is critical to complete healing and reduce inflammation at the stoma site. Sedation may be required to remove the small sutures placed at the urethrostomy stoma.

Perineal Urethrostomy

Perineal urethrostomy is the recommended site of urinary diversion for obstructions of the penile urethra in male cats.[42] Amputation of the penile urethra and exposure of the distal portion of the membranous urethra to the level of the bulbourethral glands provide adequate luminal diameter ($\approx$1.3 mm) for the creation of a permanent stoma.[42,51] Dissection and disruption of the pelvic attachments to the penile urethra, including ischiocavernosus muscles, ischiourethralis muscles, and penile ligament, are essential to provide adequate mobility of the distal urethra, creating a permanent stoma without tension.[42] Stricture of the perineal stoma is one of the most frequently reported complications.[45–47,51] Surgical revision of the urethral stoma following perineal urethrostomy was reported in 11 cats.[51] The median time from perineal urethrostomy to presentation for stoma revision was 71 days (range, 4–1623 days).[51] The perineal stoma was visibly stenotic in 8 of 11 cats. The remaining 3 cats developed hyperemia, edema, and bruising of the perineum and rear legs, indicative of extravasation of urine from the surgical site into the subcutaneous tissues immediately after surgery. At the time of surgical revision, inadequate dissection of the urethra to the level of the bulbourethral glands was identified as the cause for this complication in 8 cats. Failure to disrupt or sever the pelvic attachments of the penile urethra prevented adequate mobilization of the urethra and excessive tension at the stoma.[51] Excessive anastomotic tension results in ischemia, inflammation, separation of urethral margins, and increased formation of granulation tissue containing contractile myofibroblasts.[51] In addition, failure to adequately mobilize the urethra will create a stoma from a site more distal on the penile urethra. The size of the luminal diameter of the urethra gradually decreases distal to the bulbourethral glands.[51] Surgical intervention is recommended when stricture of a perineal urethrostomy stoma is identified. Careful incision around the stricture stoma permits dissection of the surrounding soft tissue structures to expose ischiocavernosis muscles or remnants of the penile crus to be freed from the pelvic attachments mobilizing the membranous urethra.[51] Excessive dissection along dorsolateral aspect of the pelvic urethra can disrupt vital vascular and/or nerve supply to the urethra, resulting in urinary incontinence.[45–47] Urinary incontinence due to denervation is not responsive to medical management. Endoscopic injection of submucosal urethral bulking agents has been attempted to improve the continence with very limited success.

Scrotal Urethrostomy

Scrotal urethrostomy is the procedure of choice in male dogs when creation of a new urethral orifice distal to the pelvic urethra is necessary.[5,40,41] The scrotal location positions the stoma ventrally, permitting urine flow away from the patient and thereby minimizing local skin irritation and urine scald. In the scrotal region, the urethra is more superficially located, is surrounded by less cavernous tissue, and has a wider more distensible luminal diameter than either the perineal or prescrotal sites.[5,40,41,50] Scrotal urethrostomy requires both castration and scrotal ablation. Passage of an appropriate-size urethral catheter assists in identifying the urethral lumen within the cavernous tissues of the penis. The penile urethra is palpated and exposed on ventral midline. Paired retractor penis muscles located on the ventral aspect of the penis are isolated and laterally retracted, exposing the corpus spongiosum covered by the fibrous tunica albugenia. Careful incision along ventral midline of the exposed penile urethra, using the intraluminal catheter as a guide, exposes the urethral lumen. Avoid excessive incision or dissection of the surrounding cavernous tissues. Persistent hemorrhage from the cavernous tissue is temporarily controlled with digital pressure. Suturing of the urethrostomy stoma assists with hemostasis. Both interrupted and continuous suture patterns have been recommended for scrotal urethrostomy.[40,41,43] A modified urethrostomy technique has been described because standard interrupted suturing often resulted in unacceptable peristomal bleeding and bruising.[40,43] This modified continuous suturing technique uses a small (4-0 or 5-0) nonabsorbable monofilament suture placed in a 3-needle bite sequence. The needle is inserted through the urethral mucosa followed by a bite through the fibrous tunica albugenia and a third split-thickness bite through the surrounding skin edge.[40,43] This suturing technique will produce a better seal by apposing more tissue layers and sealing the incised edge of the cavernous layer, reducing hemorrhage.[40] The outcome of simple continuous closure of canine scrotal urethrostomy was reported in 20 dogs.[43] The mean duration of active postoperative bleeding and bleeding only associated with urinations were 0.2 day and 3.1 days, respectively.[43] No other incisional complications were noted.

Prepubic Urethrostomy

Prepubic urethrostomy is a salvage procedure that can be performed in both dogs and cats when other, more appropriate sites of urinary diversion are contraindicated or have failed.[52] Prepubic urethrostomy requires a ventral midline abdominal approach, transection of the intrapelvic membranous urethra, and redirection of the transected urethra to exit the ventral abdominal wall, creating a permanent stoma. Indications to perform prepubic urethrostomy include stricture, obstruction or disruption of the intrapelvic membranous urethra, insufficient length of the urethra to perform a standard perineal urethrostomy, complications associated with previous perineal urethrostomy, and trauma or neoplasia of the pelvic canal or perineum.[52] The total urethral length is shortened in this procedure as the membranous urethra is transected to bypass the pelvic canal. Urinary continence is maintained provided local innervation to the bladder neck and urethra is preserved as well as sufficient functional urethral length. Positioning of the bladder and urethra within the abdominal cavity is critical to avoid kinking and obstruction of the proximal urethra as it makes a gentle turn to exit ventral body wall separate from the abdominal incision (**Fig. 11**). Cystopexy of the bladder apex to the lateral abdominal wall will maintain bladder position to help prevent urethral kinking following closure of the abdomen. Complications associated with prepubic urethrostomy include peristomal dermatitis, ascending infection, urinary outflow obstruction due to kinking of the proximal urethra, and incontinence.[52] Inflammation and maceration of the peristomal skin can occur as a result of chronic urine contact. Clipping the hair from the local region and application of a petroleum jelly or topical antibiotic ointment to the skin surrounding the stoma will provide a protective layer. Systemic antibiotic therapy should be considered if ulceration or maceration of the peristomal skin is identified. Oral or fecal contamination of the stoma site or surrounding skin can result in chronic or recurrent ascending urinary tract infection. Compromised urethral length may alter the patient's ability to ward off ascending pathogens. Chronically ulcerated peristomal skin that does not respond to appropriate local and systemic therapies may require resection

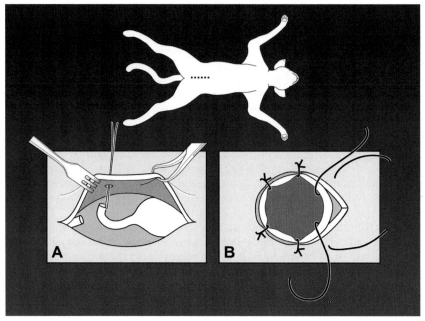

Fig. 11. Prepubic urethrostomy in a cat. Transection is performed of the intrapelvic membranous urethra to bypass the pelvic canal. Positioning of the bladder is critical to avoid kinking of the proximal urethra as it exits the ventral body wall at a site separate from the celiotomy incision. Suturing the urethral mucosa to the skin creates a permanent urethral stoma. (*Courtesy of* The Ohio State University; with permission.)

and creation of a new stoma. Management of chronic or recurrent urinary tract infections may require diligent monitoring for clinical symptoms of lower urinary tract disease, including hematuria, stranguria, and pollakiuria. Obtaining a urine sample via cystocentesis and submission of the sample for aerobic bacterial culture and sensitivity are essential to make appropriate antibiotic choices for treatment.

SUMMARY

Complications of lower urinary tract surgical procedures occur uncommonly if the basic principles of urinary tract surgery are used. Appropriate diagnosis, detailed knowledge of the regional anatomy, and surgical planning are essential for a successful outcome. Early recognition of complications is critical to avoid systemic metabolic alterations associated with accumulation of urine outside of the lower urinary tract or urinary outflow obstruction. Noninvasive interventional procedures should always be attempted before surgical correction of lower urinary tract complications.

REFERENCES

1. McLoughlin MA. Complications of urinary surgery. In: BSAVA Congress 2004: Scientific Proceedings of the 47th Annual Congress, April 2004, Birmingham, UK. Gloucester, England: Quedgeley; 2004.
2. Evans HE, Christensen GC. The urogenital system. In: Miller's anatomy of the dog. 3rd edition. Philadelphia: WB Saunders; 1993. p. 552–79.

3. McLoughlin MA, Bjorling DE. Surgery of the ureter. In: Slatter DH, editor. Textbook of small animal surgery. 3rd edition. Philadelphia: WB Saunders; 2003. p. 1619–27.
4. Pozzi A, Smeak DD, Aper R. Colonic seromuscular augmentation cystoplasty following subtotal cystectomy for treatment of bladder necrosis caused by bladder torsion in a dog. J Am Vet Med Assoc 2006;229(2):235–9.
5. Bjorling DE. Surgery of the urethra. In: Slatter DH, editor. Textbook of small animal surgery. 3rd edition. Philadelphia: WB Saunders; 2003. p. 1638–49.
6. Boothe HW. Managing traumatic urethral injuries. Clin Tech Small Anim Pract 2000; 15(1):35–9.
7. Peacock EE. Epithelialization and epithelial-mesenchymal interactions. In: Peacock EE, editor. Wound repair. 3rd edition. Philadelphia: WB Saunders; 1984. p. 29–35.
8. Peacock EE. Healing and repair of viscera. In: Peacock EE, editor. Wound repair. 3rd edition. Philadelphia: WB Saunders; 1984. p. 476–82.
9. Peacock EE. Collagenolysis and the biochemistry of wound healing. In: Peacock EE, editor. Wound repair. 3rd edition. Philadelphia: WB Saunders; 1984. p. 107–15.
10. Degner DA, Walshaw R. Healing responses of the lower urinary tract. Vet Clin North Am Small Anim Pract 1996;26(2):197–206.
11. Jens B, Bjorling DE. Suture selection for lower urinary tract surgery in small animals. Compend Contin Educ Pract Vet 2001;23:524–31.
12. Edlich RF, Rodenheaver GT, Thacker JG. Considerations in the choice of sutures for wound closure of the genitourinary tract. J Urol 1987;137(3):373–9.
13. Greensburg CB, Davidson EB, Bellmer DD, et al. Evaluation of the tensile strengths of four monofilament absorbable suture materials after immersion in canine urine with or without bacteria. Am J Vet Res 2004;65(6):847–53.
14. Rosin E, Robinson GM. Knot security of suture materials. Vet Surg 1989;18(4): 269–73.
15. Desch JP, Wagner SD. Urinary bladder incisions in dogs: comparison of dorsal vs. ventral. Vet Surg 1986;15(2):153–5.
16. Fossum TW. Surgery of the bladder and urethra. In: Fossum TW, editor. Textbook of small animal surgery. 3rd edition. St Louis: Mosby; 2007. p. 663–85.
17. Radasch RM, Merkley DF, Wilson JW, et al. Cystotomy closure: a comparison of strength of appositional and inverting suture patterns. Vet Surg 1990;19(4):283–8.
18. Rawlings CA, Mahaffey MB, Barsanti JA, et al. Use of laparoscopic-assisted cystoscopy for removal of urinary calculi in dogs. J Am Vet Med Assoc 2003;222(6):759–61.
19. Grant DC, Harper TA, Were SR. Frequency of incomplete urolith removal, complications, and diagnostic imaging following cystotomy for removal of uroliths from the lower urinary tract in dogs: 128 cases (1994–2006). J Am Vet Med Assoc 2010; 236(7):763–6.
20. Weichselbaum RC, Fenney DA, Jessen CR, et al. Urocystolith detection: comparison of survey, contrast radiographic and ultrasonographic techniques in an in vitro bladder phantom. Vet Radiol Ultrasound 1999;40(4):386–400.
21. Adams LG, Berent AC, Moore GE, et al. Use of laser lithotripsy for fragmentation of uroliths in dogs: 73 cases (2005–2006). J Am Vet Med Assoc 2008;232(11):1680–7.
22. Lulich JP, Osborne CA, Albasan H, et al. Efficacy and safety of laser lithotripsy in fragmentation of urocystoliths and urethroliths for removal in dogs. J Am Vet Med Assoc 2009;234(10):1279–85.
23. Corgozinho KB, de Souza HJ, Pererira AN, et al. Catheter-induced urethral trauma in cats with urethral obstruction. J Feline Med Surg 2007;9(6):481–6.
24. McLoughlin MA. Surgical emergencies of the urinary tract. Vet Clin North Am Small Anim Pract 2000;30(3):581–601.

25. Burrows CF, Bovee KC. Metabolic changes due to experimentally induced rupture of the canine urinary bladder. Am J Vet Res 1974;35:1083.

26. Bjorling DE. Traumatic injuries of the urogenital tract. Vet Clin North Am Small Anim Pract 1984;14(1):61–76.

27. Aumann M, Worth LT, Drobatz KJ. Uroperitoneum in cats: 26 cases (1986–1995). J Am Anim Hosp Assoc 1998;34(4):315–24.

28. Rawlings CA, Wingfield WE. Urethral reconstruction in dogs and cats. J Am Anim Hosp Assoc 1976;12:850.

29. Schulz KS, Waldron DR, Smith MM, et al. Inadvertent prostatectomy as a complication of cryptorchidectomy in four dogs. J Am Anim Hosp Assoc 1996;32(3):211–14.

30. Sereda C, Fowler D, Shmon C. Iatrogenic proximal urethral obstruction after inadvertent prostatectomy during bilateral perineal herniorraphy in a dog. Can Vet J 2002; 43(4):288–90.

31. Meige F, Sarrau S, Autefage A. Management of traumatic urethral rupture in 11 cats using primary alignment with a urethral catheter. Vet Comp Orthop Traumatol 2008; 21(1):76–84.

32. Layton CE, Ferguson HR, Cook JE, et al. Intrapelvic urethral anastomosis. A comparison of three techniques. Vet Surg 1987;16(2):175–82.

33. Anderson RB, Aronson LR, Drobatz KJ, et al. Prognostic factors for successful outcome following urethral rupture in dogs and cats. J Am Anim Hosp Assoc 2006;42(2):136–46.

34. Wood MW, Vaden S, Cerda-Gonzalez S, et al. Cystoscopic-guided balloon dilation of a urethral stricture in a female dog. Can Vet J 2007;48(7):731–3.

35. Powers MY, Campbell BG, Weisse C. Porcine small intestinal submucosa augmentation urethroplasty and balloon dilation of a urethral stricture secondary to inadvertent prostatectomy in a dog. J Am Anim Hosp Assoc 2010;46(5):358–65.

36. Bennett SL, Edwards GE, Tyrrell D. Balloon dilation of a urethral stricture in a dog. Aust Vet J 2005;83(9):552–4.

37. Bjorling DE, Petersen SW. Surgical techniques for urinary tract diversion and salvage in small animals. Comp Contin Educ Pract Vet 1990;12(12):1699–709.

38. Weisse C, Berent A, Todd K, et al. Evaluation of palliative stenting for management of malignant urethral obstructions in dogs. J Am Vet Med Assoc 2006;229(2):226–34.

39. Christensen NI, Culvenor J, Langova V. Fluoroscopic stent placement for the relief of malignant urethral obstruction in a cat. Aust Vet J 2010;88(12):478–82.

40. Smeak DD. Urethrotomy and urethrostomy in the dog. Clin Tech Small Anim Pract 2000;15(1):25–34.

41. Dean PW, Hedlund CS, Lewis DD, et al. Canine urethrotomy and urethrostomy. Comp Contin Educ Small Anim Pract 1990;12(11):1541–54.

42. Wilson GP, Harrison JW. Perineal urethrostomy in cats. J Am Vet Med Assoc 1971;159(12):1789–93.

43. Newton JD, Smeak DD. Simple continuous closure of canine scrotal urethrostomy: results in 20 cases. J Am Anim Hosp Assoc 1996;32(6):531–4.

44. Savicky RS, Jackson AH. Use of rectus abdominis muscle flap to repair urinary bladder and urethral defects in a dog. J Am Vet Med Assoc 2009;234(8):1038–40.

45. Scavelli TD. Complications associated with perineal urethrostomy in the cat. Probl Vet Med 1989;1(1):111–9.

46. Smith CW, Schiller AG. Perineal urethrostomy in the cat. A retrospective study of complications. J Am Vet Med Assoc 1978;14:225–8.

47. Gregory CR, Vasseur PB. Long-term examination of cats with perineal urethrostomy. Vet Surg 1983;12(4);210–12.

48. Johnson MS, Gourley IM. Perineal hernia in a cat: a possible complication of perineal urethrostomy. Vet Med Small Anim Clin 1980;75(2):241–3.
49. Griffin DW, Gregory CR. Prevalence of bacterial urinary tract infection after perineal urethrostomy in cats. J Am Vet Med Assoc 1992;200(5):681–4.
50. Bilbrey SA, Birchard SJ, Smeak DD. Scrotal urethrostomy: a retrospective review of 38 dogs (1973–1988). J Am Anim Hosp Assoc 1991;27:560–4.
51. Phillips H, Holt DE. Surgical revision of the urethral stoma following perineal urethrostomy in 11 cats: (1998–2004). J Am Anim Hosp Assoc 2006;42(3):218–22.
52. Baines SJ, Rennie S, White RS. Prepubic urethrostomy: a long-term study in 16 cats. Vet Surg 2001;30(2):107–13.

Complications of Gastrointestinal Surgery in Companion Animals

Gary W. Ellison, DVM, MS

KEYWORDS
- Gastric dilatation • Volvulus • Gastropexy
- Laparoscopic gastropexy • Intestinal anastomosis
- Intestinal dehiscence • Short bowel syndrome
- Subtotal colectomy

The small animal surgeon routinely creates wounds in the gastrointestinal (GI) tract for biopsy, for foreign body or neoplasm removal for correction of gastric dilatation volvulus, or to relieve intestinal and colonic obstruction. Unlike dehiscence of a skin wound, which is often easily remedied with appropriate local wound treatment, dehiscence of a wound of the GI tract often leads to generalized bacterial peritonitis and potentially death. Consequently, technical failures and factors that negatively affect GI healing are of great clinical significance to the surgeon. Surgery of the GI tract must be considered clean-contaminated at best, and as one progresses aborally down the GI tract, the bacterial population increases. Therefore, intraoperative spillage, wound dehiscence, or perforations that occur in the lower small intestine or colon tend to be associated with a higher mortality rate than those of the stomach or upper small intestine.

WOUND HEALING OF THE GI TRACT

Basic understanding of GI tract healing is essential to the surgeon since it dictates proper clinical approach in those cases in which GI complications develop. Immediately after wounding, platelets aggregate, the coagulation mechanism is activated, and fibrin clots are deposited to control hemorrhage.[1] The fibrin clot offers minimal wound strength on the first postoperative day, but the main wound support during the lag phase of healing comes from the sutures.[2] Fibrin also has adhesive properties and may increase the risk of secondary obstruction since these fibrinous adhesions may ultimately be converted to fibrous adhesions. Enterocyte regeneration begins almost immediately after wounding; however, the epithelium offers little biomechanical

The author has nothing to disclose.
Department of Small Animal Clinical Sciences, College of Veterinary Medicine, PO Box 100126, Health Science Center, University of Florida, Gainesville, FL 32610-0126, USA
E-mail address: ellisong@ufl.edu

Vet Clin Small Anim 41 (2011) 915–934
doi:10.1016/j.cvsm.2011.05.006
0195-5616/11/$ – see front matter © 2011 Elsevier Inc. All rights reserved.

vetsmall.theclinics.com

support.[2] This *lag* or *inflammatory* phase is the most critical period during GI wound healing, and most dehiscences take place within 72 to 96 hours.[2]

The *proliferative* or *logarithmic* phase of GI wound healing lasts from days 3 through 14.[1] Fibroplasia occurs logarithmically during this period. The fibroblasts produce large amounts of immature collagen, resulting in rapid gains in wound strength, but this is a dynamic process in which collagen synthesis takes place in the presence of collagenolysis. In the stomach and small intestine, collagenase activity at the wound edge is minimal and rapid gains in tensile and bursting strength occur. At the end of 14 days, gastric and small intestinal wound bursting strength is approximately 75% that of normal tissue.[1] Conversely, the colon heals much more slowly due to marked collagenase activity at the wound edge and regains only about 50% of its normal tensile strength 14 days post wounding.[1] Factors such as traumatic suturing, fecal contamination, and infection all increase the amount of local collagenase produced at the wound and hence can increase the risk of infection.[1]

The *maturation* phase of wound healing is characterized by reorganization and cross-linking of collagen fibers. This phase extends from day 14 through day 180 in the gastrointestinal tract of the dog.[1] Similar to skin wounds, the size and thickness of the scar decrease during this time without weakening the wound. The maturation phase is relatively unimportant clinically in GI wound healing, except in those cases where significant adhesions are present or in cases of sclerosing encapsulating or fibrosing peritonitis.[3,4]

COMPLICATIONS ASSOCIATED WITH GASTRIC DILATATION VOLVULUS
Predictors of Mortality and Gastric Necrosis

Mortality continues to occur in all published reports of gastric dilatation volvulus (GDV). However, over the past four decades, survival rates have improved due to early recognition, rapid gastric decompression, earlier cardiovascular resuscitation, and availability of better medical and surgical care. In older studies from the 1970s and early 1980s, *GDV-related mortality rates* ranged from 43% to 60%.[5,6] However, in a large epidemiologic study of over 1900 dogs with GVD, the mortality rate had reduced to 33% in cases evaluated during the late 1980s and early 1990s[7] and was even reported to be as low as 15% in the mid 1990s.[8] In a recent study the postoperative mortality rate of 306 dogs with GDV was 10%. Those dogs receiving gastropexy alone had mortality of only 3%, while dogs receiving partial gastrectomy with gastropexy had a rate of 9% and those receiving partial gastrectomy, splenectomy, and gastropexy had a rate of 20%.[9] That study also showed a reduction of mortality in dogs if the clinical signs occurred less than 6 hours prior to presentation. While one study suggested that reduced duration of clinical signs and shorter time from presentation to the surgery table also decreased mortality rate in 166 dogs with GDV,[10] a second study contradicted these findings.[11] Severity of clinical presentation has also been related to outcome, with recumbency at presentation increasing risk of death by 4.4 times and dogs with varying degrees of obtundation having mortality that ranged between 3% and 36%.[7–9,12]

The presence of preoperative *cardiac ventricular dysrhythmias* has been evaluated as a predictive indicator for survival in dogs with GDV since they may act as a sentinel for gastric or splenic ischemia. In one study, dogs having intermittent ventricular arrhythmia on admission had a significantly higher mortality rate than did dogs with ventricular tachycardia. Additionally, 48% of those dogs presenting with preoperative cardiac arrhythmias underwent splenectomy or partial gastrectomy, whereas just 27% of the dogs without arrhythmias required those procedures.[9] However, in another study of 295 dogs with GDV, 40% of the animals developed arrhythmias perioperatively and survival rate was unaffected by their presence.[8]

Approximately 40% of dogs with GDV also develop concurrent disseiminated intravascular coagulopathy (DIC). Reported *abnormal hemostatic profiles* with GDV include prolonged prothrombin time (PT), prolonged activated partial thromboplastin time (aPTT), reduced fibrinogen concentration, increased fibrin degradation product (FDP) concentration, reduced platelet counts, and reduced antithrombin III (ATIII) activity, and these may be useful in estimating gastric ischemia/necrosis and DIC. In a study of 20 dogs with GDV, thrombocytopenia occurred in 9 of 20 dogs, followed by decreased ATIII (8 of 20), elevated FDP (6 of 20), prolonged PT (6 of 20), hypofibrinogenemia (6 of 20), hyperfibrinogenemia (5 of 20), prolonged aPTT (5 of 20), and shortened aPTT (4 of 20). Approximately 70% of dogs with more than one abnormal hemostatic test result had gastric necrosis, whereas dogs with one or no abnormality rarely had gastric necrosis.[13]

Considerable attention has turned to *serum lactate* as predictor of gastric necrosis and increased mortality. In an original retrospective study of 102 dogs with GDV, dogs with serum lactate values less than 6 mM had a survival rate of 99%, whereas dogs with initial lactate concentrations of greater than 6 mM were associated with only a 58% survival rate.[13] A more recent study showed a positive predictive correlation between lactate values before and after intravenous fluid resuscitation. In that study, even animals with an elevated initial serum lactate less than 9 mM were likely to survive, as long as the post resuscitation value dropped to 5.6 mM or less.[14] Other factors reported to increase postoperative mortality include hypotension, concurrent peritonitis, DIC, and blood plasma transfusions.[10]

Although the timing of surgery varies between studies, what is clear is that shock therapy and gastric decompression need to be followed by definitive surgical management of GDV. Definitive management of GDV involves (1) repositioning of the stomach with resection or involution of any devitalized gastric wall and (2) a prophylactic gastropexy technique to prevent recurrence. In studies using shock therapy and gastric decompression without gastropexy, the recurrence rate of GDV was 56% to 76%, with many recurrences within 3 months after initial presentation.[15,16] Because of this we now advocate laparotomy as soon as the patient is a reasonable anesthetic risk. This allows for early assessment of gastric wall viability and gastric derotation, which increases gastric circulation and helps with cardiovascular resuscitation.

DIAGNOSIS AND MANAGEMENT OF GASTRIC NECROSIS

Intraoperative clinical criteria for determining gastric wall viability include assessment of color, peristalsis, and tissue thickness. Viable gastric wall may be discolored and blue or dark red in appearance but is normal thickness upon palpation and will often contract when pinched. Ischemic or necrotic gastric wall, on the other hand, is black, gray, or green and is thin on palpation and lacks peristalsis.[17] Fluorescein dye is not an accurate indicator of ischemia since the gastric wall is too thick to be affected by vital dyes. However, surface laser Doppler flowmetry of the gastric serosal surface has been shown to be a relatively good predictor of viability.[18]

Standard methods for gastrectomy involve ligation of branches of the left gastroepiploic arteries and veins, allowing areas along the greater curvature of the stomach to be resected. The stomach is resected back to areas of healthy bleeding. Spillage is prevented through the use of Babcock forceps or stay sutures. The mucosa and submucosa are closed with a continuous inverted Cushing pattern. The serosa and muscularis are then closed with a similar pattern. We have also used utostapling

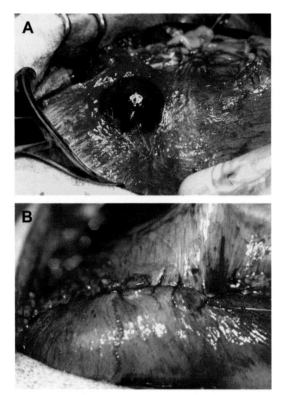

Fig. 1. (*A*) Intraoperative image of the stomach of a 3-year-old Chinese sharpei presenting for GDV. A 3 × 3 cm area of full-thickness necrosis exists along the ventral gastric fundus. (*B*) The area of gastric necrosis has been invaginated using a continuous Lembert suture pattern.

equipment for rapid gastrectomy procedures with minimum risk of spillage. The TA 90 autostapler is used with the green (4.8 mm) or blue (3.5 mm) cartridge. Often the surgeon needs to overlap the staple lines by a few mm to prevent leakage between the staples. The author has seen one clinical case in which perforation and leakage occurred between the overlapping staple lines several months after the original resection. Partial invagination of the stomach has been a useful technique for those animals with small areas of gastric necrosis (**Fig. 1A**). With this technique, ligation of some of the short gastric vessels may be necessary to allow transection of the gastrosplenic ligament.[19] The area of gastric necrosis is then invaginated using a continuous Lembert suture pattern (see **Fig. 1B**). Since the invaginated tissue will ultimately slough, an H2 antagonist such as cimetidine or mucosal protectant such as sucralfate should be given for 5 to 7 days postoperatively. While the development of a bleeding ulcer in a single dog 21 days after gastric resection prompted a recommendation for prolonged administration of gastric protectants after this procedure,[20] the author has used the invagination technique successfully on many dogs that failed to develop overt signs of gastric ulceration after surgery.

RATIONAL FOR PROPHYLACTIC GASTROPEXY

There are reports documenting the occurrence of *GDV following splenectomy* for large splenic tumors or splenic torsion in dogs.[21,22] Because of this, many veterinary surgeons in North America advocate the practice of performing a prophylactic gastropexy after a splenic mass is removed in large or giant breeds of dogs. A recent report from the United Kingdom controverts these earlier studies, suggesting that there was no increased risk of dogs with splenectomy developing GDV compared to the risk incidence for the general population of dogs.[23] The contradictory conclusions of these studies may be related to differences in breed distribution, leaving the issue of prophylactic gastropexy after splenectomy somewhat controversial.

While gastropexy is clearly indicated as a therapeutic procedure in cases of naturally occurring GDV,[11] there is now growing evidence that it may be indicated as a prophylactic procedure in dogs at risk for developing the syndrome. In 136 dogs with GDV, there was only a 4.3% recurrence rate in dogs and a 547-day median survival time in dogs receiving a gastropexy procedure. Conversely, there was a recurrence rate of 54.5% with a median survival time of 188 days in those dogs not receiving a GDV. The mortality associated with GDV recurrence was reported to be 83% in those dogs not receiving gastropexy.[11]

Breed incidence of GDV has been closely evaluated, with giant and large breeds having a lifetime probability of 22% to 24% in 1914 dogs as determined by studies using the Veterinary Medical Data Base.[7] Also, great Danes with moderate and high abdominal height-to-width ratios were approximately 5½ to 8 times as likely to develop GDV as were those with low abdominal height-to-width ratios. Breeds such as the great Dane and bloodhound had reported lifetime incidences of 53% and 39%, respectively.[24] A decision-tree analysis for prophylactic gastropexy using lifetime probability of death from GDV and expected cost savings for veterinary services as outcome measures was undertaken to determine the preferred course of action in several dog breeds.[25] Prophylactic gastropexy was the preferred choice of action for all breeds examined, with the reduction in mortality (vs no gastropexy) ranging from 2.2-fold (Rottweiler) to 29.6-fold (great Dane). Assuming a prophylactic gastropexy costs US$400, the procedure was cost effective when the lifetime risk of GDV was 34% or greater.[25]

Complications associated with gastropexy

Most North American surgeons use an antral gastropexy procedure to affix the stomach to the right abdominal wall and prevent GDV. Common antral gastropexy techniques used in North America include the tube gastrostomy,[26] the incisional gastropexy,[27] the circumcostal gastropexy,[28] the belt-loop gastropexy,[29] and the ventral midline gastropexy.[16] Recurrence rates are typically reported 5% to 29% for the tube gastrostomy and between 3% and 8% with the other techniques.[30] In most reports, recurrence is typically defined to include the occurrence of gastric dilatation without volvulus and does not necessarily indicate failure of the gastropexy site. Prophylactic gastropexy techniques may also be performed using minimally invasive techniques such as laparoscopy or endoscopy.[31]

Potential advantages of the tube gastropexy are that the tube not only creates a permanent adhesion of the gastric antrum to the abdominal wall but also allows for continued gastric decompression in the early postoperative period. In addition, slurried food or medications can be offered through the tube. The main disadvantages of the technique are the nursing care and long hospital period required for tube management and the potential for fatal peritonitis secondary to leakage around the tube or early removal by the dog (**Fig. 2**). In a study by Fox and others, complication rate of tube gastropexy was approximately 18%, with local cellulitis around the tube site being the most common complication and 2 of 24 dogs developing fatal peritonitis.[32]

Incisional gatropexy is performed by making a 3- to 4-cm longitudinal incision in the seromuscular layer of the antrum, suturing this to a similar length incision in the

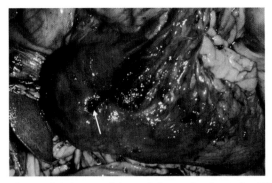

Fig. 2. Necropsy specimen of a dog receiving a tube gastrostomy for GDV that had prematurely removed its Foley catheter. Gastric spillage occurred from the open gastrostomy site, resulting in fatal septic peritonitis.

transversus muscle and peritoneum of the right ventral abdominal wall. Advantages of the incisional gastropexy are that the procedure is rapidly performed, the stomach lumen is not entered, and fibrous connective tissue enters the abdominal rectus muscle and stomach wall to form a strong mature adhesion. Pneumothorax is a potential complication if the incision in the peritoneum is made too far cranially, so the surgeon must take care to identify the caudal extent of the diaphragm before selecting the site of gastropexy. Incisional gastropexy is popular among many North American surgeons, but unfortunately few retrospective studies are available to determine the rate of failure or recurrence rate with this technique.

The circumcostal gastropexy technique uses a viable muscle flap to create a mechanically strong adhesion by wrapping the flap around one of the caudal ribs. In a clinical study by Lieb and others, circumcostal gastropexies were associated with a lower recurrent rate (2.6% at 13.7 months) than tube gastrostomy.[32,33] Use of this technique allows the surgeon to achieve proper anatomic placement of the stomach, although the complicated nature of the technique prolongs surgical time compared to other methods of gastropexy. Complications of circumcostal gastropexy include rib fracture during dissection for passage of the flap and pneumothorax because of the close proximity to the diaphragm.[32,33]

The *belt-loop gastropexy* offers similar advantages to the circumcostal and incisional gastropexies in that the gastric lumen is not entered and the risk of peritonitis if properly performed is minimal. A seromuscular flap is threaded through a tunnel in the transversus and peritoneum of the right ventral abdominal wall, before being sutured back down to the donor bed. In a series of 20 dogs receiving this technique there were no reported recurrences of GDV within 3 to 13 months after the procedure was performed. The technique can be performed by an unassisted surgeon but is technically more difficult than the incisional gastropexy and, as a result, is not as popular in the United States. Although the gastric flap has the potential to undergo necrosis if a narrow flap is created, this complication has not been recognized in clinical studies of the technique.[29] The ventral midline gastropexy is possibly the easiest gastropexy to perform. The gastric antrum is incorporated into the celiotomy closure with this technique. After the serosa is abraded with a dry surgical sponge, the seromuscular layer of the stomach is incorporated in the linea alba closure using 0 polypropylene sutures. The main disadvantage of this technique is that if a future laparotomy is performed, there is risk that an inadvertent gastrotomy might occur with secondary gastric spillage.[16]

Laparoscopy-assisted or extracorporeal gastropexy procedures have been used as elective procedures in breeds at risk for developing GDV. These elective procedures are commonly done on an outpatient basis and consistently are reported as creating less pain for the patient and good efficacy for creation of a permanent adhesion. Potential complications include perforation of the gastric lumen or any laparoscopy-related complication such as splenic laceration during insufflation. In a series of 25 client-owned dogs, 23 received laparoscopy-assisted gastropexy as an elective procedure and 2 as a treatment for GDV. None of the dogs developed GDV the year after surgery and 20 evaluated with ultrasonography were found to have intact gastropexy attachments.[31]

In summary, with the exception of the tube gastrostomy a variety of open and minimally invasivegastropexy techniques are associated with a low failure rate and minimal complications if properly performed. There are inherent advantages and disadvantages with each technique, making the choice of the procedure a matter of surgeon's preference.

COMPLICATIONS FOLLOWING PARTIAL GASTRECTOMY

Gastric resection for GDV related necrosis usually has few long-term side effects since the gastrectomy site is typically fundic in origin. Unfortunately, since most malignant neoplasms involve the pyloric antral area, resection of the pylorus is required. Pyloric resection may necessitate an end-to-side anastomosis of the duodenum to the stomach also known as a Billroth I gastroduodenostomy procedure. Alternatively, creation of a blind duodenal loop with end-to-side-to-side anastomosis of the stomach to the jejunum is known as a Billroth II gastrojejunostomy. Of these 2 procedures, there is less postoperative vomiting and morbidity associated with the gastoduodenostomy procedure.[34] The tumor mass may also invade the proximal duodenum and common bile duct, forcing the surgeon to anastomose the gallbladder to the duodenum (cholecystoduodenostomy) to reestablish bile flow back into the intestine. Ascending cholecystitis has been reported as a common sequelae to a cholecystoenterostomy. The pathogenesis is thought to be due to a reflux of duodenal contents into the gallbladder. Clinical signs include fever, abdominal pain, vomiting, neutrophilia, and elevation of liver enzymes. Patients usually respond to oral antibiotic therapy, but recurrent episodes are common. Creation of a stoma at least 2.5 cm in length may decrease gallbladder retention of ingesta and minimize the occurrence of postoperative cholecystitis (see Complications of Biliary Surgery). Other reported complications of cholecstoenterostmy in dogs include hepatic abscess, acquired portosytemic shunts, pancreatitis, and vomiting.[35]

Gastric bypass procedures are technically difficult to perform and have numerous complications associated with them, such as the dumping syndrome, marginal ulcers at the anastomosis site, and cholecystitis.[34] After gastric resection and especially gastrojejunostomy procedures, rapid gastric emptying (dumping) occurs, which may lead to abdominal bloating, pain, vomiting, and diarrhea as well as vasomotor symptoms, which also cause tachycardia.[36] Since the pyloric antrum contains the mucus-secreting cells of the stomach and is often removed during the resection, marginal ulceration of the anastomosis site may also occur.[34] Damage to the pancreatic duct may cause resultant pancreatitis after any of the aforementioned gastrectomy techniques.[35] Sporadic vomiting is usually seen during the first 24 to 72 hours after pyloric surgery and is possibly due to bilious duodenal reflux into the causing secondary gastritis. We therefore recommend treating the animal with gastric protectants such as sucralfate or using H2 blockers such as ranitidine or famotidine for 5 to 7 days postoperatively.

COMPLICATIONS ASSOCIATED WITH INTESTINAL SURGERY
Intestinal Wound Dehiscence

Wound dehiscence of intestinal biopsy, enterotomy, or intestinal resection and anastomosis sites often leads to generalized bacterial peritonitis and subsequent death. Risk of intestinal anastomotic leakage can be affected by the cause of the obstruction, failure to adequately identify ischemic tissue, improper suturing or stapling technique, and a variety of factors that negatively affect wound healing such as sepsis, malnutrition, and antineoplastic therapy. In a retrospective study of 115 cases of intestinal anastomosis in dogs and cats, leakage occurred in 13 of 90 dogs but in none of 25 cats.[37] The incidence of leakage and postoperative complications was directly related to the cause of the problem, and mortality was higher in dogs that needed intestinal surgery because of foreign body obstruction compared to those with intestinal neoplasia.[37] In this study, discriminate analysis indicated that dogs with preoperative peritonitis, intestinal foreign body, and serum albumin concentration of 2.5 g/dL or less were also most likely to have leakage from the intestinal wound.[37] A simple method of checking the anastomotic wound site for leakage is to inject the sutures site with saline to check for an adequate seal. In a recent study, 38 jejunal biopsies in dogs were performed and closed using 3 or 4 full-thickness simple interrupted sutures. Saline volumes needed to achieve intraluminal pressures of 20 and 34 cm H_2O in a 10-cm canine jejunal segment containing a closed biopsy site using 2 methods of luminal occlusion were recorded. The 95% confidence intervals for the volume of saline needed to achieve 20 and 34 cm H_2O intraluminal pressure with digital occlusion were 10.9 to 13.6 mL and 16.3 to 19.0 mL, respectively, and with Doyen occlusion, 8.5 to 11.1 mL and 12.1 to 14.8 mL, respectively. Therefore, intestinal surgical sites can be checked intraoperatively for leakage by intraluminal injection of 10 to 12 mL of saline if the loop of intestine is sealed with Doyen forceps placed 10 cm apart.[38]

FACTORS INCREASING THE RISK OF INTESTINAL LEAKAGE
Inadequate removal of ischemic tissue

Ischemic intestine is often black or gray and easily discernible from normal bowel. Determining viability in cyanotic appearing bowel is sometimes difficult. The intestine first should be decompressed with a needle and suction apparatus to relieve venous congestion. Intraoperative criteria for establishing intestinal viability are color, arterial pulsations, and the presence of peristalsis. Questionable areas of bowel should be pinched to determine whether smooth muscle contraction and peristalsis are present. If clinical criteria are inadequate to determine viability, intravenous fluorescein dye or surface oximetry can be used. A 10% fluorescein solution is given at a dosage of 1 mL/5 kg intravenously through any peripheral vein.[39] After 2 minutes, the tissues are subjected to long-wave ultraviolet light (Wood's lamp). Areas of bowel are considered viable if they have a bright green glow. Areas of bowel are not viable if they have a patchy density with areas of nonfluorescence exceeding 3 mm, have only perivascular fluorescence, or are completely nonfluorescent.[39] Oxygen saturation may also be a reliable method of determining intestinal wall viability. A sterile probe is placed on the surface of the bowel and an oxygen saturation level reading will occur. According to published reports in rabbits, saturation levels above 81% typically indicate that the bowel is viable, whereas values below 76% were consistent with mucosal necrosis and those below 64% indicated transmural intestinal necrosis.[40]

Poor wound apposition

Direct approximation of the wound edge allows for optimum rapid healing characterized by primary intestinal wound healing. Accurate apposition allows for rapid mucosal reepithelialization, and early formation occurs of young well-vascularized collagen between the submucosa, muscularis, and serosa. Other advantages of approximating patterns for intestinal anastomosis are that (1) the lumen diameter is not compromised, (2) the wound strength meets or exceeds everting or inverting wound strengths after 24 hours, and (3) the adhesions are minimal.[2] Sutures should not be tied too tight since crushing of tissue has been shown to cause more tissue ischemia directly at the suture line and is discouraged. Mucosal eversion or tissue overlap retards healing and should be avoided. Mucosal eversion results in delayed fibrin seal formation, delayed mucosal reepithelialization, increased mucocele formation, prolonged inflammatory response, and marked adhesion formation. Eversion may initially widen the intestinal lumen diameter, but the prolonged inflammatory response eventually narrows the lumen, contributing to the risk of stenosis. Everting anastomoses also have an increased tendency for leakage, especially in the face of septic peritonitis, and should never be used in the colon. Inversion of the wound edge creates an internal cuff of tissue that reduces lumen diameter. Hemodynamic compromise of the inverted submucosa occurs, resulting in mucosal edema and necrosis. After 5 days the internal cuff usually sloughs. Inverting anastomoses are characterized by a rapid serosa-to-serosa seal and minimal adhesion formation. Yet because of their safety against leakage, inverting patterns may be the preferred technique for the colon.

As an alternative to hand suturing, autostapling may be used for intestinal anastomosis. The GIA and TA auto staplers lay an overlapping double row of staples for security and, when used in combination, create a functional "end-to-end anastomosis." The GIA portion of the anastomosis is inverted, whereas the TA portion of the anastomosis is everted. Recent studies in human have shown that leakage rates are similar to hand-sewn techniques but autostapler use significantly reduces surgical time.[41] In veterinary surgery, direct comparisons between hand-sewn and stapled anastomosis are poorly documented, but in a recent study, nonspecialists were able to achieve very good results with stapling devices in 25 of 30 dogs, with anastomotic problems occurring in only 2 dogs.[42] An alternative to sutured anastomosis is the use of an AutoSuture Premium 35 skin stapler with stainless skin staples (Covidien, Norwalk, CT, USA). After triangulating the intestine with 3 stay sutures, the skin stapler is used to place staples every 2 to 3 mm around the perimeter of the wound. These closures are more rapidly done than hand-sewn anastomosis and have similar bursting strengths. However, mucosal eversion may occur between staples.[43]

Improper selection of suture material

For hand-sewn anastomoses, either continuous or interrupted patterns can be used with equal efficacy. Although both absorbable and nonabsorbable suture materials have been used successfully for anastomosis, the braided nonabsorbable suture materials such as silk may harbor bacteria and create granulomatous inflammatory reaction or draining suture sinus. Monofilament nonabsorbable sutures such as Nylon and polypropylene are safe in contaminated environments. However, polypropylene has been associated with foreign body adherence in one case series.[44] Absorbable suture materials reported in the veterinary literature for intestinal suturing include chromic gut, polyglycolic acid (Dexon), polygalactin 910 (Vicryl), polydioxanone (PDS), polyglyconate (Maxon), and poliglecaprone (Monocryl). Of these, surgical gut is not recommended for anastomosis because it is rapidly broken down by collagenase.

Polygalactin 910 and polyglycolic acid are braided and retain good tensile strength for up to 28 days. Vicryl is commonly used for intestinal anastomosis in humans with good published success and is popular in Europe for veterinary use. In North America, monofilament sutures such as polydioxanone (PDS) and polyglyconate (Maxon) are more commonly used. These polyester monofilament suture materials are absorbed by hydrolysis and therefore are unaffected by contaminated environment. They maintain up to 40% of their original tensile strength after 3 weeks. Many surgeons are also starting to use shorter acting monofilament suture such as Monocryl or Biosyn for intestinal anastomosis. They have similar handling properties to PDS but are degraded more quickly. The newer "Plus" sutures are impregnated with the antibacterial agent Triclosan. Their efficacy in reducing infection in contaminated dermal wounds may foster an increased use in intestinal anastomosis.

Omentalization

All anastomoses should be covered with a vascularized omental flap that is tacked in place. Omentum is useful in (1) restoring blood supply to a devascularized area, (2) facilitating lymphatic drainage, and (3) minimizing mucosal leakage and secondary peritonitis. The role of omentum is significant when one considers that in one study 90% mortality rates were seen with intestinal anastomoses after omental resection was performed in dogs.[45] Free omental flaps are not as effective as pedicle omental flaps and may in fact lead to anastomosis failure.[45]

OTHER FACTORS AFFECTING DEHISCENCE

Healing of visceral wounds is negatively affected by a number of other factors. Chronic weight loss of 15% to 20% due to cancer cachexia or other reasons has a negative effect on visceral wound healing. Correction of cachexia as well as early postoperative enteral feeding appears to increase collagen deposition and bursting wound strength.[46] Glucocorticoids have a negative effect on wound healing when given in large doses prior to the third day after wounding.[1] NSAIDs appear to affect the early inflammatory phase of wound healing but do not appear to interfere with the proliferative phase of wound healing or have a significant negative effect on visceral healing strength.[47] Radiation therapies interfere with fibroblast mobilization, replication, and collagen synthesis as well as causing sclerosis of microvasculature, thereby reducing oxygenation at the wound site. Whenever possible, radiation therapy should be initiated after visceral wound healing is complete. The negative effects of cancer on wound healing appear to be secondary to nutritional deficiencies rather than direct tumor impairment on wound healing. Visceral wound healing may actually be mildly augmented, owing to release growth factors by the neoplasm. Effects of chemotherapeutic agents on visceral wound healing are variable. Drugs such as vincristine, vinblastine, and azathioprine seem to be safe when used in therapeutic doses. Drugs such as cyclophosphamide, methotrexate, 5-FU, and doxorubicin have been shown to delay wound healing in both experimental and clinical studies.[46,48] Cisplatin appears to significantly impair intestinal wound healing in rats and should be used with caution after intestinal surgery.[49]

EFFECT OF EARLY POSTOPERATIVE ENTERAL FEEDING ON VISCERAL HEALING

Malnutrition induces intestinal mucosal atrophy, reduced motility, increased incidence of ileus, and the potential for bacterial translocation through the bowel wall, with resultant sepsis.[50] Impaired wound healing due to nutritional causes may be reversed by feeding an enteral or a parenteral diet that supplies energy needs in the form of fatty acids and sugars and provides essential amino acids. Feedings of high protein meals after injury can optimize conditions for normal visceral wound healing. Amino acids provided through enteral nutrition are utilized for the synthesis of structural proteins such as actin, myosin, collagen, and elastin. Early, if not immediate, postoperative enteral feeding has been shown to have a positive influence on the healing rate of intestinal anastomosis in dogs.[51] Bursting pressures and collagen levels of ileal and colorectal anastomosis were compared in beagles fed elemental diets versus those fed only electrolytes and water for 4 days.[51] The dogs fed orally had nearly twice the bursting strengths of the control group and nearly double the amount of both immature and mature collagen at the wound site.[51] Total parenteral nutrition (TPN) does not appear to ameliorate the mucosal atrophy or increase collagen deposition as did enteral nutrition.[50] In human studies, the incidence of septic complications is significantly lower in people fed between 8 and 24 hours after surgery versus those maintained on TPN. Additionally, early-fed patients had a reduced incidence of postoperative ileus and reduced hospital stay.[50]

EFFECTS OF MASSIVE SMALL INTESTINAL RESECTION

The propensity for short-bowel syndrome after massive intestinal resection depends on the amount of tissue excised, the location of the resection, and the time allowed for adaptation. Resection of up to 80% of the small intestine in puppies may allow for normal weight gain, whereas resection of 90% produces morbidity and mortality in dogs.[52] After resection of large portions of small intestine, maldigestion, malabsorption, diarrhea induced by fatty acids or bile salts, bacterial overgrowth, and gastric hypersecretion may occur. Location of the resection is important in people. High resection of the duodenum and upper jejunum may decrease pancreatic enzyme secretion because pancreatic-stimulating hormones such as secretin and cholecystokinin are produced in the mucosa of these sections. These reductions in release of pancreatic enzymes contribute to maldigestion. Maldigestion of protein, carbohydrate, and fat leads to catabolism, negative nitrogen balance, and steatorrhea. Unabsorbed sugars also may cause osmotic diarrhea. If the ileocecal valve is resected, bacteria may ascend, overgrow in the small bowel, and contribute to diarrhea. After massive resection, the remaining small intestine adapts by increasing lumen diameter, enlarging microvilli, and increasing mucosal cell number. These compensatory changes may take several weeks; during this period, parenteral fluids, electrolytes, and hyperalimentation may be necessary for the survival of the animal. With proper supportive care, the animal will be able to maintain weight even with diarrhea. Medical treatments for unresponsive diarrhea after massive resection in dogs include frequent small meals, low-fat diets such as intestinal diet (I/D Hills, Topeka, KS), elemental diet supplements, medium-chain triglyceride oils, pancreatic enzyme supplements, B vitamins, kaolin antidiarrheals, and poorly absorbed oral antibiotics such as neomycin.

A recent retrospective study determined outcome in 13 dogs and 7 cats that underwent extensive (ie, >50%) resection of the small intestine.[53] In this study, in all 7 cats and 8 of the 13 dogs, extensive intestinal resection was performed because of a foreign body. Mean ± SD estimated percentage of intestine that was removed was 68 ± 14% (range, 50%–90%). Two dogs were euthanized 3 days after surgery because of dehiscence of the surgical site and development of septic peritonitis; 1 dog died of acute respiratory distress syndrome 5 days after surgery. The remaining 10 dogs and 7 cats were discharged from the hospital, and follow-up information was available for 15 of the 17. Median survival time was 828 days, and 12 of the 15 animals for which long-term follow-up information was available had good outcomes. However, none of the factors examined, including percentage of intestine resected, were significantly associated with outcome. In summary, most dogs and cats that underwent extensive resection of the small intestine had a good outcome after a variable period of intestinal adaptation. The amount of intestine resected was not always associated with outcome.

SURGICAL MANAGEMENT OF INTESTINAL LEAKAGE

Revision of the primary surgical site, copious abdominal lavage, and broad-spectrum intravenous antibiotic therapy are the mainstays of addressing intestinal anastomotic leakage and are addressed separately in this chapter (Diagnosis and Drainage Options for Septic Abdomen). After revision of the primary anastomotic site, mechanical reinforcement if the anastomosis is typically performed. Use of an omental pedicle graft (described earliere) is sufficient in most animals; however, when the omentum is devitalized or when more substantial mechanical reinforcement is desired, intestinal serosal patching is recommended. The serosal patch technique uses the antimesenteric surface of the small bowel to cover or buttress an adjacent area of questionable tissue viability or an area that cannot be reliably sutured. Jejunum is commonly used because its freely movable mesentery allows it to be mobile. The serosal patch provides mechanical stability and will help to induce and localize a fibrin seal over the questionable area. A section of jejunum free of mesenteric tension is transposed over the perforation or area to be buttressed. It is important not to stretch, kink, or twist its mesenteric root or the vascular supply may be disrupted. The bowel chosen for the patch is then gently looped to prevent luminal bowel obstruction. Multiple perforations sometimes require patching using a back-and-forth looping of the entire segment of bowel. The lateral aspects of the bowel wall or antimesenteric border are used for the patch **(Fig. 3A)**. The patch is not sutured directly to the edges of the defect but rather 3 to 4 mm beyond its margins. Simple interrupted sutures of 4-0 nylon or polypropylene are placed 3 to 4 mm from the wound edges and 3 to 4 mm apart (see **Fig. 3B**). The sutures grasp the submucosa of the patch and bowel wall but do not penetrate the lumen.

Externalized intestinal anastomosis has been used in humans in the management of leaking colonic anastomosis, and this novel approach was successfully used to manage a leaking ileocolic anastomosis in a dog.[54] A 6-year-old, spayed female Labrador retriever was presented 48 hours after an intestinal resection and anastomosis for management of a small intestinal foreign body. Abdominal ultrasound confirmed the presence of peritoneal effusion. Cytology of fluid collected by abdominocentesis revealed a large number of degenerate neutrophils with intracellular cocci. A diagnosis of septic peritonitis was made, presumably because of dehiscence of the anastomosis. Upon repeat exploratory celiotomy, the intestinal anastomosis was found to be leaking intestinal contents into the abdomen. An end-to-end, ileocolic anastomosis was performed and subsequently exteriorized into the subcutaneous space via a paramedian incision through the abdominal wall. The anastomosis was inspected daily for 4 days before it was returned to the abdomen and the subcutaneous defect was closed. Serial cytology of the peritoneal fluid, which was performed during this 4-day postoperative period, confirmed progressive resolution of the peritonitis and the dog was discharged from the hospital with a successful recovery.

DIAGNOSIS AND DRAINAGE OPTIONS FOR SEPTIC ABDOMEN

With generalized septic peritonitis, massive fluid and protein movement to the peritoneal cavity result in a shift of fluid away from the intravascular space, causing

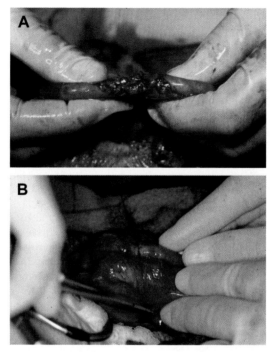

Fig. 3. (*A*) Intraoperative image of a leaking enterotomy that had been closed with chromic gut. (*B*) A loop of jejunum has been sutured in place over the previous enterotomy site to create a serosal patch.

hemoconcentration and eventual hypovolemic shock. The presence of large numbers of free bacteria or endotoxins causes massive shifts of neutrophils to the abdomen, vasodilation of the visceral vasculature, high hepatic energy demand (hypoglycemia), metabolic acidosis, and often fatal septic shock. Mortality rates with septic peritonitis secondary to leaking intestinal anastomosis may be as high as 70%. In cases where cytologic evaluation of peritoneal fluid is not diagnostic, clinicians are now using comparisons of serum versus intraperitoneal glucose and lactate values as a means of determining the diagnosis of septic peritonitis. In a study evaluating 18 dogs and 12 cats with septic effusion dogs with septic effusion, all animals had peritoneal fluid glucose concentration lower than the blood glucose concentration.[55] A blood-to-fluid glucose (BFG) difference greater than 20 mg/dL was 100% sensitive and 100% specific for the diagnosis of septic peritoneal effusion in dogs. Also, in the 7 dogs in which it was evaluated, a blood-to-fluid lactate (BFL) difference less than −2.0 mM was also 100% sensitive and specific for a diagnosis of septic peritoneal effusion. In cats, the BFG difference was 86% sensitive and 100% specific for a diagnosis of septic peritonitis. In dogs and cats, the BFG difference was more accurate for a diagnosis of septic peritonitis than was peritoneal fluid glucose concentration alone.[55]

Once diagnosed, treatment of septic peritonitis is directed toward the correction of electrolyte and colloid abnormalities, appropriate antimicrobial therapy, and exploratory celiotomy to determine and surgically correct the underlying cause of the peritonitis. After *aerobic and anaerobic culture* and correction of the offending problem, aggressive *peritoneal lavage* is performed; either the abdomen is closed primarily or closed peritoneal drainage techniques are used. Thorough peritoneal lavage of the abdominal cavity is performed with body-temperature 0.9% NaCl or lactated Ringer's solution. Lavaging a cat with 500 to 750 mL and a large dog with 3 to 5 L of fluid will help remove the bacteria and foreign debris, which are the initiators of the peritoneal inflammation. Although lavage of the peritoneum may have the theoretical disadvantage of spreading bacterial contamination, peritoneal lavage is well established as a means of reducing morbidity and mortality due to septic peritonitis. All lavage fluid should be aspirated because when bacteria are suspended in residual lavage fluid, phagocytosis is impaired. Three cycles of lavage and aspiration are recommended.

Peritoneal drains, when used, vary in their effectiveness with single-lumen passive drains such as Penrose tubes, recovering much less fluid than that collected by double-lumen active drains in most studies.[56] Gravity drains have several other disadvantages, including early occlusion of the drain by the omentum, fibrin, or exudate and mechanical irritation of the peritoneum. Last, passive drains may facilitate migration of bacteria into the peritoneal cavity. Active suction drains, such as the Jackson-Pratt drain, improve efficacy of fluid removal and maintain a closed system that minimizes bacterial contamination of the peritoneum, making them the clear choice if closed abdominal drainage is elected for following surgery. As an added benefit to the use of closed suction drains, the clinician is able to monitor changes in gross and cytologic features of peritoneal fluid on a daily basis until drain removal is performed. Intra-abdominal drains may also be used to perform a technique called intermittent peritoneal lavage. Isothermic, sterile fluids are administered via a peritoneal catheter or fenestrated tube. The fluids are then removed by gravity flow back through a separate outflow tube. Our clinical impressions are that this technique has been helpful in reducing mortality associated with diffuse peritonitis. However, experimental results suggest that good lavage of the entire abdomen is not provided.[57] The development of hypoproteinemia and hypokalemia is common, although these complications are less severe than those noted during open peritoneal drainage.

Open peritoneal drainage is a process by which the linea alba and skin are left partially or completely open and covered with sterile dressings, which are changed at frequent intervals. The main advantages of open peritoneal drainage are that it allows unimpeded drainage of fluid and exudate from the peritoneal cavity and at the same time alters the anaerobic environment of the peritoneum. Many surgeons advocate open peritoneal drainage as the optimal treatment for generalized septic peritonitis.[58–60] The mortality rate associated with open peritoneal drainage for management of septic peritonitis in dogs and cats ranges between 11% and 48%.[56–58] Most studies document that mortality is increased if sepsis is secondary to GI leakage compared to leakage from the reproductive tract.[58,59] The author facilitates open peritoneal lavage by placing continuous or interrupted Nylon or polypropylene sutures loosely in the linea alba, allowing it to gap 1 to 2 cm. The skin and subcutaneous tissues are not closed and are covered with antibiotic ointment and nonadherent gauze dressing before applying a large cotton padded bandage (**Fig. 4**). The animal is continuously observed and the bandage aseptically changed at 12- to 24-hour intervals under general anesthesia and strict aseptic technique. The abdominal wound is closed primarily in 1 to 5 days depending on when the peritoneal inflammation has resided. Common complications associated with open peritoneal drainage are patient dehydration and hypoproteinemia secondary to massive fluid and protein loss into the bandage.

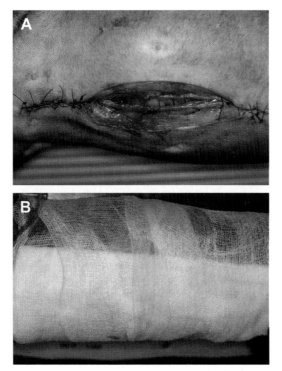

Fig. 4. (*A*) Image from a cat with multiple intestinal perforations secondary to an arrow traversing the abdomen. After repair of all intestinal wounds, the abdomen was thoroughly lavaged and open abdominal drainage was performed. The abdominal wall has been partially closed with a loosely placed polypropylene sutures. (*B*) The abdomen is covered with a sterile dressing that is changed under general anesthesia or deep sedation on a daily basis. The abdominal is typically closed within 1 to 5 days depending on the degree of inflammation.

It is unclear whether open or closed peritoneal drainage is superior in the treatment of septic peritonitis in dogs and cats. Open peritoneal drainage is a more effective technique for achieving peritoneal drainage than is tube drainage[56] and is generally recommended if contamination is diffuse and not readily removed during the initial exploratory celiotomy. With open drainage, large volumes of abdominal fluid and exudate can be removed from the abdomen and the bacterial environment can be favorably altered, therefore decreasing the number of anaerobic microorganisms. In humans it has been reported that open abdominal drainage can improve a patient's metabolic condition, reduce abdominal adhesion formation, and leave access for repeated exploration and inspection of the abdomen.[61] Yet that same study actually indicated a higher mortality rate associated with patients managed with open peritoneal drainage compared to patients managed with closed abdomens, largely due to the acquisition of nosocomial infections. Other reported complications included massive fluid and protein loss, increased nursing care, increased cost, additional anesthetic, enteric fistula formation, incisional herniation, evisceration, small bowel obstruction secondary to adhesion formation, and nosocomial infection.[61] Information provided by a limited number of retrospective studies in veterinary medicine offer guidelines as to when open peritoneal drainage may be indicated.[58–60,62,63] In general, open peritoneal drainage is considered in cases where the source of contamination cannot be identified, the contamination is severe or longstanding, or the virulence of organisms is considered high, such as that seen with fecal contamination or anaerobic infections. In these situations, open peritoneal drainage offers the possibility of reexploration and subsequent lavage. On the other hand, if the source of contamination is successfully eliminated and lavaging the abdomen is effective at removing residual debris, the abdomen may be closed with good results in a majority of the cases.[62]

Vacuum-assisted closure (VAC) (V.A.C., Kinetic Concepts, Inc, San Antonio, TX, USA) is a relatively new concept in veterinary medicine that can be adopted for use in cases of septic peritonitis. Vacuum-assisted therapy consists of placing a dressing sponge made of open-cell polyurethane ether foam over the partially closed abdominal incision. Embedded in this sponge is a noncollapsible, side-ported evacuation tube that is connected to an adjustable pump. The vacuum applied may be used intermittently or continuously. All the cells in the open cell foam communicate so the vacuum is evenly applied to all wound surfaces in contact with the sponge. A plastic adhesive drape (Ioban) is placed around the abdomen to create an air-tight seal. The excellent drainage characteristics provided by vacuum therapy appear to be a therapeutic option for the treatment of septic peritonitis. One human study compared different bandaging techniques for the management of patients with open abdomens and found a 40% reduction in mortality in patients treated with VAC therapy.[64] There are limited studies in the human literature supporting the use of VAC therapy in patients with septic peritonitis, but the positive results from these studies are encouraging.[64,65]

COMPLICATIONS AFTER SUBTOTAL COLECTOMY

Subtotal colectomy is a salvage technique for treatment of recurrent megacolon. In North America, dogs have traditionally been treated medically because of their propensity for postoperative diarrhea after removal of large segments of the colon. However, in a recent UK study, 8 dogs with acquired megacolon underwent subtotal colectomy with preservation of the ileocolic junction.[66] The diagnosis was confirmed in all animals by abdominal palpation, plain radiography, and postoperative histopathologic findings. There were no intraoperative complications, although 1 dog died postoperatively as a result of septic peritonitis. Long-term follow-up was obtained by clinical records and telephone interviews with the owners of the 7 surviving dogs. Resolution of obstipation and improved stool consistency of the remaining dogs were improved at discharge and all surviving animals eventually returned to normal defecation in 5 to 10 weeks and were alive 11 to 48 months (mean 40.5 months) after surgery. These results emphasized the long-term effectiveness of subtotal colectomy with preservation of the ileocolic junction in dogs with idiopathic megacolon.

In cats, subtotal colectomy has been a successful salvage procedure for idiopathic megacolon for more than 25 years.[67–70] Some controversy exists as to whether the cecum should be preserved and a colon-to-colon anastomosis (colocolostomy) done or whether it can be sacrificed and an ileum-to-colon anastomosis (ileocolostomy) performed. Ileocolostomy has the inherent luminal disparity to deal with but ligation of the ileocolic artery and removal of the cecum allow easy transposition of the mobile ileum down to the colonic stump. With colocolostomy, luminal disparity is kept to minimum, but the technique may be technically demanding because the relatively immobile mesocolon places considerable tension on the suture line. Studies indicate that removal of the cecum does not lead to ascending bacterial enteritis, and cats with ileocolostomies do as well clinically as those with the cecum preserved.[69,70]

Colocolostomy can also be performed using an end-to-end anastomosis autostapler, but it must be done via a typhlotomy incision (EEA; Covidien Inc).

Cats are often somewhat depressed and anorectic for 48 hours following subtotal colectomy. They will sometimes have a moderate fever of 103° to 103.5°F in the absence of leukocytosis.[68] Dark tarry liquid feces are usually noted for about 3 to 4 days. The presence of abdominal tenderness, vomiting, detection of intracellular bacteria on peritoneal fluid cytology, or significant glucose differential between peritoneal fluid and serum warrants early reexploration of the abdomen. Normally, feces remain liquid and poorly formed for 2 to 6 weeks after surgery, at which time they usually become soft and poorly formed for the remainder of the cat's life. Long-term follow-up studies indicate that most cats seem to maintain their normal body weight or even gain weight after the procedure.[67,68] After surgery, cats generally use the litter box 2 or 3 times a day, but the total amount of water loss in the feces equals that of normal cats.[63] The ileum increases it absorptive capacity by increasing villous height. Bacterial overgrowth, folic acid deficiency, and anemia are not uncommon, despite initial concerns.[70] The major complaint of cat owners is chronic perineal soiling caused by the loose feces. If this becomes a problem, it can often be managed by clipping hair in the perineal area. Occasionally cats become reconstipated and must be treated medically with lactulose and cisapride for a period of time. In recurrent cases, reexploration and removal of additional residual colon are sometimes necessary.

SUMMARY

A large number of naturally occurring disease conditions are treated by GI surgery in small animals. The GI tract is rich in blood supply and has the potential to heal in rapid fashion but GI effluent is contaminated and surgery is fraught with many pitfalls, the most notable of which is leakage of the surgical site due to technical error, patient cachexia, chemotherapy, metabolic disorders, or preexisting septic peritonitis. Once present, septic peritonitis requires reoperation, patching techniques for the leakage sites, aggressive fluid resuscitation, and appropriate antibiotic therapy based on culture and sensitivity. Innovative surgical techniques such as the VAC drainage or extra abdominal anastomosis placement may increase the survival rates in these critical patients but need further investigation.

REFERENCES

1. Peacock EE. The gastrointestinal tract. In: Surgery and biology of wound repair. 3rd edition. Philadelphia: WB Saunders; 1984. p. 78–85.
2. Ellison GW. Wound healing in the gastrointestinal tract. Semin Vet Med Surg (Sm Anim) 1989;4:287–98.
3. Boothe HW, Lay JC, Moreland KJ. Sclerosing encapsulating peritonitis in three dogs. J Am Vet Med Assoc 1991;198:267–70.
4. Hardie EM, Rottman JB, Levy JK. Sclerosing encapsulating peritonitis in four dogs and a cat. Vet Surg 1994;23:107–14.
5. Muir WW. Gastric dilatation-volvulus in the dog, with emphasis on cardiac arrhythmias. J Am Vet Med Assoc 1982;180:739–42.
6. Betts CW, Wingfield WE, Green RW. A retrospective study of gastric dilatation-torsion in the dog. J Sm Anim Pract 1974;15:727–34.
7. Glickman LT, Glickman NW, Pérez CM, et al. Analysis of risk factors for gastric dilatation and dilatation-volvulus in dogs. J Am Vet Med Assoc 1994;204:1465–71.
8. Brockman DJ, Washabau RJ. Canine gastric dilatation/volvulus syndrome in a veterinary critical care unit: 295 cases. J Am Vet Med Assoc 1995;207(4):460–4.

9. Mackenzie G, Barnhart M, Kennedy S, et al. A retrospective study of factors influencing survival following surgery for gastric dilatation-volvulus syndrome in 306 dogs. J Am Anim Hosp Assoc 2010;46:97–102.

10. Beck JJ, Staatz AJ, Pelsue DH, et al. Risk factors associated with short-term outcome and development of perioperative complications in dogs undergoing surgery because of gastric dilatation-volvulus: 166 cases (1992-2003). J Am Vet Med Assoc 2006;229: 1934–9.

11. Glickman LT, Lantz GC, Schellenberg DB, et al. A prospective study of survival and recurrence following the acute gastric dilatation-volvulus syndrome in 136 dogs. J Am Anim Hosp Assoc 1998 34:253–9.

12. de Papp E, Drobatz KJ, Hughes D. Plasma lactate concentration as a predictor of gastric necrosis and survival among dogs with gastric dilatation-volvulus: 102 cases (1995-1998). J Am Vet Med Assoc 1999;215:49–52.

13. Millis DL, Hauptman JG, Fulton RB Jr. Abnormal hemostatic profiles and gastric necrosis in canine gastric dilatation-volvulus. Vet Surg 1993;22:93–7.

14. Zacher LA, Berg J, Shaw SP, et al. Association between outcome and changes in plasma lactate concentration during presurgical treatment in dogs with gastric dilatation-volvulus: 64 cases (2002-2008) J Am Vet Med Assoc 2010;236:892–7.

15. Eggertsdóttir AV, Moe L. A retrospective study of conservative treatment of gastric dilatation-volvulus in the dog. Acta Vet Scand 1995;36:175–84.

16. Meyer-Lindenberg A, Harder A, Fehr M, et al. Treatment of gastric dilatation-volvulus and a rapid method for prevention of relapse in dogs: 134 cases (1988-1991). J Am Vet Med Assoc 1993;203:1303–7.

17. Mattheisen DT. Partial gastrectomy as treatment of gastric volvulus in 30 dogs. Vet Surg 1985;14:185–94.

18. Monnet E, Pelsue D, MacPhail C. Evaluation of laser Doppler flowmetry for measurement of capillary blood flow in the stomach wall of dogs during gastric dilatation-volvulus. Vet Surg 2006;35:198–205.

19. MacCoy DM, Kneller SF, Sundberg JP. Partial invagination of the canine stomach for treatment of infarction of the gastric wall. Vet Surg 1989;15:237–45.

20. Parton AT, Volk SW, Weisse C. Gastric ulceration subsequent to partial invagination of the stomach in a dog with gastric dilatation-volvulus. J Am Vet Med Assoc 2006;228: 1895–900.

21. Marconato L. Gastric dilatation-volvulus as complication after surgical removal of a splenic haemangiosarcoma in a dog. J Vet Med A Physiol Pathol Clin Med 2006;53: 371–4.

22. Millis DL, Nemzek J, Riggs C, et al. Walshaw R. Gastric dilatation-volvulus after splenic torsion in two dogs. J Am Vet Med Assoc 1995;207:314–5.

23. Goldhammer MA, Haining H, Milne EM, et al. Assessment of the incidence of GDV following splenectomy in dogs. J Small Anim Pract 2010;51:23–8.

24. Glickman LT, Glickman NW, Schellenberg DB, et al. Non-dietary risk factors for gastric dilatation-volvulus in large and giant breed dogs. J Am Vet Med Assoc 2000;217:1492–9.

25. Ward MP, Patronek GJ, Glickman LT. Benefits of prophylactic gastropexy for dogs at risk of gastric dilatation-volvulus. Prev Vet Med 2003;60:319–29.

26. Parks J. Surgical management of gastric torsion. Vet Clin North Am Small Anim Pract 1979;9(2):259–67.

27. MacCoy DM, Sykes GP, Hoffer RE. A gastropexy technique for permanent fixation of the pyloric antrum. J Am Anim Hosp Assoc 1982;18:763–8.

28. Fallah AM, Lumb WV, Nelson AW. Circumcostal gastropexy in the dog: a preliminary study. Vet Surg 1982;11:19–22.

29. Whitney WO, Scavelli TD, Matthiesen DT. Belt loop gastropexy: technique and surgical results in 20 dogs. J Am Anim Hosp Assoc 1989;25:75–9.

30. Hosgood G. Clinical update: gastric dilatation-volvulus in dogs. J Am Vet Med Assoc 1994;204:1742–7.

31. Rawlings CA, Mahaffey MB, Bement S, et al. Prospective evaluation of laparoscopic-assisted gastropexy in dogs susceptible to gastric dilatation. J Am Vet Med Assoc 2002;221:1576–81.

32. Fox SM. Gastric dilatation volvulus: results from 31 surgical cases of circumcostal vs tube gastrostomy. Calif Vet 1985;8:8–11.

33. Leib MS, Konde LJ, Wingfield WE, et al. Circummcostal gastropexy for preventing recurrence of gastric dilatation-volvulus in the dog: an evaluation of 30 cases. J Am Vet Med Assoc 1985;187:245–8.

34. Papageorges M, Breton L, Bonneau NH. Gastric drainage procedures: effects in normal dogs II. Clinical observations and gastric emptying. Vet Surg 1987;16:332–40.

35. Papazoglou LG, Mann FA, Wagner-Man C, et al. Long-term survival after chole-cystoenterostomy: a retrospective study of 15 cases. J Am Anim Hosp Assoc 2008;44:67–74.

36. Feikes HL, Syphers CE, Hinshaw DB, et al. Coronary blood flow in experimental dumping syndrome in the dog. J Am Med Assoc 1961;178:1012–3.

37. Ralphs SC, Jessen CR, Lipowitz AJ. Risk factors for leakage following intestinal anastomosis in dogs and cats: 115 cases (1991-2000). J Am Vet Med Assoc 2003;223(1):73–7.

38. Saile K, Boothe HW, Boothe DM. Saline volume necessary to achieve predetermined intraluminal pressures during leak testing of small intestinal biopsy sites in the dog. Vet Surg 2010;39(7):900–3.

39. Ellison GW, Jokinen MC, Park RD. End-to-end intestinal anastomosis in the dog: a comparative fluorescein dye, angiographic and histopathologic evaluation. J Am Anim Hosp Assoc 1982;18:729–36.

40. Erikoglu M, Kaynak A, Beyatli EA, et al. Intraoperative determination of intestinal viability: a comparison with transserosal pulse oximetry and histopathological examination. J Surg Res 2005;128(1):66.

41. Golub R, Golab RW, Cantu R, et al. A multivariate analysis of factors contributing to leakage of intestinal anastomosis. J Am Coll Surg 1999;184:364–72.

42. Jardel N, Hidalgo A, Leperlier D, et al. One stage functional end-to-end stapled intestinal anastomosis and resection performed by nonexpert surgeons for the treatment of small intestinal obstruction in 30 dogs. Vet Surg 2011;40(2):216–22.

43. Coolman BR, Ehrhart N, Pijanowski G, et al. Comparison of skin staples with sutures for anastomosis of the small intestine of dogs. Vet Surg 2000;29:392.

44. Milovancev M, Weisman DL, Palmisano MP. Foreign body attachment to polypropyl-ene suture material extruded into the small intestinal lumen after enteric closure in three dogs. J Am Vet Med Assoc 2005;225:1701,1713–5.

45. McLackin AD. Omental protection of intestinal anastomosis. Am J Surg 1973;125:134.

46. McCaw DL. The effects of cancer and cancer therapies on wound healing. Semin Vet Med Surg 1989;4:2817.

47. Donner GS, Ellison GW, Peyton LC. Effect of flunixin meglumine on surgical wound strength and healing in the rat. Am J Vet Res 1986;47:2247–51.

48. Laing EJ. The effect of antineoplastic agents on wound healing. Compend Contin Educ Sm Anim Pract 1989;11:136.

49. Moore AS, Kitchell BE. New chemotherapy agents in veterinary medicine. Vet Clinics Sm An Pract 2003;37:629–49.
50. Braga M. Early postoperative enteral nutrition improves oxygenation and reduces costs compared with total parenteral nutrition. Clin Nutr 2001;29:242–8.
51. Moss G, Greenstein A, Lew S, et al. Maintenance of GI function after bowel surgery and immediate full nutrition. 1. Doubling of canine colorectal anastomotic bursting pressure and intestinal wound mature collagen content. J Parenter Enteral Nutr 1980;4:535–8.
52. Chatworthy HW, Saleby R, Lovingood C. Extensive small bowel resection in young dogs: its effect on growth and development. Vet Surg 1952;32:341–6.
53. Gorman SC, Freeman LM, Mitchell SL, et al. Extensive small bowel resection in dogs and cats: 20 cases (1998-2004). J Am Vet Med Assoc 2006;228:403–7.
54. Simcock J, Kuntz CA, Newman R. Externalized ileocolic anastomosis: case report. J Am Anim Hosp Assoc 2010;46:274–80.
55. Bonczynski JJ, Ludwig LL, Barton LJ, et al. Comparison of peritoneal fluid and peripheral blood pH, bicarbonate, glucose, and lactate concentration as a diagnostic tool for septic peritonitis in dogs and cats. Vet Surg 2003;32(2):161–6.
56. Donner GS, Ellison GW. The use and misuse of abdominal drains in small animal surgery. Cont Educ Pract Vet 1986;8:705–15.
57. Hosgood G, Salisbury SK, Cantwell HD, et al. Intraperitoneal circulation and drainage in the dog. Vet Surg 1989;18:261–8.
58. Greenfield CL, Walshaw R. Open peritoneal drainage for treatment of contaminated peritoneal cavity and septic peritonitis in dogs and cats: 24 cases. J Am Vet Med Assoc 1987;191:100–5.
59. Woolfson JM, Dulisch ML. Open peritoneal drainage in the treatment of generalized peritonitis in 25 dogs and cats. Vet Surg 1986;15:27–32.
60. Orsher RJ, Rosin E. Open peritoneal drainage in experimental peritonitis in dogs. Vet Surg 1984;13:222–6.
61. Bosscha K, Hulstaert PF, Visser MR, et al. Open management of the abdomen and planned reoperations in severe bacterial peritonitis. Eur J Surg 2000;166:44–9.
62. Lanz OI, Ellison GW, Bellah JR, et al. Surgical treatment of septic peritonitis without abdominal drainage in 28 dogs. J Am Anim Hosp Assoc 2001;37:87.
63. Staatz AJ, Monnet E, Seim HB III. Open peritoneal drainage versus primary closure for the treatment of septic peritonitis in dogs and cats: 42 cases (1993-1999). Vet Surg 2002;31:174–80.
64. Grutzner KU. Role of vacuum therapy in the management of the septic abdomen. Zentralbl Chir 2006;131(Suppl 1):S115–9.
65. Hinck D, Struve R, Gatzka F. Vacuum-assisted fascial closure in the management of diffuse peritonitis. Zentralbl Chir 2006;131(Suppl 1):S108–10.
66. Nemeth T, Solymosi N, Balka G. Long-term results of subtotal colectomy for acquired hypertrophic megacolon in eight dogs. J Small Anim Pract 2008;49:618–24.
67. Bright RM, Burrows CF, Goring R, et al. Subtotal colectomy for treatment of acquired megacolon in the dog and cat. J Am Vet Med Assoc 1986;188:1412–5.
68. Rosin E, Walshaw R, Malhaff C, et al. Subtotal colectomy for treatment of chronic constipation associated with idiopathic megacolon in cats: 38 cases. J Am Vet Med Assoc 1988;193:850–3.
69. Bertoy RW, MacCoy DM, Wheaton LG, et al. Total colectomy with ileorectal anastomosis in the cat. Vet Surg 1989;18:204–10.
70. Gregory CR, Guilford WG, Berry CR, et al. Enteric function in cats after subtotal colectomy for treatment of megacolon. Vet Surg 1990;19:216–20.

Complications of Hepatic Surgery in Companion Animals

Lauren R. May, VMD*, Stephen J. Mehler, DVM

KEYWORDS
- Hepatobiliary • Liver surgery • Liver lobectomy
- Liver biopsy • Hemorrhage

The most common hepatic procedures performed in companion animals are liver biopsies and partial or complete liver lobectomies. Although these procedures are relatively simple to perform in healthy animals, surgery in clinical patients with liver disease is often complicated by the presence of significant systemic illness or by the technical challenges associated with removing massive hepatic tumors. An in-depth understanding of the possible complications that can occur with hepatic surgery helps to provide the best possible outcome for the patient by allowing the surgeon to not only take precautions to try to prevent complications but allows one to monitor for them postoperatively and treat them early if noted.

ANATOMY OF THE LIVER

The liver consists of 4 lobes including the left, right, quadrate, and caudate lobes with the caudate lobe consisting of 2 processes, the caudate process and the quadrate process; the right lobe consisting of a right medial and right lateral sublobe; and the left lobe consisting of the left medial and left lateral sublobe.[1] In some texts, the right and left medial and lateral sublobes are described as separate lobes, giving a total of 6 lobes.[2–4] The liver can be grouped into 3 subdivisions[4–6]: the right, central, and left divisions. The caudate and right lateral lobes make up the right division, the right medial and quadrate lobes make up the central division, and the left medial and lateral lobes make up the left division.

The left lateral and medial liver lobes are often completely separate from each other and the left division is clearly demarcated from the central division. In contrast, the lobes of the right and central divisions are normally fused to some degree, complicating isolation of the vascular pedicle when performing liver lobectomy in these areas.[1,5]

The liver is suspended in the abdomen by a complex series of supporting ligaments, which must be disrupted to mobilize the liver during many surgical procedures. The diaphragmatic surface of the liver is attached to the diaphragm by

Veterinary Specialists of Rochester, 825 White Spruce Boulevard, Rochester, NY 14623, USA
* Corresponding author.
E-mail address: lrmay10@hotmail.com

Vet Clin Small Anim 41 (2011) 935–948
doi:10.1016/j.cvsm.2011.05.007 **vetsmall.theclinics.com**

the coronary ligament, a thick connective tissue that is centralized at the foramen venae cavae. The triangular ligaments arise from the lateral borders of the coronary ligament and extend the diaphragmatic attachments of the liver to the central portion of the left and right liver lobes. Several attachments are also located on the visceral side of the liver. The hepatorenal ligament attaches the caudate lobe of the liver to the cranial pole of the right kidney, while the lesser omentum, containing the hepatogastric and hepatoduodenal ligaments, extends caudally from the liver to the lesser curvature of the stomach and cranial aspect of the duodenum.[1,2]

In the dog, the hepatic artery courses through the hepatoduodenal ligament to the hilus of the liver and it branches to supply the three divisions of the liver.[4,5] The portal vein approaches the hilus of the liver and divides into a left and a right branch. The right branch supplies the right division of the liver and the left branch divides to supply the central and left divisions.[5,6] In cats, the portal vein divides into the right, left and central branches.[6] In dogs, due to further branching of the hepatic arteries and portal vein, each liver lobe/sublobe is supplied by a single hepatic artery and 1 to 3 lobar portal veins. In addition, each lobe/sublobe has 1 biliary duct and up to 3 lobar hepatic veins (most commonly 1) exiting it. The hepatic artery and biliary duct are most often located ventral to the lobar portal vein.[7]

HEMORRHAGE

Hemorrhage is a common and occasionally life-threatening complication that can be encountered during hepatic surgery. It is reported that a healthy dog on average has 2 mL of blood loss from a liver biopsy.[8–10] Unfortunately, underlying hepatic disease can actually increase the risk of hemorrhage in dogs and cats undergoing surgical procedures. In one study, 4.4% of patients that underwent laparoscopic liver biopsies required a transfusion.[11] Liver lobectomy in dogs as treatment for hepatocellular carcinoma is reported to have resulted in intraoperative death in 4.8% of patients due to exsanguination with intraoperative hemorrhage reported to be major in 7.1% of patients, moderate in 2.4% of patients, and mild in 14.3% of patients.[12] The liver is the primary source of all coagulation factors, except for factor VII, and is responsible for activation of all of the vitamin K–dependent coagulation factors (II, VII, IX, and X). From 57% to 93% of dogs with hepatic disease and 82% of cats with hepatic disease have been reported to have at least one abnormal coagulation parameter.[13–15] Therefore, prior to performing liver surgery, it is recommended that prothrombin time (PT) and activated partial thromboplastin time (aPTT) be evaluated. Concentrations of specific clotting factors are not normally evaluated because this testing is not readily available, it is costly, and it would not alter the recommended treatment. Animals with prolongation of PT and PTT can be treated with preoperative vitamin K1 for 24 hours prior to surgery; when surgery is required on a more urgent basis, administration of fresh frozen plasma or cryoprecipitate will replace coagulation factor deficiencies more rapidly. Unfortunately, liver failure can cause increased the risk of surgical bleeding and preoperative coagulation testing does not accurately reflect the risk of intraoperative or postoperative hemorrhage in all cases.[14,15] In humans, risk factors for massive bleeding during major hepatectomy has been determined, but this information is not available in dogs and cats.[16]

Aside from the underlying risk of coagulopathy, hepatic anatomy presents a number of unique challenges in hemostasis. Blood supply to the liver is derived from both portal and systemic arterial sources, with the majority of the blood being derived from the large, thin-walled branches of the portal vein. In addition, the right lateral and right medial liver lobes are adhered to a lengthy section of the caudal vena cava. Dissection around these venous structures can cause laceration of the thin vessel walls, resulting in brisk hemorrhage. While discrete vessels can be repaired or ligated, fracture or incision of hepatic tissue causes parenchymal bleeding from the cut surface of the liver, which can only be addressed through topical therapies or by direct pressure, as the vessels involved are too small and numerous to allow individual ligation. These unique aspects of hepatic physiology and anatomy have led to widespread application of advanced hemostatic techniques, ranging from stapling equipment to vessel sealing devices and topical hemostatic agents. In this section, we will consider each method of hemostasis and how they can be most effectively used to control intraoperative hemorrhage during hepatic surgery.

The simplest technique to address parenchymal hemorrhage during liver surgery is to apply direct pressure. Direct pressure prevents blood from escaping while allowing vasospasm and clotting mechanisms to create a clot. Mild hemorrhage that is created from dissecting the gallbladder out of the hepatic fossa is a good example of bleeding that can often be stopped by gentle pressure. Pressure can be applied for several minutes using a moistened laparotomy sponge that is applied to the traumatized surface of the liver. It is important to allow blood to get to the site of vessel injury. If too much pressure is applied, the clotting factors and platelets will not reach the site and no clot will form. Once a clot forms, it must not be disturbed. The laparotomy sponge is slowly removed and residual blood must be blotted or dabbed with gauze rather than being wiped, which would carry away the freshly formed clot.

When direct pressure fails to stop parenchymal hemorrhage from the liver, a variety of topical hemostatic agents can be applied. Gelatin sponge (Gelfoam; Pfizer distributed by Pharmacia & Upjohn Co, New York, NY, USA; and Vetspon; Ethicon, Johnson & Johnson, Somerville, NJ, USA) is a sterile, absorbable hemostatic agent. Gelatin sponges promote clot formation by absorbing large volumes of blood and thereby applying via tamponade to the area of bleeding. The material is compressed, then applied to the bleeding tissue. Gelatin sponge is commonly used to pack off the hepatic fossa after cholecystectomy or over the cut edge of liver tissue following partial liver lobectomy. Alternatively, small pieces can be broken off and rolled to fit in a punch liver biopsy site. The material is invaded by fibrous tissue and absorbed in 4 to 6 weeks. Oxidized regenerated cellulose (Surgicel; Ethicon, Johnson & Johnson) is a similar absorbable material that aids in hemostasis by providing a matrix for clot formation. Surgicel is a clothlike material with less absorptive capacity than gelatin sponge, but it adheres better to irregular tissue surfaces because it is thin and pliable. Oxidized regenerated cellulose has inherent antibacterial properties that make it more amenable for use in animals with suspected liver abscessation or in other areas of potential bacterial contamination. Bovine-derived thrombin is a commercially available topical hemostatic agent that is often used as an adjunct to absorbable hemostatic agents in humans undergoing hepatic or cardiac surgery. Thrombin binds to fibrinogen and forms soluble fibrin monomers that go on to polymerize. Factor VIIIa links the fibrin polymers to form insoluble cross-linked fibrin and stable clot. Fibrin also promotes many other procoagulation reactions in the clotting cascade. The product is available as Thrombin-JMI (GenTrac, Middleton, WI, USA) in vials of different volumes and can be applied directly to the tissue or used to soak gelatin sponge or cellulose to further promote clotting. Development of antibodies to bovine coagulation factors is a major risk of using these products.[17] Although recent development of a recombinant human thrombin product will limit these complications in human beings, there is no canine or feline product available.

Ligatures are considered the most secure method of small vessel ligation, but placement of ligatures can be quite difficult when working in deep locations with little room to maneuver. Hemostatic clips, such as Hemoclips (RICA Surgical Products,

Inc, Chicago, IL, USA), serve the same purpose as ligatures but are easily placed in deep locations using a specially designed applicator. Hemoclips are useful for ligating the cystic artery and for occluding the cystic duct during cholecystectomy. They are also useful in closing the numerous small vessels dissected in partial liver lobectomies. They are available in various sizes, and it is recommended that the length of the compressed clip be 2 to 3 times the diameter of the vessel. Right-angled appliers are also available and are especially useful for applications deep in the body cavity of small patients. Although use of hemostatic clips has been shown to improve efficiency compared to suture ligation, proper selection of clip size and good application technique are essential, as incorrectly applied clips are easily dislodged. For this reason, some surgeons will apply a single suture ligation, then use the surgical clips as an additional hemostatic technique, rather than relying on Hemoclips alone for ligation of crucial vessels.

The thoracoabdominal stapler (TA) is useful for partial and complete liver lobectomy but is also useful to arrest hemorrhage secondary to complications associated with partial and complete lobectomy. The TA stapler (**Fig. 1**) is available in 3 staple line lengths (30, 55, and 90 mm) and 2 sizes of staples, with white staple cartridges closing to 1 mm in height, blue cartridges closing to 1.5 mm, and green cartridges closing to 2 mm. Larger staples are designed for application to thicker (parenchymal) tissue pedicles, while the smaller staples have improved hemostatic effects in isolated vascular tissues. For example, the TA 55-mm and 90-mm-long staple lines place 2 staggered rows of staples in the tissues and can be used across large tissue pedicles for either partial or complete liver lobectomy; however, oozing often persists after placement of these staples without the use of direct pressure or topical hemostatic agents. The TA 30-mm V3 is a shorter staple line but it applies 3 staggered rows of smaller staples to the tissue. Because of the small size of this unit, the V3 cartridge is most applicable for placement on the thin vascular pedicle at the hilus of the left lateral or left medial liver lobes, when little hepatic tissue is incorporated in the ligation.

TA stapler instruments are available as disposable units or as reusable stainless steel application units, which contain a safety and approximating lever and accepts disposable staple cartridges.[18,19] The reuseable units are used more commonly in veterinary medicine. The disposable cartridges contain the staples, opposing anvil, and a retaining pin. To apply a TA staple line, the safety is placed in the locked position to prevent the handle from closing. The approximating lever is elevated and the staple cartridge is inserted into the application unit. The tissue is that inserted into the opening of the staple cartridge and the approximating level is then depressed, which moves the retaining pin into place, securing the tissue within the device. At this point, the placement of the tissue positioned in the cartridge is evaluated and, if inappropriate, the approximating lever is elevated, the tissue is adjusted, and the approximating lever depressed again, moving the retaining pin into place. The safety is then released by elevating it, and the handle is squeezed, which forces the staples out of the cartridge against the anvil. Once the staples are applied, the tissue can be transected along the cartridge distal to the staples. The approximating lever is then elevated allowing the cartridge to release the staples and tissue. This allows the staple line to be visible and the cut edge should be inspected for any hemorrhage.

A variety of electrosurgical devices have been used to aid in achieving hemostasis during surgery of the liver. Electrosurgical devices use electromagnetic radiation to generate heat. The current passes from the electrode through the tissue, resulting in vaporization of intracellular water, cell rupture, and tissue incision. Alternatively, electrosurgical units can be set to generate heat that coagulates protein for hemostasis. Most

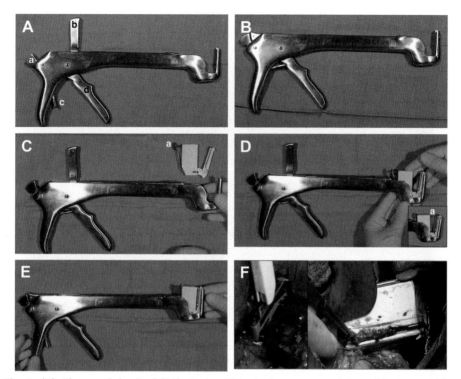

Fig. 1. (*A*). Thoracoabdominal (TA) stapler. This stapler accommodates a 30-mm cartridge with either 2 or 3 staggered rows of titanium staples. Important aspects of the stapler include the release for the approximating lever (a), the approximating lever (b), the safety (c), and the handle that deploys the staples (d). (*B*) Empty stapler with the approximating lever and safety engaged. In order to insert the cartridge, the approximating lever must be released. (*C*) A TA V3 (three 30-mm rows of staggered staples) cartridge (a) is ready to be loaded. (*D*) The cartridge is fully loaded in to the stapling instrument. *Inset:* The retaining pin (a) is being exposed as the approximating lever is being lowered. (*E*) After closing the approximating lever, and releasing the safety, the staples are ready to be deployed. (*F*) A TA 30 with 3.5-mm staples (blue cartridge) is being placed on a liver lobe for a partial liver lobectomy and a TA 30 V3 (white cartridge) is shown after deployment of staple line and manual transection of the liver lobe distal to the stapler. Notice the instrument clamped on the distal edge of the resected tissue, allowing the surgeon to inspect for hemorrhage from the cut edge after releasing the stapling device.

units use a frequency of 0.4 to 1.5 MHz and have monopolar and bipolar capability. When bipolar handpieces are used, the current passes between the 2 tips of the instrument, rather than passing through the patient to the groundplate. Bipolar handpieces are applicable only for focal hemostasis and not for cutting tissues. Both monopolar and bipolar handpieces are useful in hepatobiliary surgery.

Related devices use advanced bipolar electrosurgical handpieces with a patented feedback technology to allow sealing of arteries up to 5-mm diameter and of veins up to 7-mm diameter. The LigaSure (Valleylab, Boulder, CO, USA) is a vessel-sealing system that has gained popularity in minimally invasive surgery but is also very useful for open cholecystectomy and in partial or complete liver lobotomy. The generator is designed to sense the type of tissue within the tips and to deliver the correct amount

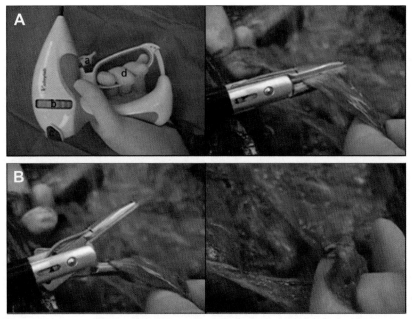

Fig. 2. (*A*) A 5-mm LigaSure handpiece including the cutting lever (a) that activates the blade at the tip of the handpiece, the rotating wheel (b) used to rotate the tip, the activating button, which can be used to activate the handpiece (c), and the ratcheting mechanism (d), which locks the tips securely once tissue has been grasped. (*B*) In the first image, a 5-mm vessel has been sealed but not cut with the LigaSure handpiece. The image on the right is the distal aspect of a sealed and transected vein.

of current to result in effective melting of collagen and elastin, creating a permanent seal after a single application. The LigaSure has been used successfully in place of titanium stapling devices, such as the TA 30 V3, in performing partial and complete liver lobectomy in experimental studies,[20–22] although the efficacy and safety of electrosurgical liver lobectomy in clinical veterinary patients have not been described. The device is unable to predictably seal the cystic duct but may be appropriate for sealing smaller hepatic ducts (**Fig. 2**).[22–24]

Other novel vessel sealing technologies include the use of ultrasound activated scalpel or LASER energy in hepatic surgery. Similar to the LigaSure device, the Harmonic Scalpel (Ethicon Endo-Surgery, Cincinnati, OH, USA) has gained popularity for providing hemostasis during both minimally invasive surgery and open procedures. This ultrasonically activated tissue-cutting device converts electrical energy to mechanical energy. Ultrasonic vibrations at the tip of various handpieces generate heat, which results in tissue coagulation. The Harmonic Scalpel is useful for laparoscopic cholecystectomy in aiding gallbladder dissection out of the hepatic fossa and as an ancillary hemostatic device incomplete and partial liver lobectomy. Although the Harmonic Scalpel is not recommended for vessels above 5-mm diameter, it does have the advantage of offering cutting tools that are useful for incision of liver parenchyma. Argon plasma coagulation (APC) involves the use of a jet of ionized argon gas (plasma) that is directed through a probe passed through an endoscope or laparoscopy port. The probe is placed at some distance from the bleeding lesion, and argon gas is emitted then ionized by a high voltage discharge

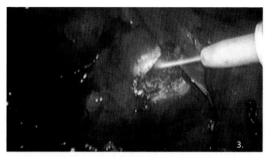

Fig. 3. Argon plasma coagulation (APC) being used to seal small hepatic vessels after a laparoscopic liver biopsy was performed.

(6 kV). High frequency electricity is then conducted through the jet of gas, resulting in coagulation of the bleeding lesion. The depth of coagulation is only a few millimeters. The authors have used APC to seal small vessels after partial liver lobectomies and to stop mild hemorrhage after liver biopsy (**Fig. 3**).

LIVER BIOPSY

Liver biopsies are performed to obtain a definitive diagnosis of lesions noted in the liver or to further evaluate a suspected hepatopathy. There are multiple ways that a liver biopsy can be performed, including a closed technique using a needle core biopsy (commonly performed under ultrasound guidance), laparoscopically, or via an open surgical approach. Laparoscopic and open surgical biopsies are commonly performed by veterinary surgeons, and complications associated with these techniques will be discussed in more detail.

Complications of Laparoscopic Liver Biopsies

Laparoscopic liver biopsies increase the accuracy of obtaining diagnostic samples compared to blind percutaneous techniques.[5] In addition, laparoscopy allows gross examination of the liver that cannot be achieved during ultrasound-guided biopsy, helping to direct where the biopsy should be obtained. Laparoscopic biopsy can be used for diffuse or focal disease and is best for lesions located near the periphery of the lobe. Laparoscopic liver biopsies are most commonly obtained using cup forceps without additional hemostatic techniques.[25,26] Complications secondary to laparoscopy have been reported to occur in 2% to 35% of cases[8,11,25] with complications of liver biopsy including hemorrhage or inadvertent damage to other organs during trocharization or manipulation. In one study, 18.8% of 45 dogs that had laparoscopic liver biopsies were considered anemic postoperatively and not preoperatively.[27] Other complications are technique related and involve inadvertent injury to the spleen or gastrointestinal tract during trocharization or instrument manipulation, with occasional significant injuries requiring conversion to an open surgical approach. In humans, these injuries are often unrecognized at the time of surgery and therefore manifest later as peritonitis, an intra-abdominal abscess, or an enterocutaneous fistula.[28] In humans, perforation of the gastrointestinal tract during diagnostic laparoscopy that required an additional procedure is reported in only 0.6% of patients.[11]

Due to the dependence upon endogenous coagulation processes when using the cup biopsy technique, coagulation status (PT, aPTT, and platelet count) are typically evaluated prior to liver biopsy.[25] In breeds with a high incidence of inherited disorders of hemostasis, additional tests may be indicated (eg, buccal mucosal bleeding time in doberman pinschers). Animals with prolongation of PT and PTT can be treated with preoperative vitamin K1 for 24 hours prior to surgery. When surgery is required on a more urgent basis, administration of fresh frozen plasma or cryoprecipitate will replace coagulation factor deficiencies more rapidly. As previously mentioned, it is important to note that in vitro coagulation testing does not necessarily predict if hemorrhage will occur after liver biopsy.[25,26]

When a liver biopsy is obtained, mild, self-limiting bleeding is expected. If spontaneous clotting does not occur, a number of techniques can be applied using laparoscopic instrumentation including placement of hemostatic agents (gelatin foam) at the biopsy site, use of monopolar electrocautery, and placement of a ligature clip or a loop ligature (pre-tied or extracoporally assembled) proximal to the biopsy site to control bleeding.[25,26,29,30] If the bleeding continues despite efforts to stop it or it is significant enough that visualization through the scope is obscured, it is recommended to open the abdomen to stop the bleeding surgically. If an animal is believed to be at an increased risk for hemorrhage, a pre-tied loop ligature or an extracorporally assembled loop ligature can be placed around the lobe prior to performing a biopsy of the tip of the lobe or a needle core biopsy can be performed under laparoscopic guidance to evaluate bleeding potential before obtaining larger biopsy samples.[29] All liver biopsy sites should be visualized prior to removing the scope from the abdomen to ensure that none are currently bleeding. If any bleeding is noted, techniques described earlier should be performed to achieve hemostasis prior to removing the scope from the abdomen.

Postoperatively, it is extremely important to monitor the patient's hemodynamic parameters, packed cell volume/total solids ratio, and abdominal comfort level. If an animal is showing signs of hypovolemic shock, it is important to evaluate the abdomen for free fluid and, if noted, perform abdominocentesis with a packed cell volume/total solids ratio on the fluid to evaluate for a hemoabdomen. If significant intra-abdominal hemorrhage is noted postoperatively, fluid therapy and blood products are administered to correct fluid deficits and any abnormalities in coagulation status. If medical therapy fails to stabilize the animals, then abdominal exploration may be required. Although bleeding typically occurs in the immediate perioperative period, hemorrhage has been reported as late as 13 days after liver biopsy.[30] Patients with a coagulation disorder may show later signs of bleeding due to slow oozing.[5]

Complications of Open Liver Biopsy

Open liver biopsies are most commonly performed when the abdomen has already been approached for another procedure. Multiple sampling techniques have been descr bed including the guillotine method, punch biopsy, overlying mattress sutures, and ultrasound-activated scalpel.[2–5,31,32] Hemorrhage is the most common complication noted after any of these techniques are used and therefore, as described for laparoscopic liver biopsies, it is important to evaluate the animal's clotting status prior to surgery and to monitor them for signs of hemorrhage during the postoperative period. In one study, the volumes of blood loss from liver biopsies obtained using a punch biopsy, biopsy needle, ligature, laparoscopic biopsy forceps, and ultrasonically activated scalpel were compared. Biopsy specimens were taken from central and peripheral locations. All techniques resulted in minimal hemorrhage, but in peripheral biopsies the ultrasonically activated scalpel and ligature methods had significantly less hemorrhage than in other methods and in central lesions the ultrasonically activated scalpel technique had significantly less hemorrhage than in other methods.[32] This is important to consider when performing a biopsy in a patient in which hemorrhage is an increased concern (eg, coagulopathic patient). Intraoperative bleeding from open liver biopsies should be controlled using a topical hemostatic agent, by ligation of the specific bleeding vessel, or by ligation of the lobe proximal to the biopsy site.

As described for laparoscopic liver biopsies, patients should be evaluated for hemorrhage postoperatively using serial monitoring of mucous membranes, heart rate, pulse quality, and packed cell volume.

LIVER LOBECTOMY

Liver lobectomies are most commonly performed in the treatment of neoplasia, abscesses, vascular anomalies, torsions, or trauma, and the location of the lesion will determine if a complete or partial liver lobectomy is performed. In a large case series of 48 dogs with primary hepatic neoplasia, intraoperative complications occurred in 26% (12 of 42) of dogs, with hemorrhage being the most common and most serious complication.[12] Three dogs experienced major intraoperative hemorrhage, 1 experienced moderate hemorrhage, and 6 experienced mild hemorrhage. Two dogs died intraoperatively as a result of exsanguination, with another 3 dogs dying in the first 5 days after surgery. In 2 dogs, resection of the left medial lobe caused ischemia of the left lateral lobe, necessitating left lateral liver lobectomy. Other potential complications such as bile peritonitis, infection, and inadvertent ligation of the portal vein or bile duct were not reported. In dogs that survived the perioperative period, median survival was longer than 1460 days, showing that although liver lobectomy can pose significant risk of surgical complications, successful lobectomy can be a very effective treatment for malignant hepatic neoplasia. Based on the frequency and seriousness of hemorrhage during liver lobectomy, this section will focus primarily on means of achieving effective hemostasis during partial and complete liver lobectomy.

Complete Liver Lobectomy

Complete liver lobectomies are indicated in the treatment of hepatic malignancy, when the disease process being treated involves the entire lobe, or when there is focal disease near the hilus. Due to the risk of significant intraoperative hemorrhage during this procedure, blood typing and crossmatching should be considered prior to surgery, in addition to coagulation testing, as already discussed. Although the rate of transfusion was not reported in the previously described case series, clinical experience would suggest that transfusion therapy is often indicated on an urgent basis, when intraoperative blood loss occurs during resection of a right-sided liver mass.[12]

Reported techniques for complete liver lobectomies in veterinary patients include an encircling ligature placed around the base of the liver, the dissection and ligation technique, or the use of a thoracoabdominal stapler.[2,5,31] The encircling ligature technique is only recommended for use in small dogs and cats for left medial or left lateral liver lobectomies, due to an increased risk of hemorrhage and bile leakage when this technique is used for other lobes or in larger dogs.[2,3,5,7,31] In contrast to the encircling ligation methods, the dissection and ligation technique involves bluntly dissecting the parenchyma at the hilus in order to allow individual ligation of the vessels and ducts, decreasing the likelihood of ligature slippage and thereby decreasing the risk of hemorrhage.[2,3,5,7,31] The use of a thoracoabdominal stapler does not require blunt dissection and isolation of the specific lobar vessels and hepatic ducts.[2,5,19,31,33] When possible, it is recommended that the TA30 V3 cartridge is applied during complete liver lobectomy due to improved hemostasis achieved using a triple row of staples; however, it is often impossible to achieve placement of the TA30 cartridge on the hilus of a lobe due to the small size of the cartridge and the thickness of the tissue in large dogs.[24]

Adequate exposure is essential to avoid iatrogenic injury to vascular structures during dissection and to achieve secure hemostasis during surgery. The standard ventral midline approach can be extended with a right paracostal approach to expose the base of the liver or through the caudal sternum if needed.[2,31,34] Ligamentous attachments to the lobe being resected must be transected to allow adequate exposure to the hilus and resection of the lobe. Most notably, the triangular ligaments are transected when removing the right or left liver lobes and the hepatorenal ligament is transected when removing the caudate liver lobe.[2,3,31] When performing lobectomy of the right or central division of the liver, the lobar attachments along the vena cava must be freed from the vena cava, being careful not to lacerate the vessel during dissection.

If severe hemorrhage is encountered during liver lobectomy, hepatic vascular supply can be temporarily occluded by using the Pringle maneuver, a technique that involves inserting a finger into the epiploic foramen in order to allow digital compression of the hepatoduodenal ligament containing the portal vein and hepatic artery. Maximum time of occlusion in normal dogs is 10 to 20 minutes.[31,34,35] Use of the Pringle technique will improve visualization of the site of hemorrhage, permitting ligation or repair of an injured vessel. Ligation of the hepatic artery or the hepatic lobar arteries to the affected lobe can also be used to decrease intrahepatic hemorrhage.[4,5,31] Prior to ligation of these arteries, the surgeon should confirm that the portal flow to the remaining lobes is normal. In addition, if this technique is used, antibiotics should be administered intraoperatively and postoperatively, because vascular occlusion can lead to rapid proliferation of endogenous clostridial organisms or fatal gangrenous necrosis of the liver.[1,5,31,36,37] If the portal flow is within normal limits and antibiotics are administered, mortality is reported to be low in normal dogs that undergo hepatic vascular occlusion.[31,38,39]

Inadvertent ligation of the portal vein or common bile duct can occur during resection of massive hepatic neoplasia due to difficulty in identifying normal anatomic structures. Ligation of the portal vein must be corrected immediately or life-threatening portal hypertension will occur rapidly. Signs of portal hypertension that can be noted intraoperatively include hypermotility of the gastrointestinal tract, cyanosis of the intestines, or edema of the pancreas. If ligation of the lobar portal vein occurs with resection, it is advisable to remove the ligature if possible. If the ligature cannot be removed, occlusion of a lobar branch of the portal vein is not life threatening but will lead to atrophy of the liver lobes supplied by the vein.[31]

Inadvertent ligation of the bile duct can occur intraoperatively with complete liver lobectomy. One can evaluate for bile duct obstruction prior to abdominal closure by manually expressing the gallbladder. If the bile duct has been ligated, it will not be able to be expressed. If ligation has occurred, the ligature should be removed if possible, and if the wall of the duct appears healthy in that area, an intraluminal bile duct stent should be placed.

If ligation of the bile duct occurs and is not noted during surgery, it will become evident early in the postoperative period. Clinical signs that may be noted include vomiting, icterus, abdominal pain, fever, anorexia, and lethargy. See Complications of Extrahepatic Biliary Tract Surgery for more in-depth discussion on the diagnostics used to identify a biliary tract obstruction. Once diagnosed, stabilization of the patient and abdominal exploration are recommended. On exploration, the ligature encircling the common bile duct should be removed, and if the wall appears healthy, placement of an intraluminal bile duct stent should be considered. If the wall appears significantly traumatized or nonviable, the bile duct is ligated and cholecystoduodenostomy is performed as a biliary diversion procedure. In animals with a large common bile duct, resection of the injured section can be performed, followed by end-to-end anastomosis of the bile duct over an intraluminal stent. In comparing these options, biliary diversion is recommended as the method of choice due to technical difficulty of bile duct anastomosis and the likelihood of postoperative leakage or stricture.[31]

Bacterial infection of the liver parenchyma can also occur following liver lobectomy, especially in an area of vascular compromise due to surgical manipulation. Anaerobes (*Clostridium*) are reported to be normal inhabitants of the liver while infection of the liver commonly consists of gram-negative aerobes.[2,3,5,31] Bacteria can migrate from the intestine to the liver by way of the portal vein. Ischemic liver due to ligation of the hepatic artery in dogs has been reported to develop fatal gangrenous necrosis due to proliferation of endogenous clostridial organisms.[5,31] Therefore, as a precautionary measure during hepatic surgery, antibiotics are recommended that are effective against the most common gram-negative aerobes of the gastrointestinal tract and anaerobic organisms. Use of postoperative antibiotics are determined on an individual basis, based on the patient's health status, the reason hepatic surgery was performed, and type of surgery that was performed.

Complications of partial liver lobectomy

Partial liver lobectomy involves removal of a liver lobe when it is transected at any portion other than at the hilus. There are many reported techniques for performing a partial liver lobectomy including the guillotine technique, placement of overlapping mattress sutures, skeletonization of the parenchyma by either finger fracture or a suction tip followed by ligation of the vessels and ducts with suture, placement of pre-tied endoscopic loops, use of an energy based sealer-divider (LigaSure), use of a Harmonic Scalpel, or use of a TA stapler placed across the parenchyma.[2–5,31,40,41] Complications noted in partial liver lobectomy are identical to those seen in complete lobectomy, with intraoperative hemorrhage being the most significant. However, the challenge of obtaining hemostasis while transecting a liver lobe through thick, well-vascularized parenchyma warrants specific discussion of the techniques that may be used. Recently, the amount of intraoperative blood loss during partial liver lobectomy was compared in an experimental dog model using 5 techniques (pretied suture, LigaSure, Harmonic Scalpel, TA stapler, and skeletonization using a Poole suction tip followed by the application of vascular clips for hemostasis).[41] Results showed that skeletonization followed by application of individual vascular clips resulted in increased blood loss compared to the other techniques, but blood loss was still less than 7.5% of total blood volume and therefore all were determined to be clinical useful techniques in dogs.[41] In a related study, the security of closure for the same 5 techniques was compared postmortem and all techniques appeared to be safe for clinical use, with leakage occurring only at supraphysiologic pressure.[40] Important to note is that both studies were performed in the same set of healthy research dogs with the largest being 26.2 kg.[40,41] Therefore, these results may not hold true for larger dogs or in dogs with clinical disease of the liver.

No significant bleeding should be noted on examination of the cut surface of the liver after partial liver lobectomy. Continued bleeding after use of a TA stapler may be caused by misfire of the instrument or by selection of a staple cartridge that is inappropriate for the tissue pedicle that is being manipulated. The staple cartridge must be wide enough to incorporate the entire tissue pedicle within the tissue retaining pin of the closed device, and the surgeon must select a cartridge that correctly matches the staple length to the thickness of the tissue that is being resected.[5,41] Similar problems can occur after use of the skeletonization or with automatic vessel sealing devices such as the LigaSure or Harmonic Scalpel. If minor bleeding is noted, electrocautery or hemostatic agents applied to the site can be used to control bleeding. If bleeding does not respond to hemostatic agents or is too severe, individual vessels are ligated using suture or vascular clips. Alternatively, absorbable sutures can be placed in a horizontal mattress pattern that is centered through the parenchyma over the site of active hemorrhage.

SUMMARY

Surgery of the liver is fraught with many potential complications; most commonly hemorrhage. The ideal therapy for these complications is avoidance and prevention by gaining a better understanding of the physiology and anatomy of the liver, which will help direct preoperative diagnostics, treatment, and surgical technique. Often, if complications occur from liver surgery, they must be treated immediately and delay in treatment could lead to an altered outcome for the patient. Therefore, it is extremely important to have a thorough knowledge base of not only the possible complications but also their treatments, prior to undertaking hepatic surgery.

REFERENCES

1. Evans HE. Miller's anatomy of the dog. Philadelphia: W.B. Saunders Company; 1993. p. 453, 456, 457.
2. Niles J. The liver and biliary tract. In: Williams J, Niles JD, editors. BSAVA manual of canine and feline abdominal surgery. Quedgeley, Gloucester: British Small Animal Veterinary Association, 2005. p. 168–79.
3. Fossum TW. Surgery of the liver. In: Fossum TW, editor. Small animal surgery. 3rd edition. St. Louis: Mosby Elsevier; 2007. p. 531–59.
4. Bjorling DE. Liver and biliary system. In: Bojrab MJ, Ellison GW, Slocum B, editors. Current techniques in small animal surgery. 4th edition. Baltimore (MD): Williams & Wilkins; 1996. p. 287–91.
5. Lipowitz A, Caywood DD, Newton CD, et al. Complications in small animal surgery: diagnosis, manamgent, prevention. Baltimore (MD): Williams & Wilkins; 1996.
6. Tobias K. Portosystemic shunts and other hepatic vascular anomalies In: Slatter D, editor. Textbook of small animal surgery. 3rd edition. Philadelphia: Elsevier; 2003. p. 727–62.
7. Covey JL, Degner DA, Jackson AH, et al. Hilar liver resection in dogs. Vet Surg 2009;38:104–11.
8. Rothuizen J, Twedt DC. Liver biopsy techniques. Vet Clin North Am Small Anim Pract 2009;39:469–80.
9. Rawlings CA, Howerth EW. Obtaining quality biopsies of the liver and kidney. J Am Anim Hosp Assoc 2004;40:352–8.
10. Rothuizen J. Diseases of the liver and biliar tract. In: Dunn J, editor. Textbook of small animal medicine. London: Saunders; 1999. p. 448–97.
11. McClaran JK, Buote NJ. Complications and need for conversion to laparotomy in small animals. Vet Clin North Am Small Anim Pract 2009;39:941–51.
12. Liptak JM, Dernell WS, Monnet E, et al. Massive hepatocellular carcinoma in dogs: 48 cases (1992-2002). J Am Vet Med Assoc 2004;225:1225–30.
13. Lisciandro SC, Hohenhaus A, Brooks M. Coagulation abnormalities in 22 cats with naturally occurring liver disease. J Vet Intern Med 1998;12:71–5.
14. Badylak SF, Dodds WJ, Van Vleet JF. Plasma coagulation factor abnormalities in dogs with naturally occurring hepatic disease. Am J Vet Res 1983;44:2336–40.

15. Prins M, Schellens CJ, van Leeuwen MW, et al. Coagulation disorders in dogs with hepatic disease. Vet J 2010;185:163–8.
16. Shirabe K, Kajiyama K, Harimoto N, et al. Risk factors for massive bleeding during major hepatectomy. World J Surg 2010;34:1555–62.
17. Lew WK, Weaver FA. Clinical use of topical thrombin as a surgical hemostat. Biologics Targets Therapy 2008;2:593–9.
18. Pavletic M. Surgical stapling devices in small animal surgery. Compend Contin Educ Pract Vet 1990;12:1724–39.
19. Tobias KM. Surgical stapling devices in veterinary medicine: a review. Vet Surg 2007;36:341–9.
20. Shamiyeh A, Schrenk P, Tulipan L, et al. A new bipolar feedback-controlled sealing system for closure of the cystic duct and artery. Surg Endosc 2002;16:812–3.
21. Shamiyeh A, Vattay P, Tulipan L, et al. Closure of the cystic duct during laparoscopic cholecystectomy with a new feedback-controlled bipolar sealing system in case of biliary obstruction: an experimental study in pigs. Hepatogastroenterology 2004;51: 931–3.
22. Romano F, Franciosi C, Caprotti R, et al. Hepatic surgery using the LigaSure vessel sealing system. World J Surg 2005;29:110–2.
23. Saiura A, Yamamoto J, Koga R, et al. Usefulness of LigaSure for liver resection: analysis by randomized clinical trial. Am J Surg 2006;192:41–5.
24. Saiura A, Yamamoto J, Koga R, et al. Liver transection using the LigaSure sealing system. HPB (Oxford) 2008;10:239–43.
25. Monnet E, Twedt DC. Laparoscopy. Vet Clin North Am Small Anim Pract 2003;33: 1147–63.
26. McCarthy T. Veterinary endoscopy for the small animal practitioner. St Louis: Elsevier Sanders; 2005.
27. Koproski AC, Kovak JR, Monette S, et al. Evalaution of laparoscopic hepatic biopsy specimens in dog and cats. In: Proceedings of the 4th Annual Meeting of the Veterinary Endoscopy Society. Hawk's Cay; 2007. p. 8.
28. McMahon AJ, Baxter JN, O'Dwyer PJ. Preventing complications of laparoscopy. Br J Surg 1993;80:1593–4.
29. Mayhew P. Surgical views: techniques for laparoscpic and laparoscopic-assisted biopsy of abdominal organs. Compend Contin Educ Pract Vet 2009;31.
30. Freeman L. Veterinary endosurgery. St Louis: Mosby; 1999.
31. Martin R, Lanz O, Tobias K. Liver and biliary system. In: Slatter D, editor. Textbook of small animal surgery. 3rd edition. Philadelphia: Elsevier, 2003. p. 708–26.
32. Vasanjee SC, Bubenik LJ, Hosgood G, et al. Evaluation of hemorrhage, sample size, and collateral damage for five hepatic biopsy methods in dogs. Vet Surg 2006;35: 86–93.
33. Lewis DD, Bellenger CR, Lewis DT, et al. Hepatic lobectomy in the dog. A comparison of stapling and ligation techniques. Vet Surg 1990;19:221–5.
34. Bellah JR. Surgical stapling of the spleen, pancreas, liver, and urogenital tract. Vet Clin North Am Small Anim Pract 1994;24:375–94.
35. Raffucci FL. The effects of temporary occlusion of the afferent hepatic circulation in dogs. Surgery 1953;33:342–51.
36. Crane SW. Evaluation and management of abdominal trauma in the dog and cat. Vet Clin North Am Small Anim Pract 1980;10:655–89.
37. Gunn C, Gourley IM, Koblik PD. Hepatic dearterialization in the dog. Am J Vet Res 1986;47:170–5.
38. Kock NG, Hahnloser P, Roding B, et al. Interaction between portal venous and hepatic arterial blood flow: an experimental study in the dog. Surgery 1972;72:414–9.

39. Richardson PD, Withrington PG. Liver blood flow. I. Intrinsic and nervous control of liver blood flow. Gastroenterology 1981;81:159–73.
40. Risselada M, Polyak MM, Ellison GW, et al. Postmortem evaluation of surgery site leakage by use of in situ isolated pulsatile perfusion after partial liver lobectomy in dogs. Am J Vet Res 2010;71:262–7.
41. Risselada M, Ellison GW, Bacon NJ, et al. Comparison of 5 surgical techniques for partial liver lobectomy in the dog for intraoperative blood loss and surgical time. Vet Surg 2010;39:856–62.

Complications of the Extrahepatic Biliary Surgery in Companion Animals

Stephen J. Mehler, DVM

KEYWORDS
- Hepatobiliary • Biliary surgery
- Extrahepatic biliary tract obstruction • Gallbladder
- Hemorrhage

The earliest documented diagnosis of gall stones dates back to the twenty-first Egyptian Dynasty (1085–945 BC), although cholelithiasis was not recognized as a clinical condition in human subjects until the 5th century AD and the earliest recorded cholecystectomy performed in a living patient did not occur for another 1300 years.[1,2] Physicians continue to struggle with the diagnosis and treatment of extrahepatic biliary disease in human patients today.

The recognition and treatment of extrahepatic biliary tract (EHBT) disease in small animals has been equally challenging. Although the vague clinical signs associated with extrahepatic biliary disease in small animals often delayed recognition and treatment of the condition in the past, the technological advances in veterinary diagnostic imaging have largely removed this obstacle. However, the recent veterinary literature continues to reflect a poor overall outcome for dogs and cats undergoing surgery of the EHBT. A conservative estimate for survival in dogs undergoing surgery of the extrahepatic biliary tract is (140/220) is 63.6% and for cats is (28/68) 41%.[3–16] The mortality rate in cats that undergo surgical intervention for EHBTO is nearly 100% when neoplasia is involved.[5] The high mortality associated with surgery of the EHBT is related not only to technical errors made during surgical procedures but is compounded by the complex pathophysiology of hepatobiliary disease, which has broad effects on wound healing, hemostasis, and sepsis. The recognition and thorough understanding of possible pathophysiologic and surgical complications associated with diseases of the extrahepatic biliary tract is the first step in achieving an improved outcome for small animals undergoing surgery of the EHBT.

ANATOMY AND PHYSIOLOGY OF THE EXTRAHEPATIC BILIARY SYSTEM

The canine extrahepatic biliary system is composed of the gallbladder, the cystic duct, hepatic ducts, the common bile duct, and the major duodenal papilla. In dogs,

Veterinary Specialists of Rochester, 825 White Spruce Boulevard, Rochester, NY 14623, USA
E-mail address: mehlerst@gmail.com

Vet Clin Small Anim 41 (2011) 949–967
doi:10.1016/j.cvsm.2011.05.009
0195-5616/11/$ – see front matter
vetsmall.theclinics.com

bile flows from the bile canniliculi into the interlobular ducts and into the lobar ducts before leaving the liver. Lobar ducts drain into hepatic ducts, through which bile passes into the common bile duct.[17,18] The gallbladder lies within a fossa between the right medial and quadrate lobes of the liver. The gallbladder is drained by the cystic duct which joins with hepatic ducts to form what is often termed the "common bile duct." It should be noted that although the term "common bile duct" is used frequently in the veterinary literature, this structure is identified simply as the "bile duct" in the standard anatomical text.[19] Throughout the following text, common bile duct and bile duct will be used interchangeably. In dogs the common bile duct terminates near the minor pancreatic duct at the major duodenal papilla. In a medium-sized dog the common bile duct is approximately 5 cm long and 2.5 mm in diameter, emptying into the duodenum 1.5 to 6 cm distal to the pylorus at the major duodenal papilla after coursing intramurally for approximately 2 cm. The blood supply to the gallbladder and common bile duct is derived from the left branch of the proper hepatic artery.[19]

Bilirubin is a byproduct of the enzymatic cleavage of the heme molecule, a central structural element in the hemoglobin molecule of erythrocytes but also in thousands of ubiquitous cellular enzymes. Unconjugated bilirubin is a hydrophobic molecule but is soluble in plasma due to a strong affinity for albumin. After traveling to the liver, bilirubin is conjugated by the enzyme UDP-GT and is released into the bile caniliculi, eventually draining into the intestine at the major duodenal papilla. Bile salts are a natural detergent for the small intestine, binding endotoxin and bacteria and rendering them ineffective. Bile salts also are important in fat emulsification and absorption, which includes the fat-soluble vitamins. The majority of bilirubin is removed from the body as stercobilinogen in the feces while a smaller portion is removed as urobilinogen in the urine.

PATHOPHYSIOLOGY OF EHBT OBSTRUCTION

The effects of EHBT obstruction are widespread and devastating. When bile is retained due to EHBT obstruction, an accumulation of bilirubin in the blood occurs and down-regulation of the reticuloendothelial system (RES) soon follows.[20,21] Lack of bile in the intestinal tract leads to diminished absorption of vitamin K in the ileum and, with time, vitamin K deficiency can lead to coagulopathies. Since factor VII has the shortest half-life of the routinely measured coagulation factors in dogs and cats, it would be expected that prothrombin time (PT) would commonly be elevated in animals with extrahepatic biliary tract obstruction; however, in many chronic cases of EHBT obstruction partial thromboplastin time (PTT) is also elevated and this finding is associated with a worse short-term outcome in dogs.[4] Prolongation in PTT may be related to the binding of coagulation factors XI and XII by endotoxin. Endotoxemia in the obstructive jaundice patient has been documented in humans and has been experimentally produced in multiple animal models.[21-29] Development of sepsis is believed to be related to the lack of a detergent effect on bacteria and endotoxin within the lumen of the small intestine, allowing delivery of unbound bacteria and endotoxin to the liver and the already failing RES. Thus, through direct and indirect effects, EHBT obstruction can produce a variety of sequelae including acute tubular necrosis, hypotension, coagulopathy, decreased wound healing, gastrointestinal hemorrhage, systemic and portal endotoxemia and bacteremia, continued gastrointestinal bacterial translocation, SIRS, sepsis, disseminated intravascular coagulation (DIC), and myocardial damage.[23-27]

CLINICAL SIGNS OF EXTRAHEPATIC BILIARY TRACT DISEASE

Clinical signs in dogs and cats with extrahepatic biliary tract obstruction include decreased appetite and lethargy in up to 100% of patients, icterus in up to 100%, vomiting in up to 92%, weight loss in up to 82%, abdominal pain on palpation in up to 50%, and fever in 38%.[5,9,30,31] The duration of clinical signs before presentation for surgery in dogs ranges from 2 hours to 210 days[8,31] and 14 to 150 days in cats[5,8,9] and signs may wax and wane for several weeks before presentation or may be acute and life threatening. Clinical signs associated with surgical complications of the biliary tree are nonspecific and mimic other abdominal disorders. Following surgery, development of abdominal pain, vomiting, anorexia, diarrhea, lethargy, icteric mucous membranes and serum, and signs of shock are all potential indicators of surgical complications that warrant further diagnostic investigations. Careful attention to daily physical examination findings in the perioperative period is an essential step in detecting complications.

COMPLICATIONS ASSOCIATED WITH A DELAY IN DEFINITIVE THERAPY

Delays in initiating definitive therapy for EHBT disease have been shown to significantly affect outcome in human patients. In the past, cholelithiasis in human beings was treated medically until the patient suffered from severe abdominal pain or when obstructive jaundice developed. Morbidity and mortality rates in human EHBT surgery were approximately 30% when surgical intervention was used as a last resort.[22,32–34] Due to these poor success rates, the current surgical trend for patients with potential surgical EHBT disease is to provide an interventional, and often definitive, surgical therapy as soon as possible, and preferentially before the patient is systemically ill. The early use of cholecystectomy to treat human patients with nonobstructive cholelithiasis has significantly lowered the morbidity and mortality rates in humans undergoing EHBT surgery.[23] Due to the influence of economics on provision of veterinary care, delays in providing definitive surgical care are also quite common in small animals with EHBT disease. Interestingly, use of surgery as a last resort has produced relatively high mortality rates in small animals, paralleling the historical results for this failed approach in human beings. Although there is no data to directly support the effects of early intervention in animals in EHBT disease, it would appear logical that adoption of this approach may show similar benefits in outcomes for animals.

Several recent publications have described the use of percutaneous biliary diversion in dogs with EHBT obstruction until the cause of the obstruction has resolved or until the patient is more stable for surgery.[35–37] Although this strategy can be effective in lowering serum bilirubin concentrations and avoiding its sequelae, it does not address the physiologic consequences that are due to the absence of bile within the small intestine. Availability of interventional and laparoscopic techniques in human medicine produced a similar use of preoperative biliary drainage and decompression or definitive extracorporeal drainage.[38] Unfortunately, most investigators concluded that preoperative biliary decompression and attempts at avoiding surgery for these diseases has led to prolonged hospitalization, increased morbidity, and, in some instances, a drastic increase in mortality.[38–42] Although there are no current veterinary studies comparing preoperative decompression to early surgical intervention, it is the opinion of the author that early surgical intervention may provide a part of the solution to many of the complications associated with surgery of the EHBT.

Surgical Complications

The diseases that lead to a need for surgery of the extrahepatic biliary system in dogs are primarily acquired conditions and include extrahepatic biliary tract obstruction (EHBTO), gall bladder mucoceles, traumatic injury, and cholecystitis. The main goals of surgery are to confirm the underlying disease process, establish a patent biliary system, and minimize perioperative complications. Despite efforts to prevent them, a number of surgical complications do occur. General complications of biliary surgery will be discussed first, followed by specific sections on each of the more commonly performed procedures.

PERIOPERATIVE HEMORRHAGE

Hemorrhage is a frequent complication associated with biliary tract surgery. Common causes of hemorrhage include failure to ligate the cystic artery, ligature slippage, and iatrogenic damage to the liver parenchyma during gallbladder dissection for chole- cystectomy. Avoidance of hemorrhage from the cystic artery is simply a matter of meticulous surgical technique. In small animals, bipolar electrocautery may be effective in coagulating this small vessel. In larger dogs, transfixation ligatures can be placed to achieve hemostasis without slippage. Hemorrhage from the surface of the liver is typically self-limiting but can be complicated by concurrent coagulopathies in patients with vitamin K deficiency. Please refer to the section on topical hemostatic agents used for hemostasis in the Complications of Liver Surgery chapter of this text.

BILE DUCT OBSTRUCTION

Postoperative bile duct obstruction can occur early or can be a latent problem. Early obstruction may occur secondary to intraoperative errors (inadvertent ligation of the bile duct, failure to recognize a source of obstruction at surgery), migrating sludge or hepatic duct choleliths not removed at surgery, or due to the development of postoperative pancreatitis. Latent obstructions are usually secondary to stricture formation at the site or previous surgery (eg, choledochotomy or choledochoenter- ostomy) or secondary to pancreatitis. In rare instances, recurrence of cholelithiasis may also result in latent postoperative bile duct obstruction. Cholecystectomy is recommended in animals with biliary stone disease to decrease the likelihood of recurrence. In animals that show evidence of continued or worsening icterus after biliary surgery, it is often difficult to discern whether the icterus is caused by an extrahepatic obstructive lesion, by the development of bile peritonitis, or by a primary hepatic parenchymal disease process. A variety of biochemical and imaging tests are used to determine a course of action when postoperative icterus is noted.

Bile duct obstruction causes an increase in total serum bilirubin with a correspond- ing bilirubinuria. Bilirubinuria may be the first sign of bile duct obstruction in dogs and may precede the development of jaundice because dogs have a low renal threshold for excretion of conjugated bilirubin and, with obstruction of the bile duct, renal excretion of bilirubin becomes important for elimination of the pigment. If the obstruction is complete, urobilinogen will be absent from the urine. Because its detection in urine is dependent upon many variables (exposure to light, drugs, sensitivity of detection methods) the absence of urobilinogen should be interpreted with caution. Changes in serum bile acid levels may be useful early in the disease but not as the disease progresses.[43,44] Based on these considerations and the ready availability of serum bilirubin measurement in small animal practice, most veterinary surgeons will use simple determinations of serum bilirubin concentrations on serial samples (eg, every 24 to 48 hours) that are obtained after surgery. In animals that

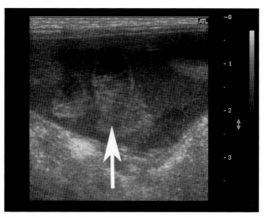

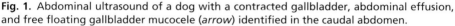

Fig. 1. Abdominal ultrasound of a dog with a contracted gallbladder, abdominal effusion, and free floating gallbladder mucocele (*arrow*) identified in the caudal abdomen.

show progressive elevation of serum bilirubin concentrations after surgery or in those that show no improvement in preoperative icterus, abdominal imaging is pursued.

As many as 50% of choleliths in dogs and cats are mineralized and, therefore, are radiopaque.[45] In patients with radiopaque cholelithis, postoperative radiographs are recommended to document the successful removal of all stones from the extrahepatic biliary tract. Gas within the biliary structures and in the peritoneal cavity may complicate interpretation of radiographic imaging, depending on the surgery performed and the amount time that has passed since surgery. Ultrasound is a sensitive and specific indicator of the cause of bile duct obstruction in the preoperative and postoperative period.[45–47] Choleliths are also readily identified with abdominal ultrasound. Abdominal ultrasound is currently the most useful and practical technique for demonstrating gallbladder and bile duct dilation associated with obstruction in small animals. Ultrasonographic findings of bile duct distention secondary to obstruction may be identified in up to 100% of cases involving dogs and cats. It is important to note that biliary obstruction may be diagnosed before the onset of clinical icterus with the use of abdominal ultrasonography and that minimal intrahepatic ductule distention is a subtle abnormality but is identified on ultrasound as early as 4 hours after experimental biliary occlusion.[48,49] The absence of gallbladder dilation does not exclude EHBTO since the gallbladder may be ruptured or contracted due to inflammation (**Fig. 1**). The degree of biliary tract dilation in obstructed dogs is variable. Therefore, duct size would allow only a crude estimation of the duration of obstruction.

Although oral, intravenous, and cholangiographic contrast studies can be performed to investigate the etiology of biliary obstruction, they are rarely used in small animals. Unfortunately, high serum bilirubin concentrations, hypoalbuminemia, icterus, hepatocellular disease, pancreatitis, peritonitis, biliary obstruction, cholecystitis, or concurrent sulfonamide and salicylate administration cause decreased hepatic concentration of the contrast resulting in poor opacification of the extrahepatic biliary system.[45]

Hepatobiliary scintigraphy in animals with hepatic and biliary disease has been used clinically in small animal patients with EHBO and may be a valuable diagnostic tool for differentiating postoperative extrahepatic biliary obstruction from hepatocellular disease or damage.[50–54] Various radiopharmaceutical agents have been used for hepatobiliary scintigraphy in both dogs and cats but most are derivatives of ^{99m}Tc iminodiacetic acid (mebrofenin or diofenin). After intravenous injection, these compounds are excreted through the biliary system, then pass into the duodenum through the major duodenal papilla. Most reports have concluded that in dogs and cats if the intestines cannot be visualized within 3 hours of the injection of the agent it is generally considered likely that EHBO is present.[50–54] The main disadvantage of scintigraphy is that it does not give accurate information as to the exact site or cause of obstruction, the patient must be housed in a radiation safe area until no longer radioactive (usually within 24 hours), and the test itself takes much longer to perform than most ultrasound exams of the biliary system.

When detected, postoperative bile duct obstruction will require surgical intervention to alleviate the source of obstruction. In rare instances, such as in dogs with postoperative pancreatitis and secondary biliary obstruction, a conservative approach may allow for spontaneous resolution of the obstruction.

POSTOPERATIVE BILE PERITONITIS

Bile peritonitis, or bilious ascites, is the inflammatory response of the peritoneum to the presence of bile. Postoperative bile peritonitis can be caused by dehiscence of a cholecystotomy incision, failure of cystic duct, bile duct, or hepatic duct ligatures, or anastomotic dehiscence of an incision in the biliary tract. Failure to identify and remove a diseased gallbladder or to recognize a damaged duct intraoperatively may also result in postoperative bile peritonitis. During cholecystoenterostomy it is possible to damage the cystic artery or twist the cystic duct leading to necrosis of the gallbladder wall or rupture of the cystic duct, respectively. If the bilirubin concentration of the abdominal effusion is greater than twice that of the serum concentration, it is diagnostic for bile peritonitis. There is a 27% to 45% survival rate for dogs with septic bile peritonitis and an 87% to 100% survival rate for dogs with sterile bile peritonitis.[3,4] The onset of clinical signs in dogs with a ruptured biliary tract and the degree of peritonitis present are likely dependent on the volume of liquid bile, the concentration of bile salts, and the presence or absence of bacteria. Clinical signs include vomiting, anorexia, diarrhea, weight loss, icterus, abdominal distention, fever, and abdominal pain.

Bile salts are toxic to tissues and cause permeability changes and tissue necrosis that encourage the growth of bacteria. Sources of bacteria are thought to be endogenous anaerobic bacteria from the liver and intestine as well as hematogenous spread. Unconjugated bile acids are cytotoxic and induce tissue inflammation, altering the permeability of vascular structures within the peritoneal membranes. Transudation of fluid, and then transmural migration of enteric organisms into the peritoneal cavity, follows. Although virtually all bile acids derived from the biliary tree are conjugated, a bacterial infection or a low pH within the biliary tree will result in bile acid deconjugation. Postoperative bile peritonitis is fatal if left untreated and requires immediate surgical intervention. Goals of reoperation included identification and repair of the source of bile leakage, maintenance of a patent biliary tree, and copious abdominal lavage. Bacterial culture of abdominal fluid is useful in guiding postoperative antibiotic therapy and animals are placed on broad-spectrum intravenous antimicrobial therapy until results of culture and sensitivity return. The use of open or closed abdominal drainage is discussed elsewhere in this text (see Complications of Gastrointestinal Surgery).

COMPLICATIONS ASSOCIATED WITH GALLBLADDER SURGERY

In dogs and cats, a cholecystectomy is the most commonly performed surgery of the gall bladder in small animals and is preferred over a cholecystotomy because it decreases the likelihood of cholelith recurrence[55] and avoids the need for a more technically demanding cholecystostomy closure. It has been our experience that the gallbladder wall does not seal well immediately after cholecystocentesis or following a cholecystotomy. There are few physiologic side effects of cholecystectomy, and although episodic abdominal pain and diarrhea associated with fat malabsorption have been described in human beings and induced in normal dogs and cats after undergoing cholecystectomy,[56,57] this technique remains the standard of care for the treatment of cholelithiasis and gallbladder mucoceles in small animals. Complications of each procedure are described more specifically next.

Cholecystotomy

Cholecystotomy may be performed to obtain a full-thickness biopsy or mucosal cultures of the gallbladder, to explore the inside of the gallbladder and cystic duct, for removal of choleliths and sludge, for antegrade flushing and assessment of patency of the extrahepatic biliary ducts and for placement of a cholecystostomy tube.[30]

Complications of cholecystostomy include recurrence of cholelith formation, dehiscence of the incision, early or accidental dislodgement of a cholecystostomy tube, or obstruction of the cystic duct or bile duct with a blood clot. In most circumstances, there is no need to remove the gallbladder from the hepatic fossa when performing a cholecystotomy incision. If the surgeon prefers to dissect the gallbladder from the hepatic fossa, great care must be taken not to damage the cystic artery supplying the gallbladder as it branches from the left hepatic artery and is found immediately adjacent to the cystic duct.

Prevention of these complications is possible with careful attention to regional anatomy and adherence to surgical principles. Closure of a cholecystotomy incision is performed with a fine synthetic monofilament suture on a tapered needle in a simple continuous or inverting pattern. Some surgeons prefer a two-layer inverting closure but this is not necessary or recommended in most cases.[30] Full thickness bites are recommended to assure that the submucosa is incorporated in the closure. A thorough local lavage of the gallbladder incision is performed and the omentum is placed over the incision.

Cholecystectomy

Indications for cholecystectomy include cholecystitis, cholelithiasis, gallbladder mucocele, gallbladder neoplasia, cystic artery infarction, or severe gallbladder trauma. Complications include bile leakage due to failure of cystic duct ligatures (3%–8%), hemorrhage secondary to failure of cystic artery ligations or from damage to the liver parenchyma during gallbladder dissection, and failure to document bile duct patency prior to cholecystectomy.[8,31] Before performing a cholecystectomy, patency of the bile duct must be assured. This is done via a duodenotomy or from a cholecystotomy incision after removal of the gallbladder contents. Assessing the patency of the biliary tract after completing the cholecystectomy defeats the purpose as the lack of a patent system may indicate the need for a cholecystoenterostomy.

Hemorrhage from the hepatic fossa can be controlled with direct pressure applied to a lap sponge or by application of a hemostatic agent (Gelfoam or Surgicel). There is some reported risk of abscess formation using hemostatic agents in this area but the authors have not observed this clinically.[58]

If a duodenotomy was used to assess patency of the biliary ducts, a small amount of sterile saline can be flushed gently into the common bile duct to assess the security of the ligatures placed on the cystic duct remnant. Aggressive flushing and excessive manipulation of a catheter in this area have led to rupture of the bile ducts and should be avoided.

Laparoscopic Cholecystectomy

In humans, laparoscopic cholecystectomy has been performed since the early 1980s and now represents the treatment of choice for gallstone disease and acute cholecystitis. Approximately 75% of all cholecystectomies are performed laparoscopically and almost all elective cholecystectomies are performed minimally invasively. This has proved to be a very safe method for cholecystectomy in human beings and has a very small percentage of conversion to open laparotomy.[59] Surprisingly, the incidence of iatrogenic common bile duct injury in human surgery has increased by 0.5% to 1.5% during laparoscopic cholecystectomy compared to a traditional open approach.[60]

Complications of laparoscopic cholecystectomy include those listed for open cholecystectomy and those that are specific to laparoscopy (see chapter on Complications of Minimally Invasive Surgery elsewhere in this text). If significant bile leakage, excessive hemorrhage or anesthetic complications occur, conversion to an open approach should be considered. Postoperative EHBTO may be more likely to develop in animals undergoing laparoscopic cholecystectomy as a result of inadequate flushing of residual biliary sludge in the bile duct compared to patients undergoing open cholecystectomy, as it is more difficult to perform a complete exploratory of the biliary tract in patients undergoing laparoscopy. Avoidance of these latter complications is based on careful case selection. Laparoscopic cholecystectomy is not currently recommended in dogs with gallbladder mucocele or cholelithiasis that have preoperative evidence of EHBO.[61,62]

COMPLICATIONS ASSOCIATED WITH SURGERY OR INJURY OF THE EXTRAHEPATIC DUCTS
Ducts (Hepatic, Cystic, and Bile Duct)

Unrecognized damage to the hepatic ducts, cystic, or bile duct during surgery leads to bile peritonitis and has potentially fatal complications. Similar consequences from dehiscence of a choledochotomy incision or failure of a cystic or hepatic duct ligature exist. Repair of ruptured hepatic ducts, the cystic duct, or bile duct can be performed, but is technically demanding and has a high rate of failure.[5,15,63–66] There are well developed intrahepatic and extrahepatic communications between divisions of the liver that allow for collateral bile drainage. Given that dogs have between two and six extrahepatic ducts,[19] sacrifice of one or more ducts can be performed without removing the liver lobe being drained by the affected duct. Choledochotomy is commonly performed in humans, especially when endoscopic retrograde choledochoscopy is unavailable or unsuccessful.[67] Complications of choledochotomy in dogs and cats are mainly dehiscence and stricture formation. A recent report of choledochotomy and primary repair of ruptured biliary ducts in dogs and cats described successful outcome in 10 cases, with only one report of dehiscence and reoperation.[68,69] Prevention of stricture formation in the postoperative choledochotomy is achieved by using a fine, monofilament, 4-0 to 6-0 suture in a simple interrupted or continuous pattern. An inverting or two-layer closure is avoided to prevent excessive narrowing of the luminal diameter. If the longitudinal incision is relatively short, it can be closed in a transverse direction to limit the narrowing of the luminal diameter. Omentum is wrapped around the closed incision. A closed suction drain can be placed as a diagnostic aid to help detect early dehiscence of the choledochotomy. The drain is pulled in 3 to 5 days or when appropriate. A ruptured hepatic duct can be sacrificed as collateral drainage will develop in the dog. If a large tear or defect exists in the cystic duct, a cholecystectomy can be performed.

There is one report of a dog that underwent repair of the bile duct using commercially available porcine submucosa.[10] Although this technique was not successful, many independent veterinary groups are currently evaluating other synthetics and biomaterials for definitive closure of bile duct tears, rents, and defects including fibrin glue, cyanoacrylates, jugular and splenic vein grafts, and serosa of local gastrointestinal tract.[70-72]

Choledochoduodenostomy

Choledochoduodenostomy was first described in 1892 and is a commonly performed rerouting procedure in human patients.[73] Because of the size of the canine common bile duct (3 mm), compared to the human bile duct (10 mm), it is significantly more challenging to perform a choledochoenteric anastomosis in dogs, increasing the risks of dehiscence or stricture formation. This procedure is performed using a routine end-to-side anastomosis or side-to-side anastomosis.[74-77] In humans, this procedure is almost exclusively, performed laparoscopically.[78,79] For the end-to-side anastomosis, the bile duct is ligated and transected as close to the duodenum as possible to limit the amount of tension on the anastomosis. Tension is a common cause of dehiscence, and because the sphincter mechanism is not routinely included in the anastomosis, enteric reflux into the bile duct is expected as another complication.

A side-to-side anastomosis can be performed as a sphincteroplasty technique or as a true side to side anastomosis. Dehiscence is avoided by limiting tension and using a fine monofilament suture material in a simple interrupted or continuous pattern. Omentum is brought to and wrapped around the surgical anastomosis following thorough lavage of the area. A closed suction drain can be placed as a diagnostic aid to help detect early dehiscence of the biliary enteric anastomosis. The drain is pulled in 3 to 5 days or when appropriate.

COMPLICATIONS ASSOCIATED WITH BILIARY REROUTING PROCEDURES

Biliary tract rerouting procedures are performed when bile duct obstructions are unable to be resolved intraoperatively, as an adjunct to removal of the proximal duodenum including the major duodenal papilla, and as a method to bypass a nonresectable malignant process involving the pancreas, bile duct, or proximal duodenum. Complications of biliary enteric anastomosis include dehiscence of the incision, stricture of the stoma, ascending cholangiohepatitis, and alterations to gastrointestinal physiology and digestion.[8,31]

Cholecystoduodenostomy is currently accepted as the simplest and most physiologic technique to achieve biliary enteric anastomoses in dogs and cats.[8] The procedure is performed using a mucosal appositional technique, creating a permanent stoma between the small bowel and the gallbladder. This can be done with hand suturing or with automatic stapling devices.[8,9] To avoid intraoperative complications, the gallbladder must be in good health and the cystic artery must not be damaged during dissection and manipulation of the gallbladder out of the hepatic fossa. If cholecystoenterostomy is being performed because of bile duct rupture or secondary to proximal duodenal resection, it is imperative that the bile duct remnant staying in the body be ligated securely. If the rerouting procedure is being performed secondary to a blockage of the bile duct and there is little chance of the bile duct rupturing or leaking, ligation of the bile duct is not needed. When rerouting is being performed to treat a temporary cause of obstruction (eg, pancreatitis), the bile duct should be preserved so that bile flow through the duct may be re-established and the rerouting procedure can be surgically reversed once the obstructive condition has resolved.

Chronic ascending cholangiohepatitis is a latent and common complication of biliary-enteric anastomosis. The most critical factor in creating a biliary-enteric anastomosis is providing a large enough opening to permit drainage of refluxed intestinal contents from the biliary tract back into the intestine. Numerous surgery texts recommend that the length of the cholecystoenterotomy opening should be 2.5 to 4 cm long to minimize stricture of the stoma and recurrent cholangitis associated with inadequate draining of refluxed intestinal contents.[58,66,80] It is recommended to make a large stoma because contraction is expected to be about 50% of the original stoma size. The author has had success in creating an incision in the gallbladder extending from the fundus to the beginning of the cystic duct, with a corresponding incision in the intestine to minimize the effect of postoperative stoma contraction.

Several factors must be considered in selecting the enteral location for the biliary stoma. It is ideal to be as proximal in the small intestine as possible without creating tension on the biliary enteric anastomosis. This will allow for bile to enter the gastrointestinal tract as close to its normal anatomic location as possible without leading to dehiscence of the anastomosis. The surgeon must be careful not to damage, twist, or stretch the cystic artery or cystic duct when removing the gallbladder from the hepatic fossa or when the gallbladder is sutured to the intestine. In balancing the pros and cons of physiologic location against potential tension and damage of the cystic artery and cystic duct, many surgeons prefer to leave the gallbladder within the hepatic fossa or partially dissect it and perform a cholecystoduo-denostomy, releasing the duodenocolic ligament will facilitate this technique.

The proposed section of bowel that will be used for the anastomosis is brought up to the gallbladder to make sure that there will not be too much tension. A full-thickness incision is made in the ventral surface of the gallbladder from the fundus to the beginning of the cystic duct at the infundibulum. A full-thickness longitudinal incision is made on the antimesenteric border of the small intestine the same length of the gallbladder incision. An absorbable, synthetic, monofilament suture, 3-0 to 5-0 is used in a simple continuous pattern to attach the gallbladder to the small intestine. Two separate suture lines are placed and the knots are made on the outside of the lumen. It is important to note that a common spot for leaking is where the knots of both suture lines come together at the oral and aboral ends of the anastomosis. Omentum is brought to and wrapped around the surgical anastomosis following thorough lavage of the area and abdomen. A closed suction drain can be placed as a diagnostic aid to help detect early dehiscence of the biliary enteric anastomosis. The drain is removed in 3 to 5 days or when appropriate.

The use of surgical stapling devices has also been described to accomplish a biliary-enteric anastomosis in dogs and cats, which may minimize some complica-tions.[8,81] The benefits of using a surgical stapling device for this procedure include minimizing the trauma and inflammation caused by multiple manipulations of the bowel, providing a rapid increase in tensile strength compared with sutured anasto-moses.[82–84] The use of stapling equipment also reduces surgical time. Bile duct anastomoses using titanium staples result in less fibrosis than sutured anastomoses, promote healing by primary intention and reduce the lag phase of healing.[84]

Another alteration in gastrointestinal physiology that occurs with biliary-enteric anastomosis is ulcerative damage to the proximal duodenum. Cholecystojejunostomy may decrease the chances of enterobiliary reflux but increases the risk of peptic ulceration of the duodenum due to the altered physiology of the gastrointestinal tract.

Bile is a major source of HCO^{3-}, which acts to neutralize gastric acid leaving the stomach and entering the duodenum. When bile is diverted from the duodenum to the jejunum via a rerouting procedure, fat digestion is decreased, gastric acid secretion is increased, and the neutralization of gastric acid in the duodenum is decreased.[85–88] Duodenal ulcers may develop as a sequel and post-operative treatment with a proton-pump inhibitor is recommended. Owners should monitor for fever, inappetence, and vomiting, and seek veterinary assistance if these signs develop. Given the potential physiologic consequences of a distal cholecystoduodenostomy or a cholecystojejunostomy in humans and small animals, other biliary-enteric anastomoses have been studied and described.

Other Biliary-Enteric Anastomoses (Roux-en-Y Cholecystojejunostomy and Cholecystojejunoduodenostomy)

Cholecystojejunostomy with isoperistaltic jejunal limb and cholecystojejunoduodenostomy were developed in an attempt to minimize the negative effects on gastrointestinal physiology that occur with simple cholecystoenterostomy. Cholecystojejunostomy with isoperistaltic jejunal limb (roux-en-Y) is an alternative technique to cholecystojejunostomy. This procedure involves creating an antireflux limb of jejunum to prevent ascension of jejunal contents into the extra and intrahepatic biliary system. Cholecystojejunoduodenostomy uses three intestinal anastomoses to accomplish the most physiologic of the described biliary rerouting procedures. The interposed jejunal limb functions as a bile duct and an antireflux tube, allowing bile to be presented to the duodenum yet preventing intestinal contents from entering the extrahepatic or intrahepatic biliary tract. In humans, cholecystojejunoduodenostomy (jejunal limb interposition) is the preferred technique for biliary re-routing, being associated with decreased enterobiliary reflux and less derangement in gastrointestinal physiology compared to the other types of cholecysto-enteric anastomosis. Historically, the veterinary literature has recommended against using any rerouting procedure that involves a roux-en-Y limb because the isoperistaltic jejunal arm that is created to prevent intestinal reflux from entering the gallbladder needs to be at least 40 to 50 cm long in human beings.[88–94] This has limited the clinical use of cholecystojejunoduodenostomy in veterinary medicine because it is suspected that small dogs and cats will develop clinical short bowel syndrome after utilizing 40 to 50 cm of jejunum for this procedure. However, recent clinical experience in human patients has led to a trend of avoiding the use of such long segments of jejunum for the isoperistaltic limb, as longer limbs may lead to stagnant chime and small intestinal bacterial overgrowth.[91,95,96] As an alternative to transecting the proximal jejunum, the distal duodenum can be transected and used to limit the amount of functional jejunum "lost" to the limb. These modifications may resolve concerns that have prevented the application of cholecystojejunoduodenostomy in small animal patients, although the safety and efficacy of this procedure will need to be further evaluated before it is recommended in small animals with naturally occurring diseases. Thus, though there are a variety of theoretical physiologic advantages to application of cholecystojejunoduodenostomy in dogs and cats, the simpler cholecystoduodenostomy technique is currently recommended as the standard of care.[58,66]

COMPLICATIONS ASSOCIATED WITH PLACEMENT OF BILIARY STENTS AND TUBES

Temporary biliary decompression can be accomplished using cholecystostomy tubes or choledochal stents in critically ill patients until they are stable enough for a more complicated procedure. However, preoperative decompression is controversial in humans, and in some studies has led to an increase in morbidity and mortality.[41,87,97–104]

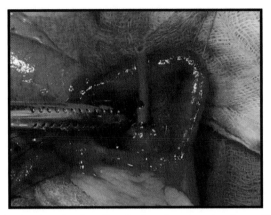

Fig. 2. Intraoperative image of a dog that had undergone stenting of its major duodenal papilla and bile duct 10 days previously to relieve an obstruction secondary to pancreatitis. The stent lumen had become obstructed with biliary sludge and concretions, causing recurrence of clinical signs. This complication may have been avoided with a more aggressive flushing of the extrahepatic biliary tract at the initial surgery and by placement of a smaller diameter stent to allow flow around the outside of the device.

Percutaneous and laparoscopic methods for biliary tract drainage have been described in a small number of veterinary patients.[35,36] Extracorporeal decompression and drainage of bile and its constituents in a patient with EHBO will facilitate the lowering of systemic bilirubin levels but will also eliminate the positive effects of enteral bile salts. As was discussed previously in this chapter, bile salts have a variety of important physiologic effects in the small intestine and biliary diversion may actually contribute to the systemic illnesses often observed in patients with EHBO.[105–108]

Complications of choledochal stenting include obstruction of the stent, premature dislodgement or migration of the stent, ascending cholangiohepatitis, and severe local inflammation caused by the stent material (**Fig. 2**). Choledochal stenting is frequently performed in humans to provide a conduit for bile flow into the duodenum across an area of obstruction or to provide support to maintain an open lumen in the face of ductal stricturing or malignant ingrowth. In dogs and cats, clinical scenarios where temporary reversible EHBT obstruction caused by pancreatitis and/or cholangiohepatitis are more frequently encountered. Candidates for stenting are those with functional EHBO (demonstrated by biochemical and imaging findings consistent with EHBO) in which a stent can be passed across the area of the obstruction. Treatment of traumatic common bile duct injury with subsequent bile leakage in addition to primary ductal repair can be supported by a choledochal stent, although it remains unclear in small animals whether stents are beneficial or detrimental to healing in these situations. Other indications for choledochal stenting may include palliation of malignancy and temporary drainage of the biliary system prior to definitive surgical repair in severely compromised animals.

Prior to considering choledochal stent placement, a thorough evaluation of the EHBT should be performed to evaluate for any evidence of biliary tract perforation, intraluminal or extraluminal masses or pancreatic abnormalities. An antimesenteric duodenotomy is performed over the anticipated location of the major duodenal papilla. A red rubber catheter of appropriate size (usually 3.5Fr to 5Fr for cats and 8Fr to 12Fr for larger dogs) is used to catheterize the major duodenal papilla to assess patency of the duct. Care should be taken not to enter the pancreatic duct. This can occur especially in cats due to the conjoined nature of the ductal systems in this species. If passage of even a small catheter is impossible, choledochal stenting is not an option in that patient and a technique for biliary re-routing should be considered. The largest stent size that does not completely fill the common bile duct lumen should be chosen. Nonmetalic stents quickly become filled with dehydrated bile concretions and bile should be allowed to passively drain around the outside of the stent if needed. A report detailing the outcome in 13 dogs where choledochal stenting was used to treat a variety of causes of EHBO no EHBT re-obstructions occurred in those that survived the perioperative period.[6] However, in a report of choledochal stenting in seven cats, two re-obstructed within 1 week of surgery.[109] The small size of the catheter lumen used in cats may predispose to early re-obstruction. Care should therefore be taken using this technique in cats as morbidity in this species may be higher than in dogs. Spontaneous passage of the stent in the feces was documented in four of five dogs and two of three cats that survived to discharge and where the fate of the stent could be confirmed. In cases where the underlying pathology resolves (especially pancreatitis) stent removal by endoscopy 2 to 4 months postoperatively is advised due to the possibility for obstruction and ascending cholangiohepatitis. Endoscopic placement of choledochal stents using a side view endoscope has been evaluated in dogs and may hold promise for minimally invasive placement of choledochal stents in the future.

Cholecystostomy tubes provide temporary diversion of bile from the gallbladder to an extracorporeal closed collection system. Similarly to choledochal stenting, cholecystostomy tubes can be used to treat a temporary and reversible cause of EHBO without resulting in the long-term anatomical alteration to the EHBT that is associated with biliary re-routing procedures. Complications include early dislodgement and bile peritonitis, obstruction, and infection. Obstruction as early as 12 hours postoperatively has been described in a cat.[36] Early dislodgement with subsequent intraperitoneal bile leakage has also been reported. Despite some suggestions that 5 to 10 days is sufficient for catheter tract maturation and leakage prevention, recent evidence suggests that maintenance of the catheters for 3 to 4 weeks may be more appropriate.[61,110] In some animals that are judged to be poor candidates for prolonged anesthesia, establishing temporary biliary drainage may be of value. If a feeding tube is in place, it may be possible to return the drained bile into the intestine through the tube, maintaining the physiologic fat absorption and endotoxin binding functions that are conveyed by bile salts in the intestinal lumen.

OTHER PERIOPERATIVE COMPLICATIONS

Excessive bleeding can occur following blunt dissection and retraction of the gallbladder from the hepatic fossa, particularly in dogs with bleeding diathesis secondary to vitamin K1 deficiency, DIC, coagulopathy, or primary hepatic disease. Assessments of coagulation factors and platelet deficiency or dysfunction should be performed preoperatively. In dogs with hemorrhage from the hepatic fossa, hemostatic agents can be placed in the fossa or an omental pedicle can be sutured over the area. In dogs with potential bleeding diathesis, freeing the gallbladder from the fossa can be partially or completely avoided, provided that a duodenal or jejunal loop can be anatomically positioned adjacent to the gallbladder and the biliary-enteric anastomosis successfully performed with minimal tension on the sutures.

Pancreatitis can result from excessive intraoperative traction and manipulation of the pancreas, which causes iatrogenic injury to the pancreatic parenchyma, ductal system, or blood supply. The pancreas is also a target organ for ischemic damage resulting from systemic disturbances such as shock and sepsis. Thus, postoperative pancreatitis may be caused by serious systemic illness in some animals, rather than by direct manipulation of the pancreas.

PROGNOSIS FOR PATIENTS WITH EHBT SURGERY

Factors affecting prognosis in humans undergoing extrahepatic biliary tract surgery include malignancy, age (>60 years), fever, leukocytosis, azotemia, hypoalbumine-mia, hyperbilirubinemia, anemia, and increased serum alkaline phosphatase (ALP).[32,33] Humans[24–27,108,111–115] and dogs[112,113,116] with obstructive jaundice are at an increased risk of acute renal failure due to bacterial endotoxemia and the mortality rate for humans with obstructive jaundice is significantly higher in patients with acute renal failure than in those without renal failure.[28,117] The absence of bile salts in the small intestine enables the absorption of endotoxin[106,108,118] and gut-derived endotoxins are powerful renal vasoconstrictors, causing a decrease in intrarenal blood flow, a fall in glomerular filtration rate, and subsequent degeneration of the renal tubular epithelium.[24–27,108,111–115]

In dogs and cats, many authors have evaluated risk factors associated with outcome in patients undergoing surgery of the EHBT.[4,5,9,14–16] Factors besides renal azotemia, include the presence of septic bile peritonitis, dyspnea, leukocystosis, prolongation of partial thromboplastin time, hypotension, sepsis, and DIC. In general, when discussing prognosis associated with surgery in dogs and cats with extraheap-tic biliary tract disease with the pet owner, a 20% to 40% and 40% to 60% mortality rate is given, respectively. However, cases in which an early diagnosis is made and surgical intervention is performed may have a much better prognosis.[6,62] Based on the complex physiology associated with biliary disorders and the potential for such broad and devastating complications, it is clear that surgeons must use all available means to avoid the occurrence of these complications.

REFERENCES

1. Gordon-Taylor G. On gallstones and their sufferers. Br J Surg 1937;25:241–51.
2. Shehadi WH. The biliary system through the ages. Int Surg 1979;64:63–78.
3. Ludwig LL, McLoughlin MA, Graves TK, et al. Surgical treatment of bile peritonitis in 24 dogs and 2 cats: a retrospective study (1987–1994). Vet Surg 1997;26(2):90–8.
4. Mehler SJ, Mayhew PD, Drobatz KJ, et al. Variables associated with outcome in dogs undergoing extrahepatic biliary surgery: 60 cases (1988–2002). Vet Surg 2004;33(6):644–9.
5. Mayhew PD, Holt DE, McLear RC, et al. Pathogenesis and outcome of extrahepatic biliary obstruction in cats. J Small Anim Pract 2002;43(6):247–53.
6. Mayhew PD, Richardson RW, Mehler SJ, et al. Choledochal tube stenting for decompression of the extrahepatic portion of the biliary tract in dogs: 13 cases (2002-2005). J Am Vet Med Assoc 2006;228(8):1209–14.
7. Mayhew PD, Weisse CW. Treatment of pancreatitis-associated extrahepatic biliary tract obstruction by choledochal stenting in seven cats. J Small Anim Pract 2008; 49(3):133–8.
8. Morrison S, Prostredny J, Roa D. Retrospective study of 28 cases of cholecystoduo-denostomy performed using endoscopic gastrointestinal anastomosis stapling equipment. J Am Anim Hosp Assoc 2008;44(1):10–8.
9. Buote NJ, Mitchell SL, Penninck D, et al. Cholecystoenterostomy for treatment of extrahepatic biliary tract obstruction in cats: 22 cases (1994–2003). J Am Vet Med Assoc 2006;228(9):1376–82.

10. Worley DR, Hottinger HA, Lawrence HJ. Surgical management of gallbladder mucoceles in dogs: 22 cases (1999–2003). J Am Vet Med Assoc 2004;225(9): 1418–22.

11. Pike FS, Berg J, King NW, et al. Revision to gallbladder mucocele article. J Am Vet Med Assoc 2004;224(12):1916–7.

12. Pike FS, Berg J, King NW, et al. Gallbladder mucocele in dogs: 30 cases (2000-2002). J Am Vet Med Assoc 2004;224(10):1615–22.

13. Bacon NJ, White RA. Extrahepatic biliary tract surgery in the cat: a case series and review. J Small Anim Pract 2003;44(5):231–5.

14. Fahie MA, Martin RA. Extrahepatic biliary tract obstruction: a retrospective study of 45 cases (1983–1993). J Am Anim Hosp Assoc 1995;31(6):478–82.

15. Martin RAM, et al. Surgical management of extrahepatic biliary tract disease: A report of eleven cases. J Am Anim Hosp Assoc 1986;22:301–7.

16. Amsellem PM, Seim HB 3rd, MacPhail CM, et al. Long-term survival and risk factors associated with biliary surgery in dogs: 34 cases (1994–2004). J Am Vet Med Assoc. 2006;229(9):1451–7.

17. Center S. Diseases of the gallbladder and biliary tree. In: Guilford WG, Strombeck DR, Williams DA, Meyer DJ, editors. Strombeck's small animal gastroenterology. 3rd edition. Philadelphia: WB Saunders; 1996.

18. Center SA. Diseases of the gallbladder and biliary tree. Vet Clin North Am Small Anim Pract 2009;39(3):543–98.

19. Evans HE, editor. Miller's anatomy of the dog. Philadelphia: W.B. Saunders Company; 1993. p. 453, 456, 457.

20. Drivas G, James O, Wardle N. Study of reticuloendothelial phagocytic capacity in patients with cholestasis. Br Med J 1976;1(6025):1568–9.

21. Pain JA, Collier DS, Ritson A. Reticuloendothelial system phagocytic function in obstructive jaundice and its modification by a muramyl dipeptide analogue. Eur Surg Res 1987;19(1):16–22.

22. Pitt HA, Cameron JL, Postier RG, et al. Factors affecting mortality in biliary tract surgery. Am J Surg 1981;141(1):66–72.

23. Pitt HA, Murray KP, Bowman HM, et al. Clinical pathway implementation improves outcomes for complex biliary surgery. Surgery 1999;126(4):751–756 [discussion: 756–8].

24. Pain JA. Reticulo-endothelial function in obstructive jaundice. Br J Surg 1987;74(12): 1091–4.

25. Pain JA, Bailey ME. Prevention of endotoxaemia in obstructive jaundice–a comparative study of bile salts. HPB Surg 1988;1(1):21–7.

26. Pain JA, Bailey ME. Measurement of operative plasma endotoxin levels in jaundiced and non-jaundiced patients. Eur Surg Res 1987;19(4):207–16.

27. Pain JA, Bailey ME. Experimental and clinical study of lactulose in obstructive jaundice. Br J Surg 1986;73(10):775–8.

28. Pain JA, Cahill CJ, Bailey ME. Perioperative complications in obstructive jaundice: therapeutic considerations. Br J Surg 1985;72(12):942–5.

29. Pain JA, Cahill CJ, Gilbert JM, et al. Prevention of postoperative renal dysfunction in patients with obstructive jaundice: a multicentre study of bile salts and lactulose. Br J Surg 1991;78(4):467–9.

30. Martin R, Lanz O, Tobias K. Liver and biliary system. In: Slatter D, editor. Textbook of small animal surgery. 3rd edition. Philadelphia: Elsevier; 2003. p. 708–26.

31. Mehler SJ, Mayhew PD, Drobatz KJ, et al. Variables associated with outcome in dogs undergoing extrahepatic biliary surgery: 60 cases (1988-2002). Vet Surg 2004;33(6):644–9.

32. Dixon JM, Armstrong CP, Duffy SW, et al. Factors affecting morbidity and mortality after surgery for obstructive jaundice: a review of 373 patients. Gut 1983;24(9):845–52.

33. Dixon JM, Armstrong CP, Duffy SW, et al. Factors affecting mortality and morbidity after surgery for obstructive jaundice. Gut 1984;25(1):104.

34. Dixon JM, Armstrong CP, Duffy SW, et al. Upper gastrointestinal bleeding. A significant complication after surgery for relief of obstructive jaundice. Ann Surg 1984;199(3):271–5.

35. Herman BA, Brawer RS, Murtaugh RJ, et al. Therapeutic percutaneous ultrasound-guided cholecystocentesis in three dogs with extrahepatic biliary obstruction and pancreatitis. J Am Vet Med Assoc 2005;227(11):1753,1782–6.

36. Murphy SM, Rodriguez JD, McAnulty JF. Minimally invasive cholecystostomy in the dog: evaluation of placement techniques and use in extrahepatic biliary obstruction. Vet Surg 2007;36(7):675–83.

37. Mayhew PD. Advanced laparoscopic procedures (hepatobiliary, endocrine) in dogs and cats. Vet Clin North Am Small Anim Pract 2009;39(5):925–39.

38. Nakeeb A, Pitt HA. The role of preoperative biliary decompression in obstructive jaundice. Hepatogastroenterology 1995;42(4):332–7.

39. Pitt HA. The use of percutaneous decompression in the jaundiced patient. Curr Surg 1986;43(6):460–3.

40. Pitt HA. General surgery: preoperative biliary tract drainage. West J Med 1985; 142(4):541.

41. Nagino M, Takada T, Kawarada Y, et al. Methods and timing of biliary drainage for acute cholangitis: Tokyo guidelines. J Hepatobiliary Pancreat Surg 2007; 14(1):68–77.

42. Sung JJ, Leung JC, Tsui CP, et al. Biliary IgA secretion in obstructive jaundice: the effects of endoscopic drainage. Gastrointest Endosc 1995;42(5):439–44.

43. Washizu T, Ikenaga H, Washizu M, et al. Bile acid composition of dog and cat gall-bladder bile. Nippon Juigaku Zasshi 1990;52(2):423–5.

44. Washizu T, Ishida T, Washizu M, et al. Changes in bile acid composition of serum and gallbladder bile in bile duct ligated dogs. J Vet Med Sci 1994;56(2):299–303.

45. Smith SA. Diagnostic imaging of biliary obstruction. Compend Contin Educ Vet 1998;20:1225–34.

46. Nyland TG, Koblik PD, Tellyer SE. Ultrasonographic evaluation of biliary cystadenomas in cats. Vet Radiol Ultrasound 1999;40(3):300–6.

47. Nyland TG, Hager DA, Herring DS. Sonography of the liver, gallbladder, and spleen. Semin Vet Med Surg (Small Anim) 1989;4(1):13–31.

48. Nyland TGG, Sonographic evaluation of experimental bile duct ligation in the dog. Vet Radiol Ultrasound 1982;23:252–60.

49. Zeman RK, Taylor KJ, Rosenfield AT, et al. Acute experimental biliary obstruction in the dog: sonographic findings and clinical implications. AJR Am J Roentgenol 1981;136(5):965–7.

50. Boothe HW, Boothe DM, Komkov A, et al. Use of hepatobiliary scintigraphy in the diagnosis of extrahepatic biliary obstruction in dogs and cats: 25 cases (1982–1989). J Am Vet Med Assoc 1992;201(1):134–41.

51. Newell SM, Graham JP, Roberts GD, et al. Quantitative hepatobiliary scintigraphy in normal cats and in cats with experimental cholangiohepatitis. Vet Radiol Ultrasound 2001;42(1):70–6.

52. Newell SM, Selcer BA, Mahaffey MB, et al. Gallbladder mucocele causing biliary obstruction in two dogs: ultrasonographic, scintigraphic, and pathological findings. J Am Anim Hosp Assoc 1995;31(6):467–72.

53. Newell SM, Selcer BA, Roberts RE, et al. Hepatobiliary scintigraphy in the evaluation of feline liver disease. J Vet Intern Med 1996;10(5):308–15.
54. Newell SM, Selcer BA, Roberts RE, et al. Use of hepatobiliary scintigraphy in clinically normal cats. Am J Vet Res 1994;55(6):762–8.
55. Harkema JR, Mason MJ, Kusewitt DF, et al. Cholecystotomy as treatment for obstructive jaundice in a dog. J Am Vet Med Assoc 1982;181(8):815–6.
56. Friman S, Radberg G, Bosaeus I, et al. Hepatobiliary compensation for the loss of gallbladder function after cholecystectomy. An experimental study in the cat. Scand J Gastroenterol 1990;25(3):307–14.
57. Mahour GH, Wakim KG, Soule EH, et al. Effect of cholecystectomy on the biliary ducts in the dog. Arch Surg 1968;97(4):570–4.
58. Matthiesen DT. Complications associated with surgery of the extrahepatic biliary system. Probl Vet Med 1989;1(2):295–315.
59. Sicklick JK, Camp MS, Lillemoe KD, et al. Surgical management of bile duct injuries sustained during laparoscopic cholecystectomy: perioperative results in 200 patients. Ann Surg 2005;241(5):786–92 [discussion: 793–5].
60. Vazquez RM. Common sense and common bile duct injury: common bile duct injury revisited. Surg Endosc 2008;22(8):1743–5.
61. Mayhew PD. Advanced laparoscopic procedures (hepatobiliary, endocrine) in dogs and cats. Vet Clin North Am Small Anim Pract 2009;39(5):925–39.
62. Mayhew PD, Mehler SJ, Radhakrishnan A. Laparoscopic cholecystectomy for management of uncomplicated gall bladder mucocele in six dogs. Vet Surg 2008; 37(7):625–30.
63. Martin WF, Page GD. Carcinoma of the extrahepatic bile duct; review of recent literature and a case report. South Med J 1951;44(2):109–14.
64. Breznock EM, Wisloh AL, Gienapp I. A chronically implantable gallbladder cannula for dogs. Am J Vet Res 1975;36(08):1255–7.
65. Harvey AM, Holt PE, Barr FJ, et al. Treatment and long-term follow-up of extrahepatic biliary obstruction with bilirubin cholelithiasis in a Somali cat with pyruvate kinase deficiency. J Feline Med Surg 2007;9(5):424–31.
66. Matthiesen DT, Rosin E. Common bile duct obstruction secondary to chronic fibrosing pancreatitis: treatment by use of cholecystoduodenostomy in the dog. J Am Vet Med Assoc 1986;189(11):1443–6.
67. Pitt HA. Role of open choledochotomy in the treatment of choledocholithiasis. Am J Surg 1993;165(4):483–6.
68. Baker SGM, Mehler PD, et al. Choledochotomy and primary repair of extrahepatic biliary duct tears in dogs and cats. Proceedings of the American College of Veterinary Surgeons Veterinary Symposium. Washington DC, October 8–10, 2009.
69. Baker SG, Mayhew PD, Mehler SJ. Choledochotomy and primary repair of extrahepatic biliary duct rupture in seven dogs and two cats. J Small Anim Pract 2011;52(1):32–7.
70. Zografakis JG, Jones BT, Ravichardran P, et al. Endoluminal reconstruction of the canine common biliary duct. Curr Surg 2003;60(4):437–41.
71. Karaayvaz M, Ugras S, Guler O, et al. Use of an autologous vein graft and stent in the repair of common bile defects: an experimental study. Surg Today 1998;28(8):830–3.
72. Mutter D, Aprahamian M, Evrard S, et al. Biomaterials for primary closure of a choledochotomy in dogs. Eur Surg Res 1996;28(1):32–8.
73. Kraus MA, Wilson SD. Choledochoduodenostomy: importance of common duct size and occurrence of cholangitis. Arch Surg 1980;115(10):1212–3.
74. Allen AW. A technique of choledochostomy. AMA Arch Surg 1956;72(3):532–543.
75. Barner HB. Technique of side-to-side choledochoduodenostomy. Surgery 1968; 63(6):1037–8.

76. Schein CJ, Shapiro N, Gliedman ML. Choledochoduodenostomy as an adjunct to choledocholithotomy. Surg Gynecol Obstet 1978;146(1):25–32.

77. Lopez-Cantarero M, Arcelus JI. A side-to-end choledochoduodenostomy between the common bile duct and the stump of the transected duodenum. Int Surg 1990;75(4):247–8.

78. Khalid K, Shafi M, Dar HM, et al. Choledochoduodenostomy: reappraisal in the laparoscopic era. ANZ J Surg 2008;78(6):495–500.

79. Campbell-Lloyd AJ, Martin DJ, et al. Long-term outcomes after laparoscopic bile duct exploration: a 5-year follow up of 150 consecutive patients. ANZ J Surg 2008;78(6):492–4.

80. Blass CE, Seim HB 3rd. Surgical techniques for the liver and biliary tract. Vet Clin North Am Small Anim Pract 1985;15(1):257–75.

81. Lehur PA, Gaillard F, Visset J. [Value of absorbable stapling in digestive surgery? Experimental study comparing TA metallic stapling, TA absorbable stapling and manual sutures]. J Chir (Paris) 1986;123(10):563–9 [in French].

82. Singer M, Cintron J, Benedetti E, et al. Hand-sewn versus stapled intestinal anastamoses in a chronically steroid-treated porcine model. Am Surg 2004;70:151–6.

83. Hess JL, McCurnin DM, Riley MG. Pilot study for comparison of chromic catgut suture and mechanically applied staples in enteroanastomoses. J Am Anim Hosp Assoc 1981;17:409–14.

84. Ballantyne G, Benjamin J, Rogers G, et al. Accelerated wound healing with stapled enteric suture lines Ann Surg 1985;20:360–4.

85. Davies HA, Wheeler MH, Psaila J, et al. Bile exclusion from the duodenum. Its effect on gastric and pancreatic function in the dog. Dig Dis Sci 1985;30(10):954–60.

86. Shin CS, Enquist IF. Effect of cholecystojejunostomy, Roux-Y, on intestinal absorption of labelled fat, labelled protein and Xylose. Bull Soc Int Chir 1970;29(1):21–7.

87. Tsuchiya T, Sasaki I, Imanura M, et al. [The influence of biliary diversion on canine gastric acid secretion and gut hormones]. Nippon Geka Gakkai Zasshi 1986;87(6):659–70.

88. Tatsumi M. [Influences of the biliary reconstructions by Roux-en Y method and jejunal interposition method on the gastric acid secretion in dogs]. Nippon Geka Gakkai Zasshi 1984;85(7):705–18 [in Japanese].

89. Lally KP, Kanegaye J, Matsumura M, et al. Perioperative factors affecting the outcome following repair of biliary atresia. Pediatrics 1989;83(5):723–6.

90. Hillis TM, Westbrook KC, Caldwell FT, et al. Surgical injury of the common bile duct. Am J Surg 1977;134(6):712–6.

91. Gustavsson S, Ilstrup DM, Morrison P, et al. Roux-Y stasis syndrome after gastrectomy. Am J Surg 1988;155(3):490–4.

92. Martin RA. Liver and biliary system. In: Slatter D, editor. Textbook of small animal surgery. 2nd edition. Philadelphia: WB Saunders; 1993. p. 645–59.

93. Donovan IA, Fielding JW, Bradby H, et al. Bile diversion after total gastrectomy. Br J Surg 1982;69(7):389–90.

94. Rokkjaer M, Marqversen J. Intestino-gastric reflux in dogs: spontaneous, after gastrojejunostomy, and after roux-en-Y gastrojejunostomy with various lengths of the defunctioning loop. Scand J Gastroenterol 1979;14(2):199–3.

95. Le Blanc-Louvry I, Ducrotte P, Lemeland JF, et al. Motility in the Roux-Y limb after distal gastrectomy: relation to the length of the limb and the afferent duodenojejunal segment—an experimental study. Neurogastroenterol Motil 1999;11(5):365–74.

96. Ramus NI, Williamson RC, Jonhston D. The use of jejunal interposition for intractable symptoms complicating peptic ulcer surgery. Br J Surg 1982;69(5):265–8.

97. Lawrence D, Bellah JR, Meyer DJ, et al. Temporary bile diversion in cats with experimental extrahepatic bile duct obstruction. Vet Surg 1992;21(6):446–51.
98. Pitt HA, Gomes AS, Lois JF, et al. Does preoperative percutaneous biliary drainage reduce operative risk or increase hospital cost? Ann Surg 1985;201(5):545–53.
99. Lois JF, Gomes AS, Grace PA, et al. Risks of percutaneous transhepatic drainage in patients with cholangitis. AJR Am J Roentgenol 1987;148(2):367–71.
100. Lane TC, Johnson HC, Walker HS Jr. Extrahepatic biliary decompression in traumatized canine livers. Surgery 1967;62(6):1039–43.
101. Tazawa J, Sanada K, Sakai Y, et al. Gallbladder aspiration for acute cholecystitis in average-surgical-risk patients. Int J Clin Pract 2005;59(1):21–4.
102. Sewnath ME, Birjmohun RS, Rauws EA, et al. The effect of preoperative biliary drainage on postoperative complications after pancreaticoduodenectomy. J Am Coll Surg 2001;192(6):726–34.
103. Sewnath ME, Karsten TM, Prins MH, et al. A meta-analysis on the efficacy of preoperative biliary drainage for tumors causing obstructive jaundice. Ann Surg 2002;236(1):17–27.
104. Nagino M, Takada T, Miyazaki M, et al. Preoperative biliary drainage for biliary tract and ampullary carcinomas. J Hepatobiliary Pancreat Surg 2008;15(1):25–30.
105. Wells CL, Jechorek RP, Erlandsen SL. Inhibitory effect of bile on bacterial invasion of enterocytes: possible mechanism for increased translocation associated with obstructive jaundice. Crit Care Med 1995;23(2):301–7.
106. Bailey ME. Endotoxin, bile salts and renal function in obstructive jaundice. Br J Surg 1976;63(10):774–8.
107. Cahill CJ, Bailey ME. Preoperative administration of bile salts. Br J Surg 1983;70(4):248.
108. Cahill CJ, Pain JA, Bailey ME. Bile salts, endotoxin and renal function in obstructive jaundice. Surg Gynecol Obstet 1987;165(6):519–22.
109. Mayhew PD, Weisse CW. Treatment of pancreatitis-associated extrahepatic biliary tract obstruction by choledochal stenting in seven cats. J Small Anim Pract 2008;49(3):133–8.
110. Murphy SM, RodríGuez JD, McAnulty JF. Minimally invasive cholecystostomy in the dog: evaluation of placement techniques and use in extrahepatic biliary obstruction. Vet Surg 2007;36(7):675–83.
111. Wardle EN. The importance of anti-lipid A (anti-endotoxin): prevention of "shock lung" and acute renal failure. World J Surg 1982;6(5):616–23.
112. Wardle EN. Endotoxin and acute renal failure. Nephron 1975;14(5):321–332.
113. Wardle EN, Wright NA. Endotoxin and acute renal failure associated with obstructive jaundice. Br Med J 1970;4(5733):472–4.
114. Cahill CJ, Pain JA. Obstructive jaundice. Renal failure and other endotoxin-related complications. Surg Annu 1988;20:17–37.
115. Center SA. Chronic liver disease: current concepts of disease mechanisms. J Small Anim Pract 1999;40(3):106–14.
116. Brady CA, King LG. Postoperative management of the emergency surgery small animal patient. Vet Clin North Am Small Anim Pract 2000;30(3):681–98, viii.
117. Wilkinson SP, Moodie H, Stamatakis JD, et al. Endotoxaemia and renal failure in cirrhosis and obstructive jaundice. Br Med J 1976;2(6049):1415–8.
118. Deitch EA, Sittig K, Li M, et al. Obstructive jaundice promotes bacterial translocation from the gut. Am J Surg 1990;159(1):79–84.

Complications of Upper Airway Surgery in Companion Animals

Andrew Mercurio, DVM, MS

KEYWORDS

- Brachycephalic airway syndrome • Laryngeal paralysis
- Tracheostomy • Laryngeal stenosis • Complications

Surgery of the upper airway is performed in dogs for the correction of brachycephalic airway syndrome and laryngeal paralysis and for temporary or permanent tracheostomy. Although technically simple to perform, upper airway surgeries can lead to the development of significant postoperative complications. This article reviews complications associated with common surgical conditions of the upper airway. It involves a discussion of brachycephalic airway syndrome and associated respiratory and gastrointestinal complications. It also covers laryngeal paralysis with a focus on unilateral arytenoid lateralization (UAL) and the complication of aspiration pneumonia. The condition of acquired laryngeal webbing/stenosis and potential treatment options is also discussed. Finally, tracheostomies and associated complications in dogs and cats are reviewed.

BRACHYCEPHALIC AIRWAY SYNDROME

Brachycephalic breeds, such as English and French bulldogs, the Boston terrier, pug, Pekingese, Shih Tzu, and boxer, have a shortened skull, resulting in a compressed nasal passage and altered pharyngeal anatomy. The compressed upper respiratory anatomy causes increased negative pressure during inspiration, leading to inflammation, deformation of pharyngeal tissues, and obstruction.[1–3] The primary components of brachycephalic airway syndrome include stenotic nares, elongated soft palate, and hypoplastic trachea. Secondary components, resulting from the increased negative pressure, include everted laryngeal saccules, laryngeal collapse, and everted tonsils, which further contribute to the increased airway resistance and obstruction. Dogs with brachycephalic airway syndrome typically present with clinical signs of stertorous breathing, inspiratory dyspnea, exercise intolerance, and collapse episodes.

The author has nothing to disclose.

Department of Small Animal Surgery, The Ohio State University Veterinary Medical Center, 601 Vernon L. Tharp Street, Columbus, OH 43210, USA

E-mail address: mercurio.19@osu.edu

Vet Clin Small Anim 41 (2011) 969–980

doi:10.1016/j.cvsm.2011.05.016

Dogs may also present with signs related to the gastrointestinal tract, such as difficulty eating, gagging, vomiting, and regurgitation.

Surgical treatment of brachycephalic airway syndrome is aimed at reducing airway resistance and alleviating obstruction. The components of the syndrome that are amenable to definitive surgical correction are stenotic nares, elongated soft palate, and everted laryngeal saccules. The most commonly performed surgical procedures are staphylectomy, nasal fold resection, and everted laryngeal saccule resection. Complications associated with nasal fold resection are relatively uncommon and may include dehiscence or severe suture reaction leading to revision.[1,2,4] More common complications seen after brachycephalic airway surgery are related to pharyngeal or laryngeal surgery and include excessive respiratory noise, staphylectomy dehiscence, regurgitation/vomiting, aspiration pneumonia, severe dyspnea, and perioperative death.[1–3] It is important to recognize that these patients are at a relatively high anesthetic risk. They already have respiratory compromise and an associated increase in vagal tone, making them prone to bradyarrythmias intraoperatively. Although postoperative dyspnea occurs in up to 20% of dogs undergoing staphylectomy,[3] sudden death prior to recovery is a less common complication.[2] A number of factors contribute to the development of dyspnea after surgery. Pharyngeal and laryngeal inflammation and edema secondary to surgical trauma may produce increased airway resistance. Many of these patients have some degree of laryngeal collapse that may be complicated by reduced pharyngeal and laryngeal muscle tone secondary to anesthesia.[3] Laryngeal collapse is a progressive condition characterized by loss of support of the laryngeal cartilages. While it has been reported in young brachycephalic dogs,[5] it is more commonly seen in middle-aged to older dogs with severe brachycephalic airway syndrome.[2,3,6] Progressive laryngeal collapse may contribute to an increased risk of complications in older patients, especially bulldogs, which undergo surgery for brachycephalic airway syndrome. In all cases, careful monitoring of the patient is critical to ensure that postoperative complications do not become life-threatening. In patients with moderate to severe dyspnea, temporary tracheostomy should be considered to bypass the airway obstruction. In fact, some authors suggest the placement of a temporary tracheostomy tube in all cases to allow the safest poss ble recovery.[7] In addition to providing an alternate airway, it allows the placement of a tracheal oxygen catheter and the provision of ventilatory support if necessary. As a way to prevent excessive airway swelling, most surgeons advocate the administration of fast-acting corticosteroids (eg, dexamethasone sodium phosphate, 0.1–0.25 mg/kg iv) immediately prior to surgery and continued up to 1 to 2 days postoperatively.[6–8]

The traditional staphylectomy procedure is performed with sharp excision followed by oral and nasal palatal mucosal apposition using absorbable suture material.[6] In an effort to decrease postoperative complications, other methods including carbon dioxide laser and electrothermal bipolar sealing devices have been used for soft palate resection.[9,10] These methods have the purported advantages of eliminating the need for suture and minimizing intraoperative hemorrhage. In a prospective trial comparing laser resection and traditional soft palate resection, no significant difference was found in clinical outcome with the 2 techniques, although a shorter operative time was reported for the laser resection group.[11] In comparing CO_2 laser resection and the bipolar sealing device, both had short operative times with excellent hemostasis and similar depths of tissue injury on histopathology.[12] While both techniques have been successfully used clinically, a distinct advantage over traditional soft palate resection with respect to postoperative airway complications has not been demonstrated.

Interestingly, postoperative gastrointestinal signs, such as vomiting and regurgitation, are also relatively common following surgery for brachycephalic airway syndrome, occurring in up to 18% of cases.[1,3,4] Many functional and anatomical abnormalities of the gastrointestinal tract have been described in brachycephalic dogs, including dysphagia, gastroesophageal reflux, hiatal hernia, pyloric stenosis, and cardiac atony.[4,13] In 1 study, a very high prevalence of gastrointestinal problems was identified clinically, endoscopically, and histologically in brachycephalic dogs presenting for upper respiratory problems.[13] Of the dogs that had endoscopic biopsies performed, over 98% had inflammatory lesions of the distal esophagus, stomach, or duodenum that were likely contributing to the functional gastrointestinal problems observed.[13] Additional information suggests that combining medical management of gastrointestinal disorders with upper respiratory surgery decreases the complication rate and improves the prognosis of dogs presenting for brachycephalic airway syndrome.[4] In these studies, the medical management for gastrointestinal disease included the use of omeprazole, cisapride, sucralfate, and corticosteroids, when appropriate. In our experience, treatment with cisapride (0.5 mg/kg po q8h) and omeprazole (0.5–1.0 mg/kg po q24h) along with an easily digestible gastroenteric diet for 2 to 4 weeks is beneficial in managing affected patients prior to surgery.

Effective client communication is essential to successful surgical management of brachycephalic airway syndrome, especially when performed on an elective basis. Owners must be made aware of the perioperative risks associated with anesthesia and airway surgery, with the treatment plan being tailored to the individual patient. Brachycephalic dogs with evidence of concomitant gastrointestinal disorders should be appropriately managed medically before or in combination with airway corrective surgery to improve prognosis and decrease the risk of complications.

LARYNGEAL PARALYSIS

Acquired laryngeal paralysis is a common disorder and an important cause of upper airway obstruction in middle-aged to older large and giant breed dogs, such as Labrador retrievers, Chesapeake Bay retrievers, great Danes, Irish setters, and Afghan hounds.[14–17] Congenital laryngeal paralysis is also recognized in certain breeds, including Bouvier des Flandres, Siberian husky, bull terrier, dalmatian, and rottweiler.[14] In acquired laryngeal paralysis, degeneration of the recurrent laryngeal nerves leads to neurogenic atrophy of the cricoarytenoideus dorsalis muscles and loss of abduction of the arytenoid cartilages. Potential underlying causes include neoplasia, hypothyroidism, trauma, and various neuromuscular diseases.[14,16–18] In the majority of cases, a specific underlying cause is not identified, and the condition is considered "idiopathic." The clinical hallmarks of idiopathic acquired laryngeal paralysis are related to laryngeal dysfunction and upper airway obstruction, including loss of phonation, stridorous breathing, dyspnea, exercise intolerance, coughing, and gagging. Various treatment methods for laryngeal paralysis have been described, including bilateral arytenoid lateralization, UAL, partial arytenoidectomy, unilateral and bilateral ventriculocordectomy, and castellated laryngofissure.[14] These procedures all aim to alleviate the upper airway obstruction by relocating or removing obstructing laryngeal tissue.

UAL is currently the standard treatment for canine laryngeal paralysis.[15,16] UAL involves fixation of the arytenoid cartilage to the thyroid or cricoid cartilage using 1 or 2 strands of nonabsorbable suture material. Despite its acceptance by many as the treatment of choice for laryngeal paralysis, the reported complication rate with UAL is high, ranging from 10% to 58%.[15,16] Potential complications associated with surgery for laryngeal paralysis include continued dyspnea, stridor, coughing, gagging when eating/drinking, failure of the surgical repair, and seroma formation.

Respiratory complications in the immediate postoperative period may be related to airway swelling from surgical trauma and can be minimized by having a detailed knowledge of the regional anatomy, practicing meticulous soft tissue handling, and avoiding inadvertent penetration into the laryngeal lumen. Perioperative corticosteroid administration (eg, dexamethasone sodium phosphate, 0.1–1.0 mg/kg IV) has been advocated to help reduce inflammation.[14] In our practice, 2 strands of 2-0 monofilament nonabsorbable suture are used. Excessive abduction of the arytenoids may contribute to the risk of postoperative aspiration pneumonia. Use of an assistant to observe per os the size of the laryngeal opening is described to optimize outcome.[19] Unfortunately, intraoperative visualization of the larynx requires removal of the endotracheal tube during general anesthesia, causing a temporary loss of airway control. In some cases, the arytenoid cartilages may be mineralized, and fragmentation of the cartilage can occur upon passage of the suture.[14] Breaking or pullout of the suture after surgery will lead to recurrence of the initial signs of laryngeal paralysis. In that case, arytenoid lateralization may be performed on the contralateral side.[14]

The most common complication following UAL is aspiration pneumonia, occurring in 18 to 28% of dogs after surgery.[15–17] Aspiration pneumonia results from inhalation of oropharyngeal or gastrointestinal contents into the respiratory tract, causing chemical, bacteriologic, and immunologic damage to the airways. Aspiration pneumonia is potentially life-threatening, with up to 23% of affected dogs not surviving to discharge.[20] In dogs that are successfully treated medically, pneumonia can significantly complicate recovery, leading to prolonged hospitalization, rehospitalization, and increased cost of care. The occurrence of this complication must be taken seriously, and decreasing the incidence of aspiration pneumonia should be a goal when considering the future of laryngeal paralysis treatment.

The risk of aspiration pneumonia is not linked to any one factor associated with UAL surgery. The cause of laryngeal paralysis, the complexity of laryngeal and pharyngeal anatomy and physiology, and the effects of surgical techniques and perioperative care must all be scrutinized to evaluate the risk of aspiration and develop a new direction for laryngeal surgery. Surgical technique does have an effect on postoperative outcome and the complication of aspiration pneumonia. It has been shown that bilateral arytenoid lateralization is associated with a significantly higher postoperative complication rate and higher incidence of aspiration pneumonia.[16] In 1 study, the complication rate following bilateral arytenoid lateralization was 89% and the mortality rate was 67%, with aspiration pneumonia being an important cause of death.[16] Bilateral arytenoid lateralization is thought to place dogs at higher risk of aspiration pneumonia by increasing the diameter of the rima glottis, allowing aspiration during swallowing. Coughing and gagging, especially after eating or drinking, are common sequelae of arytenoid lateralization and are probably associated with the minor incidents of aspiration.

A recently study prospectively evaluated esophageal dysfunction in dogs with idiopathic laryngeal paralysis compared to a breed- and age-matched control population of dogs.[21] The dogs were evaluated with esophageal studies including esophagrams in which oropharyngeal and esophageal function were observed under fluoroscopic guidance. Approximately 70% of dogs with idiopathic laryngeal paralysis were found to have some degree of esophageal dysfunction, with the cervical and cranial thoracic esophagus most notably affected. Furthermore, gastroesophageal reflux occurred in 62% of study dogs and only 6% of controls. Following initial evaluation, dogs with idiopathic laryngeal paralysis were treated with left UAL. The incidence of aspiration pneumonia among these

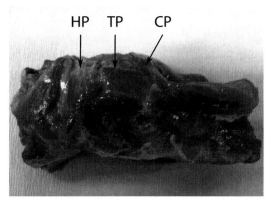

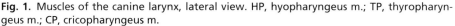

Fig. 1. Muscles of the canine larynx, lateral view. HP, hyopharyngeus m.; TP, thyropharyngeus m.; CP, cricopharyngeus m.

dogs was 18.5% and the degree of preoperative esophageal dysfunction was significantly higher in dogs that developed aspiration pneumonia.

The high incidence of esophageal dysfunction in dogs with idiopathic laryngeal paralysis may be related to the presence of generalized neuromuscular disease. There is an increasing body of evidence accumulating to support an underlying neuromuscular disease process involved in the etiology of acquired laryngeal paralysis.[18,22,23] Generalized neuromuscular disease that affects normal swallowing and airway protective mechanisms may significantly increase the risk of aspiration pneumonia. Affected dogs may have generalized signs of muscle weakness and associated gait abnormalities with deficits in segmental spinal limb reflexes consistent with lower motor neuron paresis.[18] Based on this information, it is recommended that all dogs evaluated for suspected acquired laryngeal paralysis undergo a complete neurologic examination prior to surgery and a thorough clinical history should involve an inquiry regarding clinical signs consistent with esophageal dysfunction. Discussion of the possible etiologies of acquired laryngeal paralysis, goals of surgery, and the risk of postoperative complications is an essential part of client education prior to surgery.

Degree of increase in glottal area is probably not the only aspect of surgical technique that is associated with the risk of aspiration pneumonia. The surgical approach itself for arytenoid lateralization should be considered, especially with respect to anatomy and physiology of the upper esophageal sphincter. Functionally, the upper esophageal sphincter is the intraluminal high-pressure zone that lies between the pharynx and cervical esophagus. The role of the upper esophageal sphincter is to prevent air from entering the digestive tract during inspiration, as well as to prevent esophageal contents from refluxing into the hypopharynx.[24] Anatomically, it is composed primarily of the cricopharyngeus and thryropharyngeus muscles (**Fig. 1**). The cricopharyngeus muscle arises from the lateral surface of the cricoid cartilage and inserts on the median dorsal raphe of the pharynx. It is responsible for constriction of the caudal-middle part of the pharynx. The thyropharyngeus originates from an oblique line on the outside lamina of the thyroid cartilage and inserts on the median dorsal raphe. It is involved in constriction of the middle of the pharynx. These pharyngeal constrictor muscles, along with hyopharyngeus, stylopharyngeus, pterygopharyngeus, and palatopharyngeus, are innervated by the nerves of the pharyngeal plexus. The pharyngeal plexus is composed of branches from the glossopharyngeal nerve and pharyngeal branch of the vagus nerve.[25] The cricopharyngeus muscle makes up the caudal third of the functional upper esophageal sphincter. The thyropharyngeus muscle is the thickest of the three pharyngeal constrictor muscles and contributes to the cranial two thirds of the upper esophageal sphincter. These muscles are composed of both slow and fast twitch fibers, which enable them to maintain a constant basal tone and still quickly relax in response to a swallow or belch reflex.[24] The upper esophageal sphincter relaxes/opens during swallowing, vomiting, and eructation. As part of the normal swallowing reflex, the relaxed and open upper esophageal sphincter actively contracts as the pharyngeal peristaltic wave reaches the sphincter.[24]

After the occurrence of a gastroesophageal reflux event, the upper esophageal sphincter is the only remaining physical barrier against entry of the refluxate into the pharynx and potentially the larynx and airway.[24,26] In addition to the swallowing reflex, a number of other reflexes that augment the protective function of the upper esophageal sphincter have been identified. They include the esophago–upper esophageal sphincter contractile reflex, the esophagoglottal closure reflex, and the pharyngeal (secondary) swallows reflex.[26] Studies in people and animals have identified a strong relationship between upper esophageal sphincter pressure and esophageal intraluminal pressure and pH changes during reflux events.[26]

Interestingly, the thyropharyngeus muscle is routinely transected as part of the lateral surgical approach for arytenoid lateralization. The consequence of transecting this muscle on upper esophageal sphincter function has not been evaluated. It is possible that the trauma to this muscle impairs its function as a sphincter and increases the risk of aspiration after surgery. This is an important consideration, especially in light of the evidence suggesting a high incidence of underlying esophageal dysfunction in dogs with acquired laryngeal paralysis.[21]

In addition to the factors already described, general anesthesia alone places laryngeal paralysis patients at increased risk for aspiration. The reported incidence of gastroesophageal reflux under general anesthesia varies from 17% to greater than 50%.[27,28] These events are usually clinically inapparent when they occur in otherwise healthy animals. In approximately one fourth of the dogs that develop gastroesophageal reflux, the refluxed contents reach the pharynx in sufficient quantity to place the patient at risk for aspiration.[29] There may be ways that we can improve upon anesthesia and perioperative care protocols to decrease the incidence of aspiration pneumonia, especially since that is a time period of relatively increased risk. In a prospective clinical trial, the effects of 2 doses of metoclopramide on the incidence of gastroesophageal reflux were evaluated in healthy dogs undergoing elective orthopedic surgery.[29] In this study, use of high-dose metoclopramide (1.0 mg/kg bolus followed by 1.0 mg/kg/hr CRI) resulted in a 54% reduction in the relative risk of developing gastroesophageal reflux. A single retrospective study has evaluated the use of metoclopramide in dogs undergoing surgical treatment for laryngeal paralysis, suggesting that dogs receiving metoclopramide had a lower prevalence of aspiration pneumonia than did dogs that did not receive metoclopramide.[30] Additional studies are indicated to evaluate the effect of metoclopramide, both perioperatively and long-term, on the development of aspiration pneumonia in dogs treated for laryngeal paralysis.

ACQUIRED LARYNGEAL STENOSIS

Acquired laryngeal webbing and stenosis can occur following traumatic intubation, tracheal foreign body trauma, and iatrogenic tracheal mucosal injury. In veterinary patients, it occurs most commonly after bilateral arytenoidectomy or ventriculocordectomy (vocal

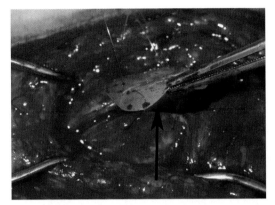

Fig. 2. Intraoperative photograph demonstrating the placement of a keel stent (*arrow*) through a ventral laryngotomy.

cordectomy).[31] Transluminal webs of mucosa-covered granulation tissue cause a progressive obstruction of the glottic lumen with associated dyspnea. Patients may compensate for as much as 60% decrease in lumen diameter with only mild dyspnea that remains unchanged for weeks.[31] Acute inflammation or mucus accumulation, however, can lead to sudden decompensation and life-threatening obstruction. The best treatment is to prevent stenosis with good surgical technique. Unfortunately, ventriculocordectomy is associated with substantial risk for the development of stenosing web formation and raises strong ethical concerns.[32] In cases of therapeutic arytenoidectomy or laryngeal trauma, surgical goals should include accurate anatomic reconstruction and direct mucosal apposition.[31]

Various surgical treatments for laryngeal webbing have been described. Unfortunately, mechanical dilation and simple surgical excision often result in rapid transverse regrowth of the scar tissue and recurrence of clinical signs.[31–34] Good success has been reported when the scar tissue is excised via a ventral laryngotomy and direct mucosal apposition over the defect is achieved.[32–34] This can be accomplished by elevating and advancing local mucosal flaps from laryngeal wall adjacent to the defects. The use of a temporary silicone "keel" type of stent inserted through the laryngotomy has been described to separate adjacent healing surfaces following web resection (**Fig. 2**).[31,33] The stent is soft enough to allow laryngeal motion without damaging tissue while it resists the transverse growth of granulation tissue, and is typically kept in place for 2 to 3 weeks.[31]

TRACHEOSTOMIES

Tracheostomies are performed when it is necessary to divert airflow directly into the trachea due to an obstruction in the more rostral sections of the airway. Tracheostomies can be used temporarily in the management of complications resulting from upper airway surgery, as discussed previously. Permanent tracheostomy may also serve as a more definitive palliative treatment for obstructive disease of the nasopharynx, larynx, or proximal trachea that cannot be addressed using other modalities. Unfortunately, tracheostomies themselves are not without complications.

Temporary tracheostomy (or tube tracheostomy) can be performed according to several previously described techniques, including transverse, vertical, and flap variations.[35] Transverse temporary tracheostomy is advantageous because no tissue is removed from the tracheal wall and the cartilage rings are not disrupted.[35] Patients with temporary tracheostomy tubes must be monitored closely until the tube is removed. Obstruction or displacement of the tube can result in asphyxiation and rapid death. Complications following temporary tracheostomy are common and approach 50% in small animals.[36] The most common complications include gagging, vomiting, and coughing. Tube obstruction and displacement also occur somewhat frequently and are potentially life-threatening. Significant tracheal stenosis is uncommonly encountered, and routine healing of a transverse tracheotomy should result in less than 5% stenosis after 1 month.[37] Selection of tube type and size is important. Stenosis is more likely to occur with a tube that is too large or with a cuff that is overinflated, causing pressure erosion of the tracheal wall. The resulting lesions heal by the formation of granulation tissue and subsequent contracture.[38,39]

Patients with temporary tracheostomies must be monitored very closely until the tube is removed. The accumulation of mucus or blood obstructing the opening of the tube occurs commonly, causing moist stridor, dyspnea, and anxiety. Tube cleaning using sterile technique should be performed at least 3 to 6 times a day to avoid obstruction.[40] This may include sterile suctioning, the use of sterile cotton-tipped applicators, replacing the inner cannula of cannulated tubes, or completely replacing tubes that cannot be cleaned adequately. The placement of encircling sutures around the cartilage rings cranial and caudal to a transverse tracheotomy is helpful to dilate the site and facilitate rapid tube reinsertion.[35,40]

Permanent tracheostomy is performed according to previously described techniques.[35,41] While the majority of owners are satisfied with their pet's response after permanent tracheostomy in terms of improved breathing and increased activity,[42] it is important to be aware of potential associated complications.[42] Over half of animals with permanent tracheostomy lose their ability to vocalize normally, even when laryngectomy is not performed.[42] Surgery site swelling, excessive exudation, and partial dehiscence occur more often in obese animals.[41] Skin-fold occlusion of the tracheostoma is the most common reported long-term complication following permanent tracheostomy.[42] This can be minimized by carefully assessing and excising adjacent skin in animals with loose skin folds in order to leave a smooth even transition between the skin surface and tracheal mucosa at the anastomosis (**Fig. 3**).[35,40] While some stenosis of the tracheostoma is expected after permanent tracheostomy, the degree of stenosis can be minimized by practicing good surgical technique with minimal manipulation of the tracheal mucosa and precise mucosa to skin apposition.[42,43]

As with temporary tracheostomy, permanent tracheostomy patients must be monitored very closely after surgery for signs of obstruction and to provide appropriate care of the stoma.[40] Mucus secretion and accumulation around the stoma are expected in the short term, and the mucus can be gently removed with a saline-moistened sterile cotton-tipped applicator or gauze square. Care must be taken to avoid irritating the tracheal mucosa and disrupting the suture line, and a water-impermeable ointment (petrolatum) should be applied around the stoma to prevent secretions from adhering and crusting.[40]

Several recent studies have demonstrated a relatively higher complication rate associated with tracheostomies in cats. In 1 study, 87% of cats experienced complications associated with temporary tracheostomies.[44] Major complications occurred in 44% of the cats, with more instances of tube occlusion and tube dislodgement than has been reported previously. Another retrospective study of permanent tracheostomies described that 67% of cats had major complications, with postoperative dyspnea from mucus plug obstruction occurring most commonly.[45]

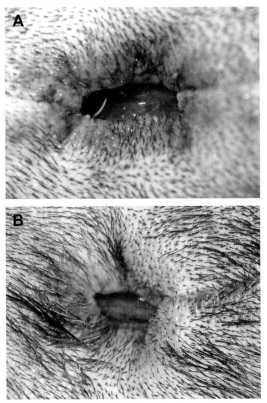

Fig. 3. Postoperative image of canine tracheostoma (*A*). Note the significant contraction of the same stoma and growth of the surrounding hair at a subsequent recheck examination (*B*).

Over half of the cats in that study died suddenly, either in the hospital or at home, with all documented causes of death being asphyxiation associated with mucus plugs. In cats, the high risk of mucus plugs causing occlusion of the respiratory tract is thought to be associated with the relatively small size of the trachea and tracheal stoma and the previously reported propensity of cats to develop thick airway secretions.[46] While successful treatment of upper airway disease with tracheostomy is possible in cats, owners must be made aware of the high risk of complications.

SUMMARY

Surgery of the upper airway has the potential to significantly improve patient quality of life but is associated with a relatively high incidence of complications. Surgical correction of brachycephalic airway syndrome carries the substantial risk of postoperative respiratory compromise in dogs that are inherently at high anesthetic risk and often have concomitant gastrointestinal disorders. Surgery for laryngeal paralysis is associated with a relatively high risk of aspiration pneumonia. That risk is likely related to the static increase in glottic diameter, the presence of underlying neuromuscular disease and esophageal dysfunction, as well as surgical trauma to the upper esophageal sphincter. The complication of stenosing laryngeal web formation is encountered commonly after ventriculocordectomy or arytenoidectomy, and treatment must be aimed at restoring mucosal integrity and preventing regrowth of scar tissue. Temporary or permanent tracheostomies are useful in bypassing the upper airway and alleviating obstruction but are associated with their own set of complications that are especially prevalent in cats. When assessing surgical problems of the upper airway, the clinician must understand the potential complications associated with surgery, and the perioperative plan should focus on decreasing those complications. Furthermore, effective client communication is essential to the clinical decision-making process and helps in the successful management of complications when they occur.

REFERENCES

1. Fasanella FJ, Shivley JM, Wardlaw JL, et al. Brachycephalic airway obstructive syndrome in dogs: 90 cases (1991–2008). J Am Vet Med Assoc 2010;237(9): 1048–51.
2. Riecks TW, Birchard SJ, Stephens JA. Surgical correction of brachycephalic syndrome in dogs: 62 cases (1991–2004). J Am Vet Med Assoc 2007;230(9):1324–8.
3. Torrez CV, Hunt GB. Results of surgical correction of abnormalities associated with brachycephalic airway obstruction syndrome in dogs in Australia. J Small Anim Pract 2006;47(3):150–4.
4. Poncet CM, Dupre GP, Freiche VG, et al. Long-term results of upper respiratory syndrome surgery and gastrointestinal tract medical treatment in 51 brachycephalic dogs. J Small Anim Pract 2006;47(3):137–42.
5. Pink JJ, Doyle RS, Hughes JM, et al. Laryngeal collapse in seven brachycephalic puppies. J Small Anim Pract 2006;47(3):131–5.
6. Monnet E. Brachycephalic airway syndrome. In: Slatter D, editor. Textbook of small animal surgery. Philadelphia (PA): Saunders; 2003. p. 808–13.
7. Hendricks JC. Brachycephalic airway syndrome. Vet Clin North Am Small Anim Pract 1992;22(5):1145–53.
8. Wykes PM. Brachycephalic airway obstructive syndrome. Probl Vet Med 1991;3(2): 188–97.
9. Brdecka DJ, Rawlings CA, Perry AC, et al. Use of an electrothermal, feedback-controlled, bipolar sealing device for resection of the elongated portion of the soft palate in dogs with obstructive upper airway disease. J Am Vet Med Assoc 2008; 233(8):1265–9.
10. Clark GN, Sinibaldi KR. Use of a carbon dioxide laser for treatment of elongated soft palate in dogs. J Am Vet Med Assoc 1994;204(11):1779–81.
11. Davidson EB, Davis MS, Campbell GA, et al. Evaluation of carbon dioxide laser and conventional incisional techniques for resection of soft palates in brachycephalic dogs. J Am Vet Med Assoc 2001;219(6):776–81.
12. Brdecka D, Rawlings C, Howerth E, et al. A histopathological comparison of two techniques for soft palate resection in normal dogs. J Am Anim Hosp Assoc 2007; 43(1):39–44.
13. Poncet CM, Dupre GP, Freiche VG, et al. Prevalence of gastrointestinal tract lesions in 73 brachycephalic dogs with upper respiratory syndrome. J Small Anim Pract 2005;46(6):273–9.
14. Monnet E. Laryngeal paralysis and devocalization. In: Slatter D, editor. Textbook of small animal surgery. Philadelphia (PA): Saunders; 2003. p. 837–45.
15. Hammel SP, Hottinger HA, Novo RE. Postoperative results of unilateral arytenoid lateralization for treatment of idiopathic laryngeal paralysis in dogs: 39 cases (1996–2002). J Am Vet Med Assoc 2006;228(8):1215–20.

16. MacPhail CM, Monnet E. Outcome of and postoperative complications in dogs undergoing surgical treatment of laryngeal paralysis: 140 cases (1985–1998). J Am Vet Med Assoc 2001;218(12):1949–56.
17. Millard RP, Tobias KM. Laryngeal paralysis in dogs. Compend Contin Educ Vet 2009;31(5):212–9.
18. Jeffery ND, Talbot CE, Smith PM, et al. Acquired idiopathic laryngeal paralysis as a prominent feature of generalised neuromuscular disease in 39 dogs. Vet Rec 2006; 158(1):17.
19. Weinstein J, Weisman D. Intraoperative evaluation of the larynx following unilateral arytenoid lateralization for acquired idiopathic laryngeal paralysis in dogs. J Am Anim Hosp Assoc 2010;46(4):241–8.
20. Kogan DA, Johnson LR, Sturges BK, et al. Etiology and clinical outcome in dogs with aspiration pneumonia: 88 cases (2004–2006). J Am Vet Med Assoc 2008;233(11): 1748–55.
21. Stanley BJ, Hauptman JG, Fritz MC, et al. Esophageal dysfunction in dogs with idiopathic laryngeal paralysis: a controlled cohort study. Vet Surg 2010;39(2): 139–49.
22. Shelton GD. Acquired laryngeal paralysis in dogs: evidence accumulating for a generalized neuromuscular disease. Vet Surg 2010;39(2):137–8.
23. Thieman KM, Krahwinkel DJ, Sims MH, et al. Histopathological confirmation of polyneuropathy in 11 dogs with laryngeal paralysis. J Am Anim Hosp Assoc 2010; 46(3):161–7.
24. Sivarao DV, Goyal RK. Functional anatomy and physiology of the upper esophageal sphincter. Am J Med 2000;108(Suppl 4a):27S–37S.
25. Venker-van Haagen AJ, Hartman W, Wolvekamp WT. Contributions of the glosso-pharyngeal nerve and the pharyngeal branch of the vagus nerve to the swallowing process in dogs. Am J Vet Res 1986;47(6):1300–7.
26. Shaker R, Hogan WJ. Reflex-mediated enhancement of airway protective mechanisms. Am J Med 2000;108(Suppl 4a):8S–14S.
27. Galatos AD, Raptopoulos D. Gastro-oesophageal reflux during anaesthesia in the dog: the effect of age, positioning and type of surgical procedure. Vet Rec 1995; 137(20):513–6.
28. Wilson DV, Evans AT, Miller R. Effects of preanesthetic administration of morphine on gastroesophageal reflux and regurgitation during anesthesia in dogs. Am J Vet Res 2005;66(3):386–90.
29. Wilson DV, Evans AT, Mauer WA. Influence of metoclopramide on gastroesophageal reflux in anesthetized dogs. Am J Vet Res 2006;67(1):26–31.
30. Greenberg MJ, Reems MR, Monet E. Use of perioperative metoclopramide in dogs undergoing laryngeal paralysis: 43 cases (1999–2006). Vet Surg 2007;36(6):E11.
31. Nelson WA. Laryngeal trauma and stenosis. In: Slatter D, editor. Textbook of small animal surgery. Philadelphia (PA): Saunders; 2003. p. 845–57.
32. Mehl ML, Kyles AE, Pypendop BH, et al. Outcome of laryngeal web resection with mucosal apposition for treatment of airway obstruction in dogs: 15 cases (1992–2006). J Am Vet Med Assoc 2008;233(5):738–42.
33. Peterson SL, Smith MM, Senders CW. Evaluation of a stented laryngoplasty for correction of cranial glottic stenosis in four dogs. J Am Vet Med Assoc 1987;191(12): 1582–4.
34. Matushek KJ, Bjorling DE. A mucosal flap technique for correction of laryngeal webbing. Results in four dogs. Vet Surg 1988;17(6):318–20.
35. Nelson WA. Diseases of the trachea and bronchi. In: Slatter D, editor. Textbook of small animal surgery. Philadelphia (PA): Saunders; 2003. p. 858–80.

36. Harvey CE, O'Brien JA. Tracheotomy in the dog and cat: analysis of 89 episodes in 79 animals. J Am Anim Hosp Assoc 1982;18:563.
37. Harvey CE, Goldschmidt MH. Healing following short term duration transverse incision tracheostomy in the dog. Vet Surg 1982;11:77.
38. Bardin J, Boyd AD, Hirose H, et al. Tracheal healing following tracheostomy. Surg Forum 1974;25:210.
39. Westgate HD, Roux KL. Tracheal stenosis following tracheostomy: Incidence and pre-disposing factors. Anesth Analg 1970;49:393.
40. Hedlund CS. Tracheostomies in the management of canine and feline upper respiratory disease. Vet Clin North Am Small Anim Pract 1994;24(5):873–86.
41. Dalgard DW, Marshall PM, Fitzgerald GH, et al. Surgical technique for a permanent tracheostomy in Beagle dogs. Lab Anim Sci 1979;29(3):367–70.
42. Hedlund CS, Tanger CH, Waldron DR, et al. Permanent tracheostomy: Peri-operative and long-term data from 34 cases. J Am Anim Hosp Assoc 1988;24:585.
43. Hedlund CS, Tanger CH, Montgomery DL, et al. A procedure for permanent tracheostomy and its effects on tracheal mucosa. Vet Surg 1982;11(1):13–17.
44. Guenther-Yenke CL, Rozanski EA. Tracheostomy in cats: 23 cases (1998–2006). J Feline Med Surg 2007;9(6):451–7.
45. Stepnik MW, Mehl ML, Hardie EM, et al. Outcome of permanent tracheostomy for treatment of upper airway obstruction in cats: 21 cases (1990–2007). J Am Vet Med Assoc 2009;234(5):638–43.
46. Colley P, Huber M, Henderson R. Tracheostomy techniques and management. Compend Contin Educ Pract Vet 1999;21:44–54.

Management of Complications Associated with Total Ear Canal Ablation and Bulla Osteotomy in Dogs and Cats

Daniel D. Smeak, DVM

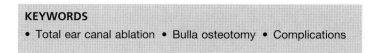

KEYWORDS

- Total ear canal ablation • Bulla osteotomy • Complications

Early reports of surgical treatment for end-stage ear canal disease described very high complication rates when total ear canal ablation (TECA) was performed without consistently accomplishing wide tympanic bulla exposure, drainage, or curettage of the tympanic cavity.[1,2] Overall complication rates ran as high as 82% and chronic deep wound infection, abscessation, and debilitating fistula formation developed in up to 10% of the cases in early studies.[1–4] Since that time, the underlying cause for most persistent infections following TECA has been determined to be retained epithelium and debris within the osseous ear canal and/or tympanic bulla.[5–7] Furthermore, middle ear disease is now identified in over 50% of dogs afflicted with long standing otitis externa, so a thorough examination of the tympanic cavity during ear canal ablation has been emphasized.[8–10]

Currently, ear canal ablation with some means of wide tympanic cavity exposure (such as lateral [LBO] or ventral bulla osteotomy [VBO] to ensure complete evacuation of the middle ear) is considered the gold standard treatment for end-stage ear canal disease and concurrent middle ear involvement.[8,9] With meticulous surgical technique and complete removal of epithelium from the bulla and ear canal, significant complications now are encountered infrequently, and most do not affect long-term success.[11,12] Ear canal ablation and bulla osteotomy are now expected to permanently resolve the signs of chronic ear disease in up to 93% of dogs.[11] Nevertheless, a thorough review of the variety of complications previously encountered in retrospective studies is important so that when surgeons encounter these problems, they can be identified early and managed appropriately. The purpose of this article is to review the rates and causes of complications related to TECA BO and the expected outcome after management of these postoperative problems. In addition, suggested

The author has nothing to disclose.
Department of Veterinary Clinical Sciences, Colorado State University, College of Veterinary Medicine and Biomedical Sciences, Veterinary Teaching Hospital, 300 West Drake Road, Fort Collins, CO 80523, USA
E-mail address: dan.smeak@colostate.edu

Vet Clin Small Anim 41 (2011) 981–994
doi:10.1016/j.cvsm.2011.05.011

strategies are offered to help surgeons improve their surgical success and to help prevent these complications.

For the purposes of discussion in this article, complications involving TECA and BO are organized into three time frames: intraoperative, early postoperative (within the first 2 weeks of the procedure), and late postoperative complications. The documented types and rates of complications in previous case series involving dogs and cats are shown in **Table 1**.[1–5,11–18] The table shows the overall trend toward a decrease in the rate of most complications over time, particularly in early wound-related problems. Fewer permanent facial nerve injuries in dogs occur now, but late complications such as chronic pinna dermatitis continue to plague some animals.

INTRAOPERATIVE COMPLICATIONS
Significant Hemorrhage

Severe hemorrhage during surgery is rare but has been reported and may result in death of the patient.[1–3,9,11,13] There are several sources for significant hemorrhage during ear canal ablation, including the retroarticular vein, the external carotid artery and maxillary vein, and the internal carotid artery. The retroarticular vein lies just rostral to the external auditory meatus and is most often damaged during detachment of the horizontal ear canal epithelium from the bone, or excessive curettage in this area[8,13] (**Fig. 1**). This hemorrhage is difficult to contain because the vein often retracts dorsally within the foramen. In most cases, bleeding can be controlled with bone wax forced into the retroarticular foramen.[8,9,13] The external carotid artery and maxillary vein lie immediately ventral to the tympanic bulla, and damage to these structures is best avoided by careful elevation of soft tissue from the entire ventral bulla, meticulous teasing of epithelium along the ventrolateral wall of the bulla, and ensuring that only bone is included within the jaws of rongeurs during LBO.[8] Hemorrhage deep *within* the tympanic bulla is thought to come from damage to the internal carotid artery on the medial bulla wall[8] (**Fig. 1**). The internal carotid can be damaged if the thin bone between the carotid canal and tympanic cavity is disrupted by curettage in a medial direction or when the medial wall of the bulla has been eroded by the disease process and is damaged during epithelial stripping.[8] Ligation of the left common carotid artery with blood transfusion was successful in controlling hemorrhage from this source in one report.[3] In the author's experience, this deep inaccessible source of bleeding is difficult to control, but packing the bulla tightly with gauze stripping is usually successful. The gauze packing is exited adjacent to the incision and is slowly pulled from the bulla on the day following surgery.

Severed Facial Nerve

In most reports, facial nerves were deliberately severed during surgery in an attempt to completely remove a neoplastic process.[13] Less frequently (<4%–6% of procedures), the nerve was accidently transected during deep dissection of the horizontal ear canal.[1–3] Isolation and protection of the facial nerve should be attempted as early in the procedure as possible. Severing the facial nerve embedded in an invasive neoplasm with curative intent provides little if any patient benefit since it is nearly impossible to obtain clean margins through this limited approach.

EARLY POSTOPERATIVE COMPLICATIONS
Incisional Problems

Most complications related to surgery (wound infection/dehiscence, neurologic deficits) are short-lived and resolve within 2 weeks.[1,3,5] Extensive contamination during surgery to remove deep-seated chronically infected ears is inevitable despite

Table 1
Reported rate of complications following ear canal ablation and bulla osteotomy

Study	Smeak 1986[1]	Mason 1988[2]	Matthieson 1990[3]	White 1990[13]	Sharpe 1990[4,a]	Beckman 1990[14]	Devitt 1997[15]	Doyle 2004[11]	Mathews 2006[12,b]	Hardie 2008[5]	Williams 1992[16,d]	Marino 1994[17]	Bacon 2003[18,d]
No. of dogs, cats	28 dogs, 3 cats	30 dogs	38 dogs	71 dogs	13 dogs	44 dogs	59 dogs	37 dogs	18 dogs, 1 cat	19 dogs	15 cats	16 cats	44 cats
No. of TECA operations	39 ears	39 ears	52 ears	100 ears	14 ears	72 ears	47 ears	47 ears	24 ears	18 ears	18 ears	16 ears	52 ears
Overall Complication Rate	82%		29%		38%[d]	21%[d]	44%[d]	34%		53%[c]			
Intraoperative Complications													
Significant hemorrhage	3%	3%	2%	3%				13%					
Severed facial nerve	5%	3%	6%	4%									
Early Postoperative Complications		57%[d]					32%[d]						
Incisional	31%									21%[c]			
Drainage		28%											
Dehiscence		15%	6%	11%				15%			7%		
Hematoma		4%											
Seroma						7%							
Cellulitis/infection	28%		19%		8%								
Neurologic													
Facial nerve injury	23% temp., 13% perm.	5% temp., 13% perm.	21% temp., 15% perm.	9% temp., 4% perm.	8% temp., 21% perm.	3% temp.	27% temp., 5% perm.	6% temp., 4% perm.	21% temp.		27% temp., 47% perm.		50% temp., 20% perm.
Hypoglossal nerve injury		3%			8%								

(table continued)

Table 1
(continued)

Study	Smeak 1986[1]	Mason 1988[2]	Matthieson 1990[3]	White 1990[13]	Sharpe 1990[4,a]	Beckman 1990[14]	Devitt 1997[15]	Doyle 2004[11]	Mathews 2006[12,b]	Hardie 2008[5]	Williams 1992[16,d]	Marino 1994[17]	Bacon 2003[18,d]
Inner ear injury/ vestibular	8%	8%	8%			3%	3%	6%	4%				
Horner's syndrome	Cats only, 67% temp.			1% temp., 1% perm.							27% temp., 13% perm.	temp.	46% temp., 7% perm.
Pinna necrosis			4%										
Dyspnea- airway obstruction													
Pain													
Aspiration pneumonia			2%				2%						
Late postoperative complications		40%[d]					22%[d]						
Pinna dermatologic problem	15%		19%	6%		6%	9%	13%	21%	21%[c]			
Owner complaint: hearing loss	5%		13%	2%		7%[d]		2%					
Owner complaint: poor ear carriage	3%		10%				6%						
Deep infection, abscessation, fistula	10%	8%	2%	None	14%	3%	7%	4%		53%			

Abbreviations: per, permanent; Temp, temporary.
[a] TECA and ventral bulla osteotomy.
[b] Subtotal ear canal ablation, LBO.
[c] Complications listed for all procedures to treat cholesteatomas.
[d] Percentages are noted when indicated in study; when no values are listed for the complication, the value could not be determined from data provided. In some studies, complications were described as "% complications per case," not per procedure.

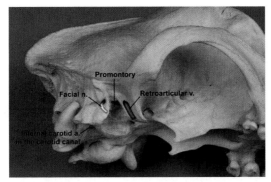

Fig. 1. Lateral view of right bulla osteotomy showing retroarticular vein just rostral to the external auditory meatus, the dorsally located promontory within the tympanic cavity, and the location of the internal carotid artery on the medial wall of the tympanic bulla. (*From* Smeak DD, Inpanbutr N. Lateral approach to subtotal bulla osteotomy in dogs. Compend Contin Ed Pract Vet 2005;27:377–84, with permission.)

proper wound preparation.[19] Debris and contaminated exudate within the ear canal spill into the deep wound during horizontal ear canal removal. It is not surprising that acute wound complications are reported commonly in the literature (ranging from 8% to 31%) and include acute cellulitis/abscessation, incisional hematoma, incisional dehiscence, and extended wound drainage.[1–3,13] To combat incisional complications, early reports advocated routine passive wound drainage following TECA LBO because the wounds are left with dead space, and they are usually highly contaminated and inflamed.[1–3,6] However, there was no difference in wound complication rates when TECA LBO procedures were closed primarily with or without drainage in a subsequent large retrospective study.[15] If wound complications develop, most are treated successfully with appropriate antibiotic therapy and local wound care until second intention healing occurs. When drainage and signs of infection persist beyond several weeks, deeper sources of infection, such as otitis media should be investigated.[1,6,7]

Appropriate perioperative antibiotic administration, meticulous wound dissection to avoid tissue devitalization, copious lavage during surgery to help remove contamination and debris from the wound, and careful apposition of the wound edges help to prevent serious early wound-related complications.[6,15]

Neurologic Problems

While facial nerve damage is the most common neurologic complication following TECA LBO in dogs (13%–36% of procedures), Horner's syndrome is rarely, if ever, encountered[1–3,13,15] (see **Table 1**). Most facial nerve deficits are temporary (range 3%–27% of procedures in dogs) and fully resolve within several weeks; in general, fewer than half are found to be permanent in dogs.[1,13] Temporary deficits are thought to occur from overzealous nerve retraction to expose the bulla during deep dissection.[6] Dogs that present with facial nerve deficits before surgery (about 15%) often do not show improvement after the procedure.[1,13] Surgeons should attempt to limit retractor placement directly around the facial nerve and consider "indirect" retraction, in which the nerve is pulled away from the line of dissection by retracting tissue lateral or more superficial to the course of the nerve.[8] Early isolation and protection of the facial nerve during deep dissection of the horizontal ear canal and bulla are important to help avoid permanent damage to the nerve.[8]

A higher frequency of Horner's syndrome and facial nerve damage has been seen in cats following TECA and LBO.[16–18] Horner's syndrome may appear in up to 53% and facial nerve damage occurs in as many as 74% of cats after this procedure.[16,18] Increased risk of nerve damage after surgery is thought to be attributed to the greater fragility of the feline tympanic plexus and facial nerve compared to the dog.[18] Although many affected cats have temporary nerve damage, 7% to 27% develop permanent Horner's syndrome and 20% to 47% of procedures result in permanent facial nerve dysfunction.[16,18] Cats with otic neoplasia in the Bacon et al study[18] were twice as likely to have facial nerve paralysis postoperatively compared to cats with other aural diseases, presumably due to the more extensive deep dissection and retraction necessary to help remove the neoplastic process. Full recovery after facial nerve damage from traumatic ear canal avulsion in cats appears to be inconsistent following TECA treatment.[20,21]

During the immediate postoperative period, all patients with facial nerve deficits should be treated with corneal protectants.[6,12] Significant decrease in tear production occurs after anesthesia, and the effect is prolonged when anesthetic duration is longer than 2 hours.[22] Complete deficits do not require specific long-term treatment provided that normal tear flow is present and that the eye is not predisposed to exposure keratitis from exopthalmia.[6,13] Most dogs and cats with complete facial nerve deficits following TECA LBO have no long-term sequelae[2–4,13]; however, loss of the globe occurred in one dog that developed corneal perforation.[1] Distribution of the corneal film is maintained in dogs with facial nerve deficits since passive third eyelid movement by retraction of the globe (cranial nerve VI) is unaffected.[6,13]

Temporary signs of hypoglossal nerve dysfunction (excessive drooling, dysphagia) occur rarely in the early postoperative period (<8% of TECA LBO) and have only been documented in dogs.[2,4] Meticulous dissection and avoidance of aggressive retraction in tissues deep to the tympanic bulla should help avoid this complication.

Vestibular signs and significant head tilt (inner ear damage) occur after TECA LBO surgery in 3% to 8% of dogs, but have not been documented in cats after this procedure.[1–3,11–15] Damage to the inner ear structures is thought to occur during exploration and removal of tissue/debris from the epitympanic recess and promontory areas.[8] Dogs with vestibular signs or head tilts before surgery had exacerbation of these signs after surgery in one study.[1] Head tilts and vestibular signs that persist longer than 2 to 3 weeks are usually permanent or improve slowly but incompletely over time.[1,3,13,14] Adequate exposure and avoidance of curettage in the dorsal aspect of the tympanic cavity are important technical steps to avoid inner ear damage during TECA LBO.[6,8,14]

Pinna Necrosis

Pinna necrosis occurs from damage to the pinna vasculature during medial dissection of the vertical ear canal, and is most often found along the caudal pinna margin[1] (**Fig. 2**). Total pinna necrosis has been reported in one dog after TECA LBO and this dog eventually died of other complications in the early postoperative period.[3] Therapy for this complication consists of debridement of devitalized tissue and open wound management until second intention healing occurs. Avoid damage to the blood supply of the pinna by incising just medial to the cartilage of the vertical ear canal during detachment of the ear canal from the pinna.

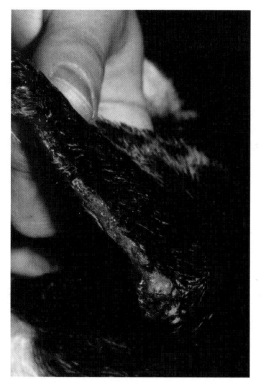

Fig. 2. Caudal pinna necrosis of the right ear following TECA.

Dypnea-Airway Obstruction

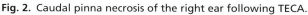

Significant pharyngeal swelling can occur if TECA AND LBO are preformed bilaterally and in dogs with preexisting airway obstruction (bulldogs).[6] If the surgical site is to be bandaged after surgery, be careful to inspect that it is placed loosely. Encircling head bandages can further constrict the pharynx, and this can cause suffocation in the early postoperative period.[6] Closely monitor respiration after TECA LBO, particularly in the first 24 hours after surgery. Remove bandages immediately if respiratory compromise is witnessed.

Pain

TECA LBO is a highly aggressive salvage procedure and postoperative pain is difficult to control without causing deleterious drug-induced side effects.[23,24] Systemic narcotic administration with or without local nerve blocks for the first 24 to 48 hours has been recommended, and nonsteroidal anti-inflammatory drugs and Tramadol are often effective for analgesia during the following 3 to 5 days postoperatively. Local anesthetic delivery systems (**Fig. 3**) alone have been shown to be viable option to reduce pain following TECA, with minimal side effects.[24]

Aspiration Pneumonia

Pneumonia developed in two dogs within days following TECA in two retrospective studies.[3,14] One Yorkshire terrier with an untreated concurrent tracheal collapse

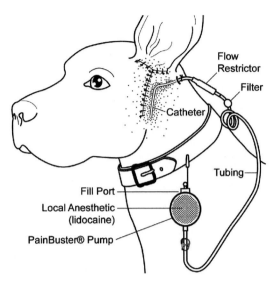

Fig. 3. Example of a constant rate local anesthetic delivery system used in a dog after TECA. (*From* Wolfe TM, Bateman SW, Cole LK, et al. Evaluation of a local anesthetic delivery system for the postoperative analgesic management of canine total ear canal ablation-a randomized, controlled, double-blinded study. Vet Anaesth Analg 2006;33:328–39, with permission.)

condition developed pneumonia and died, while a second dog died soon after anesthesia from aspiration of vomitus.[15] Treatment of concurrent disease processes before surgery is an appropriate goal before any aggressive elective surgical procedure, as well as careful postoperative monitoring to help reduce perioperative deaths.

LATE POSTOPERATIVE COMPLICATIONS
Pinna Dermatitis

Most ear diseases in cats are not associated with a systemic skin condition as they are in dogs.[25,26] So, it is not surprising that persistent ear pinna dermatitis has not been documented in cats undergoing TECA but is seen frequently in dogs (**Fig. 4**; see

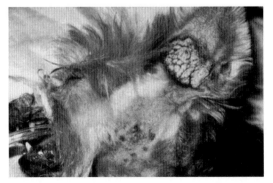

Fig. 4. Example of chronic dermatitis at the base of the left pinna after TECA.

Table 1). Chronic dermatitis of the pinna is observed in up to 21% of dogs after TECA, and this complication results from progression of an underlying dermatologic problem and/or incomplete removal of proliferative tissue at the base of the pinna when making the medial incision around the vertical ear canal opening. Persistent head shaking and self-mutilation of the pinna may plague the patient despite removal of the entire ear canal.[6] Strive to remove any chronically affected pinna tissue during TECA, even though this can result in poor ear carriage after surgery. In addition, diagnosis and proper ongoing treatment of concurrent generalized skin conditions should be recommended after TECA.

Owner Complaint of Hearing Loss

It is likely that most dogs with chronic external and middle ear infection have diminished hearing ability even *before* surgery.[6] Subjectively, if owners are made aware of their pet's auditory deficits in the preoperative evaluation, there are a low percentage of owners (generally <7%) who complain that the auditory function decreased in the postoperative period.[1,3,6,13,14,16] Whether or not TECA LBO contributes to hearing loss has been objectively examined. In one study, 100% of normal dogs were "deaf" after experimental TECA LBO (when the tympanic membrane and ossicles were purposely removed) as determined by electronic measurements of air-conducted brain stem auditory evoked potentials (BSAEP).[9] Two dogs retained some hearing but were subsequently found to have retained tympanic membranes and ossicles. In previous experimental studies, many dogs retained some hearing ability but the tympanic membrane and ossicles were routinely not found or removed during the surgery.[27,28] While air-conducted sound detection is lost, dogs do retain bone-conducted BSAEP after TECA LBO, because the surgery disrupts the sound conduction mechanisms but not the sensorineural components of the auditory pathway. However, it should be noted that bone-conducted hearing alone is not likely to be clinically relevant.[9] Retention of the tympanic membrane promotes reformation of the tympanic cavity, impedance of soft tissue ingrowth, and formation of epithelialized cavities and accumulated keratinized cellular debris, and this likely will increase the risk of late deep infection after TECA.[9] Therefore, it is recommended to remove the tympanic membrane with the epithelial lining of the osseous ear canal, despite the risk of diminished hearing after TECA LBO.[8,9]

Owner Complaint of Poor Ear Carriage

Before surgery, owners tend to be most concerned about the appearance of their pet and whether their animal will be deaf after surgery. The appearance in floppy-eared dogs, such as cocker spaniels, is unchanged after surgery, even if the ear canal excision is extended well up into the base of the pinna.[6] The author prefers to remove all diseased ear tissue, despite the potential for poor ear carriage in erect-eared dogs and cats since continued head shaking and scratching can be expected if proliferative ear tissue remains after TECA.[2,3,14] A modified technique that preserves part of the dorsal vertical ear canal (hence it maintains ear carriage in erect-eared dogs and cats), called a subtotal ear canal ablation, may be indicated when the disease process is limited to the horizontal ear canal and any systemic skin disease is expected to be controlled[12] (**Fig. 5**). A ventrally based advancement skin flap has also been proposed to maintain ear carriage after TECA in cats.[29] The primary goals of TECA LBO are to remove all diseased tissue (neoplasia or chronic deep-seated canal infection) and control or eliminate signs of ear disease, so preserving ear carriage should take second priority.

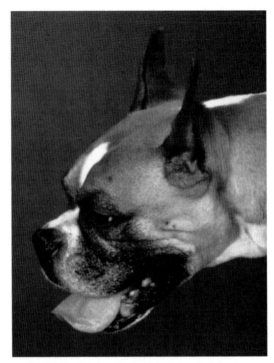

Fig. 5. Excellent ear carriage after subtotal ear canal ablation and lateral bulla osteotomy to remove an isolated left horizontal ear canal tumor.

Deep Infection/Abscessation/Fistula Formation

The most troubling long-term complication encountered after TECA LBO involves recurrent otitis media in dogs.[5,6] Deep wound infections are less common in cats after TECA LBO than in dogs presumably since severe, deeply infected, ear canal and middle ear disease are more rarely encountered in cats.[16,18] This complication can be

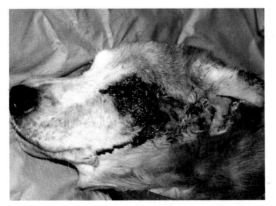

Fig. 6. Chronic draining fistula from a deep left middle ear infection 2 years after TECA.

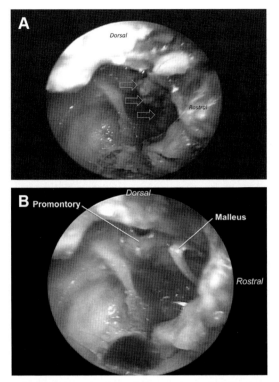

Fig. 7. (A) Intraoperative videoscopic view of tympanic cavity after aggressive lateral bulla osteotomy showing epithelial remnant in the rostral aspect (arrows). (B) Tympanic cavity view after removal of the epithelial remnant and loose bone seen around the margins of the bulla osteotomy site in (A); the malleus is now visible in the epitympanic recess. Note the excellent exposure and clarity of tympanic cavity structures when viewed through the videoscope. Inner ear structures are housed in the identified promontory.

manifested by signs of pain upon opening the mouth, diffuse swelling on the affected side, and when this infection becomes fulminate, draining tracts develop that usually drain cranial and ventral to the initial incision[5,7,30] (Fig. 6). Clinical signs can appear from 1 month to several years (mean 5.5–10 months) after TECA LBO.[1,2,5,30] The most common underlying reason for recurrent infection is incomplete removal of the secretory epithelium lining the tympanic bulla or osseous ear canal[5,7,13,14,30] (Fig. 7). Other factors purported in the literature that may be implicated in deep infection after TECA include retained infected ear canal cartilage, osteomyelitis of the ossicles, inadequate drainage of the middle ear through the eustachian tube, and parotid salivary gland damage.[3,6,14] Even when a LBO and proper curettage of the tympanic bulla is performed, the rate of recurrent deep infection is between 2% and 10%.[1-3,14] Sharpe[4] performed a VBO with TECA and found this alternative approach to the middle ear did not reduce the risk of deep infection (see **Table 1**). When TECA LBO is performed for aural cholesteatoma, recurrence of deep infection approaches 50%.[5] Risk factors for recurrence identified in this case series included inability to open the mouth or neurologic signs on admission, and lysis of any portion of the temporal bone on CT imaging.[5] Long-term antibiotic therapy is usually not successful for treatment of recurrent deep infection after TECA LBO, and surgical exploration of the region is recommended.[5,7] Surgical approaches used for reexploration of the middle ear include a lateral approach and VBO.[7,30] The lateral approach may result in more facial nerve deficits after surgery since anatomic structures are obscured by scar tissue from the original surgery, although in most cases, the deficits are temporary.[30] The author prefers the ventral approach if the nidus of infection is isolated within the middle ear, since this approach offers excellent exposure and ventral drainage. Anatomy in this approach has not been altered by previous surgery so identification of structures and dissection is easier.[7] When radiographic imaging shows that a portion of the horizontal ear canal remains, the lateral approach is chosen because removal of tissue lateral to the bulla is very difficult from the ventral approach. Regardless of the approach used to explore for the nidus of chronic infection after TECA, recurrence of deep infection approaches 30% to 71%, and reoperation is often necessary.[7,30] In the author's experience and those of others, using an operative 30-degree videoscope during exploration of the bulla greatly improves identification and complete removal of debris and epithelial remnants[31] (**Fig. 7**).

SUMMARY

In most cases, owners report high satisfaction (over 90%) after TECA LBO is performed on their pets.[11,14] Owners should be reminded that this procedure is considered elective and rare but serious complications such blood loss, upper airway obstruction, inner ear damage, recurrent deep infection, and death have been reported during and after surgery.[1–3,9]

TECA and BO remains an important and successful salvage procedure recommended for chronic inflammatory ear disease (particularly those that are end-stage and are deemed unresponsive to medical management), neoplasia, and severe trauma. Due to the anatomic complexity of the procedure, and inherent poor exposure, there is significant risk for neurologic damage and for retained ear canal or middle ear epithelium, even for the most experienced surgeon. The risk of complications can be reduced by achieving appropriate antibiotic levels in the tissue during the operation, minimizing trauma during dissection and retraction, controlling hemorrhage, thorough lavaging of the surgical site to remove bone debris and contamination, meticulous isolation of the facial nerve, obtaining wide exposure to the tympanic cavity, complete evacuation of all epithelium particularly within the tympanic bulla, and proper postoperative management.

Complication risk after TECA LBO now appears to be most associated with the nature, extent and severity of the ear canal and middle ear disease. Aggressive disease processes such as middle ear neoplasia and cholesteatoma remain difficult to control and recurrence is common.[5,32,33]

REFERENCES

1. Smeak DD, Dehoff WD. Total ear canal ablation: clinical results in the dog and cat. Vet Surg 1986;15:161–70.
2. Mason LK, Harvey CE, Orsher RJ. Total ear canal ablation combined with lateral bulla osteotomy for end-stage otitis in dogs. Results in thirty dogs. Vet Surg 1988;17:263–8.
3. Matthieson DT, Scavelli T. Total ear canal ablation and lateral bulla osteotomy in 38 dogs. J Am Anim Hosp Assoc 1990;26:257–67.
4. Sharp NJH. Chronic otitis externa and otitis media treated by total ear canal ablation and ventral bulla osteotomy in thirteen dogs. Vet Surg 1990;19:162–6.
5. Hardie EM, Linder KE, Pease AP. Aural cholesteatoma in twenty dogs. Vet Surg 2008;37:763–70.

6. Smeak DD, Kerpsack SJ. Total ear canal ablation and lateral bulla osteotomy for management of end stage otitis. Semin Vet Med Surg (Sm Animal) 1993;8:30–41.
7. Smeak DD, Crocker CB, Birchard SJ. Treatment of recurrent otitis media that developed after total ear canal ablation and lateral bulla osteotomy in dogs: nine cases (1996-1994) J Am Vet Med Assoc 1996;209:937–42.
8. Smeak DD, Inpanbutr N. Lateral approach to subtotal bulla osteotomy in dogs. Compend Contin Educ Pract Vet 2005;27:377–84.
9. McAnulty JF, Hattel A, Harvey CE. Wound healing and brain stem auditory evoked potentials after experimental total ear canal ablation and lateral bulla osteotomy in dogs. Vet Surg 1995;24:1–8.
10. Doust R, King A, Hammond G, et al. Assessment of middle ear disease in the dog: a comparison of diagnostic imaging modalities. J Small Anim Pract 2007;48:188–92.
11. Doyle R, Skelly C, Bellenger CR. Surgical management of 43 cases of chronic otitis externa in the dog. Vet J 2004;57:22–30.
12. Mathews KG, Hardie EM, Murphy KM. Subtotal ear canal ablation in 18 dogs and one cat with minimal distal ear canal pathology. J Am Anim Hosp Assoc 2006;42:371–80.
13. White RAS, Pomeroy CJ. Total ear canal ablation and lateral bulla osteotomy in the dog. J Sm Anim Pract 1990;31:547–53.
14. Beckman SL, Henry WB, Cechner P. Total ear canal ablation. Combining bulla osteotomy and curettage in dogs with chronic otitis externa and media. J Am Vet Med Assoc 1990;196,84–90.
15. Devitt CM, Seim HB, Willer R, et al. Passive drainage versus primary closure after total ear canal ablation-lateral bulla osteotomy in dogs: 59 dogs (1985-1995). Vet Surg 1997;26:210–6.
16. Williams JM, White RAS. Total ear canal ablation combined with lateral bulla osteotomy in the cat. J Small Anim Pract 1992;33:225–7.
17. Marino DJ, MacDonald JM, Matthieson DT, et al. Results of surgery in cats with ceruminous gland adenocarcinoma. J Am Anim Hosp Assoc 1994;30:54–8.
18. Bacon NJ, Gilbert RL, Bostock DE, et al. Total ear canal ablation in the cat: indications, morbidity and long-term survival. J Small Anim Pract 2003;44,430–4.
19. Vogel PL, Komtebedde J, Hirsch DC, et al. Wound contamination and antimicrobial susceptibility of bacteria cultured during total ear canal ablation and lateral bulla osteotomy in dogs. J Am Vet Med Assoc 1999;214:1641–3.
20. Smeak DD. Traumatic separation of the annular cartilage from the external auditory meatus in a cat. J Am Vet Med Assoc 1997;211:448–50.
21. Clark SP. Surgical management of acute ear canal separation in a cat. J Feline Med Surg 2004;6:283–6.
22. Herring IP, Pickett JP, Champagne ES, et al. Evaluation of aqueous tear production in dogs following general anesthesia. J Am Anim Hosp Assoc 2000;36:427–30.
23. Buback JL, Boothe HW, Carroll GL, et al. Comparison of three methods for relief of pain after ear canal ablation in dogs. Vet Surg 1996;25:380–5.
24. Wolfe TM, Bateman SW, Cole LK, et al. Evaluation of a local anesthetic delivery system for the postoperative analgesic management of canine total ear canal ablation-a randomized, controlled, double-blinded study. Vet Anaesth Analg 2006;33: 328–39.
25. Saridomichelakis MN, Farmaki R, Leontides LS, et al. Aetiology of canine otitis externa: a retrospective study of 100 cases. Vet Dermatol 2007;18:341–7.
26. Matousek JL. Diseases of the ear pinna. Vet Clin N Am Small Anim Pract 2004;34: 511–40.
27. Payne JT, Shell LG, Flora RM, et al. Hearing loss in dogs subjected to total ear canal ablation. Vet Surg 1989;18:60.

28. Krahwinkel DJ, Pardo AD, Sims MH, et al. Effect of total ablation of the external auditory meatus and bulla osteotomy on auditory function in dogs. J Am Vet Med Assoc 1993;202:949–52.

29. McNabb AH, Flanders JA. Cosmetic results of a ventrally based advancement flap for closure of total ear canal ablations in 6 cats: 2002–2003. Vet Surg 2004;33:435–9.

30. Holt D, Brockman DJ, Sylvestre AM, et al. Lateral exploration of fistulas developing after total ear canal ablations: 10 cases (1989-1993). J Am Anim Hosp Assoc 1996;32:527–30.

31. Haudequet PH, Gauthier O, Renard E. Total ear canal ablation associated with lateral bulla osteotomy with the help of otoscopy in dogs and cats: retrospective study of 47 cases. Vet Surg 2006;35:E1–20.

32. Little C, Pearson GR, Lane JG. Neoplasia involving the middle ear cavity of dogs, Vet Rec 1989;124:54–7.

33. Trevor PB, Martin RA. Tympanic bulla osteotomy for treatment of middle-ear disease in cats: 19 cases (1984-1991). J Am Vet Med Assoc 1993;202:123–8.

Complications of Reconstructive Surgery in Companion Animals

Pierre Amsellem, Docteur Vétérinaire, MS

KEYWORDS
- Complications • Skin Reconstructive surgery • Maxillectomy
- Hemipelvectomy • Radiation therapy

Reconstructive surgery may be needed after extensive traumatic injuries or after wide excision of neoplasms. The goals of reconstructive surgery in veterinary medicine are completion of wound healing and ultimately return to function, while preserving cosmesis if possible. A clear understanding of the factors that affect wound healing is thus needed to predict and prevent the occurrence of complications after reconstructive surgery.

FACTORS THAT AFFECT WOUND HEALING

Wound healing can be affected by the general health of the patient, nutritional intake, and a variety of exogenous factors in animals undergoing therapy for malignant neoplasia. Although delayed wound healing is rare in animals undergoing resection of skin or subcutaneous neoplasias, careful consideration of risk factors is indicated.

Patient Factors

Endogenous factors including hypoproteinemia,[1] uremia,[2] wound infection,[3] and hyperadrenocorticism[4] have all been shown to delay wound healing. Nutritional intake can also be affected by daily sedation for bandage changes, anesthesia for radiation therapy, or gastrointestinal complications from chemotherapeutic drugs. Calorie and protein intake should be quantified to ensure that nutritional requirements are met in patients with large healing wounds and increased metabolic demand. In animals with preexisting medical conditions, attempts should be made to stabilize the underlying condition prior to performing an aggressive oncologic resection and reconstructive surgery. In addition to the judicious use of perioperative fluid therapy, colloids, and prophylactic antibiotics, clinicians should proactively consider placement of an esophageal or gastric feeding device at the time of definitive surgery to avoid any negative nutritional balance during the early phases of healing.

Wey Referrals, 125-129 Chertsey Road, Woking GU21 5BP, United Kingdom
E-mail address: pierreamsellem@hotmail.com

Vet Clin Small Anim 41 (2011) 995–1006
doi:10.1016/j.cvsm.2011.05.005
0195-5616/11/$ – see front matter © 2011 Elsevier Inc. All rights reserved.

Effects of Oncologic Therapy

Chemotherapy drugs target rapidly dividing cells and cause delays in wound healing in experimental models.[5] Preoperative chemotherapy within the first 5 days after surgery is most likely to affect fibroblast proliferation and wound strength.[6] Based on these experimental studies, it may be wise to delay suture removal until 14 to 21 days after surgery in an animal that received chemotherapeutic drugs during the early phases of wound healing.

Radiation effects on skin and on wound healing have been reviewed.[11,12] Radiation has been shown to reduce fibroblast proliferation, decrease collagen production, and delay the maturation phase of wound healing.[13] Radiation therapy also has a variety of detrimental effects on local wound vasculature, causing endothelial cell damage, thrombosis, obliterative arteritis, and reduced neovascularization.[14] Mechanical testing of preirradiated wounds has been performed in experimental models to determine the effect of radiation dose, timing in relation to wounding, and fractionation. In mice,[13] a single 18-Gy fraction given before or up to 5 days after wounding resulted in a 50% to 66% reduction in wound strength at 3 months. The effects on wound healing could be decreased by using a lower radiation dose per fraction.[15] Radiation effect on healing seems to be long lasting, as wounds created 65 days after irradiation also had a 50% to 66% reduction in strength compared to controls. In contrast, if radiation was administered more than 12 days after wounding, wound strength was less affected. Although lab animals were used, these studies represent a guideline to optimize modalities of cancer treatment with a combination of surgery and radiation. In a veterinary clinical study, three settings were described when a combination of radiation and reconstructive surgery was used[16]: preoperative irradiation, planned postoperative irradiation, and reconstructive surgery to treat complications of irradiation. Preoperative irradiation lead to more healing complications than postoperative irradiation.[16] Reconstructive surgery for complications of radiation had the highest complication rate.[16] If possible, reconstruction to treat a radiation wound should be based on skin flaps (random or ideally axial pattern) outside of the radiation field.[16,17] Due to frequent complications associated with skin grafts after radiation therapy, this technique is not recommended to treat radiation wounds in human beings.[18]

Tumor Type

Some clinical and experimental data suggest that tumor type can affect the risk of dehiscence after surgical incision, with a specific increase in wound healing complications associated with mast cell tumor (MCT) resection. For example, one clinical study reported a 10% dehiscence after excision of MCT.[7] Although this dehiscence rate is subjectively high, there was no control group for statistical comparison. Delayed wound healing and dehiscence following excision of a MCT may be related to the release of proteolytic enzymes and vasoactives substances by the tumor.[8] In mice, release of histamine by mast cells has been shown to reduce fibroplasia and delay wound healing.[9] Inhibition of epithelialization is also suspected in vitro. Histamine and human mast cell leukemia lysates reduced keratinocyte proliferation in vitro.[10] This could translate into inhibition of epithelialization in vivo. Although clear clinical evidence in dogs and cats is still lacking, the use of both H1 and H2 blockers before and after mast cell tumor excision may be helpful in reducing the effect of mast cell tumors on wound healing.

Species

Wound healing in cats has only been studied recently as it was assumed to be similar to dogs. Bohling and colleagues[19] have shown that sutured wounds were twice as strong in dogs than in cats when tested 7 days after wounding. It was suspected that a slower rate of collagen formation or maturation occurs in cats. Based on these data, the authors recommended leaving skin sutures longer in cats than in dogs, especially if the wound is under tension. When secondary healing was evaluated, cats had less granulation tissue formation and total wound healing (reduction in open wound area from contraction and epithelialization) was slower in cats than in dogs.[19]

COMPLICATIONS OF RECONSTRUCTIVE SURGERY
Seromas and Hematomas

Surgical manipulations as skin is detached form the underlying tissues will result in the creation of an abnormal space or pocket within a wound that is termed dead space. A seroma is the accumulation of serosanguineous fluid within that space. Fluid accumulation is a result of capillary bleeding and vascular leakage secondary to postoperative inflammation. Motion at the surgical site and excessive activity may also increase risks of seroma formation.[20] In humans, use of electrocautery to elevate skin flaps has been associated with an increased incidence of seroma formation.[21] Following Halsted's principles of gentle tissue handling, meticulous hemostasis, and closure of dead space will reduce the risk of seroma formation. Reducing the activity of the patient and, if indicated, limb immobilization may help reduce seroma formation.[22] Seromas are nonpainful and often can be differentiated from abscesses during physical examination. If the differentiation cannot be made, cytology can be performed. A seroma shows a variable number of red blood cells but very few white blood cells.[23] In most cases, seromas will resolve in 1 to 2 weeks with conservative treatment. Exercise restriction should be reinforced and additional use of warm compress application or therapeutic ultrasound may aid in fluid removal. In general, aspiration of seromas should be avoided as this may increase the risk of abscess formation. Large seromas may require treatment with aspiration and compressive bandage but recurrence rate in high.[23] Drainage can be provided by removing some of the skin sutures to allow drainage or by inserting a drain. The goal of the drain is to allow the cavity to collapse so the skin can reattach to the underlying tissues. Regardless of the technique chosen, strict asepsis should be maintained to prevent secondary infectious complications.

Hematomas usually form as a result of incomplete hemostasis. Hematomas and seromas increase tension on the incision line after reconstructive surgery and can predispose to dehiscence. In addition to the indirect effect on wound tension, there is experimental evidence that postoperative hematoma formation can directly affect flap survival.[24] In a rat model, the presence of hematomas under a skin flap resulted in decreased blood supply to the tip of the flap and a mean of 45% necrosis versus 2% necrosis in control flap where the hematoma was replaced with a saline injection under the flap.[24] Interestingly, treatment with vasodilator isoxuprine reversed the effects.[24] A hematoma-mediated vasoconstriction was thus suspected. This phenomenon has not been reported in dogs but may go unrecognized in many cases. Consequently, this reemphasizes the need for adequate hemostasis during skin flap elevation. If a hematoma occurs under a skin flap, drainage should be considered to avoid complications. Following free skin grafting, a hematoma or seroma under the graft can prevent adhesion of the graft, resulting in partial or complete graft loss. Consequently, it is recommended to either use a mesh graft or an active drain under an unmeshed graft.[25]

Seromas and hematomas after tumor excision can dissect and contaminate into adjacent tissue planes. If an incomplete excision of a neoplasm is performed and a seroma occurs, the entire area is contaminated with tumor cells and further treatment (reexcision or radiation) should include the seroma. Drain placement to prevent seroma formation should also be done, keeping in mind the principles of surgical oncology. The drain entry site should be fairly close to the incision and additional undermining should be avoided. This will help minimize contamination by tumor cells of adjacent tissue, should the excision be incomplete.

Wound Infection

Infection prolongs the inflammatory phase of wound healing. Consequently, the strength of the wound will remain low and dehiscence is more likely to occur. Wound infection causes a local release of toxins and inflammatory mediators, inducing cell death and vascular thrombosis. Bacteria and leukocytes use oxygen, which reduces the amount of oxygen available to the cellular elements of wound healing. Minimizing tissue trauma, the amount of foreign material left in the wound, and the amount of dead space may help reduce the risk of infection. The vast majority of tumor resections would be considered clean procedures and may not require prophylactic use of antibiotics. However, perioperative administration of a first-generation cephalosporin antibiotic is considered in immunocompromised patients or when clean procedures last longer than 90 minutes.[26]

Contamination of Adjacent Tissues with Neoplastic Cells

When reconstructive surgery is needed following excision of neoplasia, the possible contamination of adjacent tissues should be considered. This is especially important if complete surgical margins are not obtained during the resection, causing contamination of the flap donor site.[27,28] In humans, frozen sections are used intraoperatively until complete surgical margins are obtained.[29] Reconstruction is performed only after clean resection is achieved. In veterinary medicine, frozen sections are rarely available and several alternative options have been proposed. One group has descrbed a two-step process in which the mass is excised the resulting wound in bandaged while histopathologic results are pending.[30] Reconstructive surgery is performed as a staged procedure after confirmation of clean excision.[30] Other authors have used a one-step process with immediate reconstruction after the wound was lavaged and gloves, instruments, and drapes were changed.[16] A clinical study using the latter technique reported no recurrence in the flap donor area in 26 dogs that underwent cutaneous or mucosal flap reconstruction in combination with radiation therapy.[16] These authors recommended treating the axial pattern flap and the tumor excision sites as separate surgical fields and not going from one site to the other.[16]

Complications due to Wound Tension

Dehiscence is a common complication of wound healing when a wound is closed under tension. Tension is not measured objectively. Part of the art of surgery is to be able to decide how much tension is too much when closing a surgical wound.[31] Excessive tension can lead to tissue ischemia and necrosis, wound dehiscence, and skin suture pull-out.[32] With axial pattern flaps, the vascular pedicle gets smaller toward the tip of the flap and thus is most sensitive to tension. Consequently, when an axial pattern is sutured to the recipient site, one can start with suturing the base in place, progressively moving toward the tip to minimize tension on the distal end of the flap (Nick Bacon, personal communication, 2010).

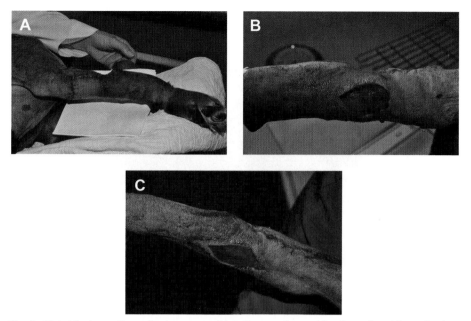

Fig. 1. Distal limb swelling after a transposition flap on the proximal antebrachium of a dog, causing a tourniquet effect (*A*). A longitudinal releasing incision was performed (*B*) allowing resolution of the swelling 2–3 days later (*C*).

In the extremities, tension on a surgical wound can create a tourniquet effect.[33] Local tissue constriction results in lymphatic and venous compression. This can cause distal limb swelling (**Fig. 1**). If the occlusion is severe enough, secondary collapse of arterial circulation can occur with ensuing ischemic necrosis. As soon as distal limb swelling is detected, prompt intervention is required. Skin sutures need to be removed to allow the wound to heal by second intention.[32] Alternatively, a releasing incision can be made parallel to the limb axis and the primary incision can be left intact.

Skin Flap Necrosis

Skin flaps (also called pedicle grafts) have been classified as either subdermal or axial pattern flaps depending on their blood supply.[34] When necrosis of skin flap occurs, it usually involves the tip and is called distal tip necrosis (**Fig. 2**). Necrosis of the entire flap is uncommon. In one study, distal necrosis occurred in 9 of 19 axial pattern flaps, with necrosis of 5% to 30% of the flap.[35] Distal tip necrosis can be managed conservatively in some cases.[35] The caudal superficial epigastric seems to be one of the most robust flaps with complete survival in 9 of 10 dogs and a minor area of necrosis in the remaining dogs.[28] Complications with the thoracodorsal flap appear to be far more common, with only 3 of 10 dogs having complete flap survival in a recent clinical study.[27] Due to the frequency of partial flap necrosis, clients should be warned of the possible need for an additional procedure to débride the necrotic tissue and close the wound when reconstruction with a skin flap is planned. The most likely cause of distal flap necrosis is a lack of blood flow to the tip of the flap.[36] In one study in dogs, subdermal flap elevation resulted in a 95% to 99% decrease in blood flow in

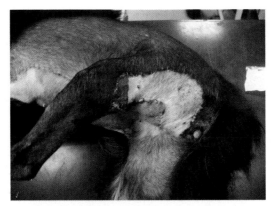

Fig. 2. Distal tip necrosis of a caudal superficial epigastric flap.

the tip of the flap.[37] For axial pattern flaps, it is critical to include and preserve the direct cutaneous vessel. Identification and preservation of the primary vascular supply can be facilitated via transillumination of the skin to find the vascular pedicle. If regional trauma has occurred, the integrity of the direct cutaneous vessel can be verified preoperatively using ultrasonography and Doppler examination.[38] All flaps should be elevated below the cutaneous trunci muscle or under the deep subcutaneous tissue to preserve the subdermal plexus.[39] Tension on the flap should be avoided at all cost. Tension causes increased interstitial pressure and secondary circulatory blockage due to a combination of venous and arterial insufficiency. It may be preferable to have a flap of adequate length that may necrose at its tip rather than a flap that is too small and is sutured under tension.[35] The flap is not tacked to the recipient bed as this could damage its blood supply. Instead, an active drain is placed to prevent seroma formation. When a flap is over a bony protuberance, like the elbow after a thoracodorsal flap, a well-padded bandage should be applied to avoid pressure necrosis.[27] Predicting flap necrosis based on flap color and temperature may be difficult. Some flaps that are purple at day 6 will eventually necrose whereas others will survive.[34] Objective methods available to evaluate viability of a skin flap include fluorescein testing[34] and measurement of hematocrit of the blood from a stab incision in the area of concern.[40] Experimental treatments to rescue a failing flap using dextrans, vasodilators, pentoxifylline, and hyperbaric oxygen have shown some encouraging results but clinical data in small animals are lacking.[34,41] In humans, if the transposed flap becomes congested, leeches can be placed on the flap, decreasing venous congestion and possibly reducing the risk of necrosis.[42,43] The effect of alpha agonists (routinely used for sedation) on skin flap survival has not been clearly evaluated. Dexmedetomidine causes a massive decrease in cutaneous blood flow.[44] Consequently, this class of drug should be used with caution after reconstruction with skin flaps.

Free Skin Graft Failure

Causes of graft failure include lack of immobilization, infection, and an inadequately vascularized graft bed.[45,46] The graft needs to be immobilized to the recipient bed until fibrous union occurs. It takes approximately 10 days for a complete union to occur.[45] Until then, graft movement may damage the fibrin and fibrous bond, impairing graft nutrition and revascularization.[45] Most authors recommend bandaging with a nonadherent contact layer and immobilization using a splint or cast. The bandage is not replaced for the first 48 to 72 hours to avoid disrupting the graft. In cats, one study showed that 14 of 17 grafts survived completely.[47] Several authors have recommended waiting 4 to 6 days before bandage change in cats to minimize complications associated with a new dressing.[47,48] Alternatively, the use of vacuum-assisted closure (VAC) has been reported to help immobilize the graft in a case report in one cat and eight dogs with distal extremity wounds. All wounds healed completely with this technique.[49,50] In humans, the use of VAC has eased skin grafting of high motion areas like the heel.[51] To survive, skin grafts require a vascular bed that will provide new blood vessel connections with the graft. This can be a fresh surgical bed or, more commonly, healthy granulation tissue. Grafts will not take over bone, cartilage, tendons, nerve, irradiated tissues, avascular fat, chronic ulcers, and chronic granulation tissue.[45]

Self-trauma and Paresthesia of a Skin Flap or Free Graft

Self-trauma is likely related to the postoperative inflammation of tissues and should be prevented with the use of appropriate analgesics and anti-inflammatory drugs in combination with an Elizabethan collar or bandage. Delayed self-trauma has also been reported and may be related to paresthesia during reinnervation of free graft or skin flap.[52] Reinnervation of skin flaps occurs from the periphery to the center in rats.[53] Reinnervation of skin grafts in humans is a slow process and does not always occur.[54,55] Delayed self-trauma of a graft has been described in a dog at 3 to 4 weeks after surgery.[52] This uncommon behavior can be temporary or persistent and could be a sign of paresthesia.[52] In animals with persistent signs, prolonged maintenance of an Elizabethan collar is recommended. Gabapentin, a GABA analogue, is used for the treatment of chronic neuralgia in human beings and could be considered as an adjunctive therapy for dogs with suspected paresthesia.

COMPLICATIONS OF SELECTED RECONSTRUCTIVE PROCEDURES
Maxillectomy

Maxillectomy is commonly performed to excise oral neoplasms in dogs and occasionally in cats. Postoperative function is excellent, with most patients able to eat the day after surgery. Complications of maxillectomy include local tumor recurrence, intraoperative hemorrhage,[56] subcutaneous emphysema, wound dehiscence, ulceration of the upper lip,[56] and zygomatic sialocele.[57] Dehiscence is one of the most common complications (**Fig. 3**). Reoperation is often needed because of the oronasal communication and subsequent rhinitis. Reconstruction after maxillectomy is based on the creation of a labial mucosal advancement flap that is undermined and sutured to the hard palate. Most authors recommend a two-layer closure with or without drilling holes in the hard palate to anchor sutures. Because of the need for reconstruction using the lip, tumors that extend beyond the midline of the hard palate are usually deemed not resectable with this technique. Dehiscence has been reported in up to 33% of cases, resulting in the formation of an oronasal fistula.[58] In most cases, dehiscence occurred caudal to the canine teeth.[58] Use of electrocoagulation at the wound edges resulted in partial dehiscence in four of four cases in one study.[59] Consequently, cautery should not be used near the mucosal edges.[60] Another critical factor associated with dehiscence is the presence of tension on the labial flap. Tension can be minimized by preserving as much lip and hard palate mucoperiosteum as possible, without compromising margins for tumor excision. Maximal undermining of the labial flap can nearly double the length of the labial mucosal flap and help reduce tension at the wound site. If dehiscence occurs, treatment with oral antibiotics should

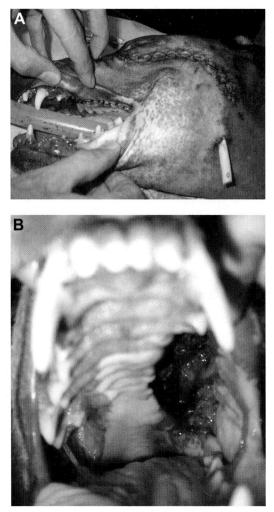

Fig. 3. Closure of a maxillectomy was performed using a labial advancement flap (*A*). Complete dehiscence of the flap occurred, producing a large oronasal fistula (*B*). This dog had received full course radiation therapy prior to tumor excision, which likely affected wound healing.

be initiated. Additional surgery should be delayed if possible to first allow maximal contraction of the fistula. Small oronasal fistulas may not require treatment if the animal is asymptomatic. Surgical treatment options include further undermining and repeat closure, the use of random buccal mucosal flaps, or the application of an axial pattern flap based on the angularis oris vessels.[61,62] An island flap using the mucoperiosteum of the hard palate has also be described to treat orosasal fistula after maxillectomy.[63] Alternatively, a prosthodontic dental appliance may be used to fill the defect.[64,65] Function is very good after maxillectomy as most animals will be able to eat the day after surgery. Occasionally, irritation of the upper lip by the lower canine tooth occurs after maxillectomy. This can be treated by extraction or by filing down the tooth in combination with endodontic treatment.[60]

Hemipelvectomy

Hemipelvectomy may be classified as total, mid-to-caudal partial, mid-to-cranial partial, or caudal partial.[66] In humans, hemipelvectomy has been additionally categorized as external (limb is removed) and internal (the limb is preserved).[67] Hemipelvectomy is most commonly used for treatment of neoplasia. Preoperative CT scan is essential to determine resectability of a pelvic neoplasm. The medial extent is usually the limiting factor in respectability.[66,68] In most cases, tumors extending past midline of the lumbar vertebra or sacrum are deemed nonresectable as excision would likely result in contralateral neurologic dysfunction or fecal/urinary incontinence.[66,68]

Intraoperative complications include hemorrhage and trauma to the urinary or gastrointestinal tract. Continuous blood loss is common, especially in large dogs, due to the extent of soft tissue dissection. It will often result in a need for a blood transfusion.[66] Placement of a urinary catheter at the time of induction is strongly recommended to facilitate identification of the urethra intraoperatively and to avoid iatrogenic damage.[66]

Early postoperative complications include seroma, infection, pain, and reduced mobility. Recovery after surgery is usually slower than after a standard hindlimb amputation. In a study in nine dogs and two cats, most animals required 1 to 2 days before they could stand or walk unassisted.[68] Postoperative analgesia is essential. A urinary catheter may be left in place postoperatively to facilitate nursing care until the animal is ambulatory.[66] Despite initial difficulties, long-term function was rated as good to excellent in all cases.[68]

Late complications include decubital ulcer formation and tumor recurrence. To avoid decubital sores, bony prominences should be covered with thick subcutaneous tissues or using a muscle flap.[66] Reconstruction after hemipelvectomy typically requires closure of the caudal abdominal wall. Muscle flaps can also be used to cover the pelvic contents, although in most cases only subcutaneous tissues and skin are closed over this area.[68] Herniation of the urinary bladder is a rare complication following hemipelvectomy in humans,[69] but this complication has not been reported in dogs.

REFERENCES

1. Perez-Tamayo R, Ihnen M. The effect of methionine in experimental wound healing: a morphologic study. Am J Pathol 1953;29:233.
2. Nayman J. Effect of renal failure on wound healing in dogs. Response to hemodialysis following uremia induced by uranium nitrate. Ann Surg 1966;164:227.
3. Bucknall TE. The effect of local infection upon wound healing: an experimental study. Br J Surg 1980;67:851.
4. Ehrlich HP, Hunt TK. Effects of cortisone and vitamin A on wound healing. Ann Surg 1968;167:324.
5. Cornell K, Waters D. Impaired wound healing in the cancer patient: effects of cytotoxic therapy and pharmacologic modulation by growth factors. Vet Clin North Am Small Anim Pract 1995;25:111.
6. McCaw DL. The effects of cancer and cancer therapies on wound healing. Semin Vet Med Surg (Small Anim) 1989;4:281.
7. Séguin B, Leibman N, Bregazzi V, et al. Clinical outcome of dogs with grade-II mast cell tumors treated with surgery alone: 55 cases (1996–1999). J Am Vet Med Assoc 2001;218:1120.

8. Thamm DH, Vail DM. Mast cell tumors. In: Withrow SJ, Vail DM, editors. Withrow and MacEwen's small animal clinical oncology. 4th edition. St Louis: Saunders Elsevier; 2006. p. 402.

9. Kenyon AJ, Ramos L, Michaels EB. Histamine-induced suppressor macrophage inhibits fibroblast growth and wound healing. Am J Vet Res 1983;44:2164.

10. Huttunen M, Hyttinen M, Nilsson G, et al. Inhibition of keratinocyte growth in cell culture and whole skin culture by mast cell mediators. Exp Dermatol 2001;10:184.

11. Dernell WS. Surgical management of radiation injury. Part 1. Comp Cont Educ Pract Vet 1995;17:181.

12. Tibbs MK. Wound healing following radiation therapy: a review. Radiother Oncol 1997;42:99.

13. Gorodetsky R, McBride W, Withers H. Assay of radiation effects in mouse skin as expressed in wound healing. Radiat Res 1988;116:135.

14. Doyle JW, Li YQ, Salloum A, et al. The effects of radiation on neovascularization in a rat model. Plast Reconstr Surg 1996;98:129.

15. Gorodetsky R, Mou X, Fisher D, et al. Radiation effect in mouse skin: dose fractionation and wound healing. Int J Radiat Oncol Biol Phys 1990;18:1077.

16. Seguin B, Mcdonald DE, Kent MS, et al. Tolerance of cutaneous or mucosal flaps placed into a radiation therapy field in dogs. Vet Surg 2005;34:214.

17. Dernell W, Wheaton L. Surgical management of radiation injury. II. The Compendium on Continuing Education for the Practicing Veterinarian (USA); 1995.

18. Rudolph R. Complications of surgery for radiotherapy skin damage. Plast Reconstr Surg 1982;70:179.

19. Bohling MW, Henderson RA, Swaim SF, et al. Cutaneous wound healing in the cat: a macroscopic description and comparison with cutaneous wound healing in the dog. Vet Surg 2004;33:579.

20. Remedios A. Complications of wound healing. In: Fowler D, Williams JM, editors. Manual of canine and feline wound management and reconstruction. Shurdington (UK): BSAVA; 1999. p. 137.

21. Porter K, O'Connor S, Rimm E, et al. Electrocautery as a factor in seroma formation following mastectomy. Am J Surg 1998;176:8.

22. Dawson I, Stam L, Heslinga J, et al. Effect of shoulder immobilization on wound seroma and shoulder dysfunction following modified radical mastectomy: a randomized prospective clinical trial. Br J Surg 1989;76:311.

23. Pavletic MM. Common complications in wound healing. In: Atlas of small animal wound management and reconstructive surgery. 3rd edition. Ames (IA): Wiley-Blackwell; 2010. p. 128.

24. Hillelson R, Glowacki J, Healey N, et al. A microangiographic study of hematoma-associated flap necrosis and salvage with isoxsuprine. Plast Reconstr Surg 1980;66:528.

25. Pope E, Swaim S. Wound drainage from under full-thickness skin grafts in dogs, Part I. Quantitative evaluation of four techniques. Vet Surg 1986;15:65.

26. Vasseur PB, Levy J, Dowd E, et al. Surgical wound infection rates in dogs and cats. Data from a teaching hospital. Vet Surg 1988;17:60.

27. Aper R, Smeak D. Complications and outcome after thoracodorsal axial pattern flap reconstruction of forelimb skin defects in 10 dogs, 1989–2001. Vet Surg 2003;32:378.

28. Aper R, Smeak D. Clinical evaluation of caudal superficial epigastric axial pattern flap reconstruction of skin defects in 10 dogs (1989–2001). J Am Anim Hosp Assoc 2005;41:185.

29. Holder K, Yeh I. Intraoperative evaluation of margin status: how much is enough? Pathol Case Rev 2010;15:148.

30. Liptak J. The principles of surgical oncology: diagnosis and staging. Comp Cont Educ Pract Vet 2009;31:(9):E1–14.

31. Johnston DE. Tension-relieving techniques. Vet Clin North Am Small Anim Pract 1990;20:67.

32. Pavletic MM. Tension relieving techniques. In: Atlas of small animal wound management and reconstructive surgery. 3rd edition. Ames (IA): Wiley-Blackwell; 2010. p. 242.

33. Swaim SF, Henderson RA. Management of skin tension. In: Small animal wound management. 2nd edition. Batimore (MD): Williams and Wilkins; 1997.

34. Pavletic MM. Pedicle grafts. In: Slatter DH, editor. Textbook of small animal surgery, vol. 1. 2nd edition. Philadelphia: W.B. Saunders; 2002. p. 292.

35. Trevor P, Smith M, Waldron D, et al. Clinical evaluation of axial pattern skin flaps in dogs and cats: 19 cases (1981–1990). J Am Vet Med Assoc 1992;201:608.

36. Myers M. Wound tension and vascularity in the etiology and prevention of skin sloughs. Surgery 1964;56:945.

37. Nathanson SE, Jackson RT. Blood flow measurements in skin flaps. Arch Otolaryngol Head Neck Surg 1975;101:354.

38. Reetz JA, Seiler G, Mayhew PD, et al. Ultrasonographic and color-flow Doppler ultrasonographic assessment of direct cutaneous arteries used for axial pattern skin flaps in dogs. J Am Vet Med Assoc 2006;228:1361.

39. Pavletic MM. Misapplication of subcutaneous pedicle flaps in the dog. Vet Surg 1982;11:18.

40. Kerrigan CL, Daniel RK. Monitoring acute skin-flap failure. Plast Reconstr Surg 1983;71:519.

41. Kerwin S, Hosgood G, Strain G, et al. The effect of hyperbaric oxygen treatment on a compromised axial pattern flap in the cat. Vet Surg 1993;22:31.

42. Batchelor A, Davison P, Sully L. The salvage of congested skin flaps by the application of leeches. Br J Plast Surg 1984;37:358.

43. Whitlock M, O'hare P, Sanders R, et al. The medicinal leech and its use in plastic surgery: a possible cause for infection. Br J Plast Surg 1983;36:240.

44. Lawrence C, Prinzen F, De Lange S. The effect of dexmedetomidine on nutrient organ blood flow. Anesth Analg 1996;83:1160.

45. Swaim SF. Skin grafts. In: Slatter DH, editor. Textbook of small animal surgery, vol. 1. 2nd edition. Philadelphia: W.B. Saunders; 2002. p. 321.

46. White RAS. Skin grafting. In: Fowler D, Williams JM, editors. Manual of anine and feline wound management and reconstruction. Shurdington (UK): BSAVA; 1999. p. 83.

47. Shahar R, Shamir M, Brehm D, et al. Free skin grafting for treatment of distal limb skin defects in cats. J Small Anim Pract 1999;40:378.

48. Siegfiried R, Schmokel H, Rytz U, et al. Treatment of large distal extremity skin wounds with autogenous full-thickness mesh skin grafts in 5 cats. Schweizer Archiv fur Tierheilkunde 2004;146:277.

49. Guille AE, Tseng LW, Orsher RJ. Use of vacuum-assisted closure for management of a large skin wound in a cat. J Am Vet Med Assoc 2007;230:1669.

50. Ben-Amotz R, Lanz O, Miller J, et al. The use of vacuum-assisted closure therapy for the treatment of distal extremity wounds in 15 dogs. Vet Surg 2007;36:684.

51. Schneider AM, Morykwas MJ, Argenta LC. A new and reliable method of securing skin grafts to the difficult recipient bed. Plast Reconstr Surg 1998;102:1195.

52. Swaim SF. Surgery of the traumatized skin: management and reconstruction in the dog and cat. Philadelphia: W. B. Saunders, 1980.

53. Waris T. Degeneration and regeneration of nerves in a dorsal skin flap in the rat. Scand J Plast Reconstr Surg Hand Surg 1978;12:95.
54. Waris T, Astrand K, Hamalainen H, et al. Regeneration of cold, warmth and heat-pain sensibility in human skin grafts. Br J Plast Surg 1989;42:576.
55. Weiss-Becker C, Fruhstorfer H, Friederich HC, et al. Reinnervation of split skin grafts in humans: comparison of two different methods of operation. Scand J Plast Reconstr Surg Hand Surg 1998;32:157.
56. Lascelles B, Thomson M, Dernell W, et al. Combined dorsolateral and intraoral approach for the resection of tumors of the maxilla in the dog. J Am Anim Hosp Assoc 2003;39:294.
57. Clarke B, L'Eplattenier H. Zygomatic salivary mucocoele as a postoperative complication following caudal hemimaxillectomy in a dog. J Small Anim Pract 2010;51:495.
58. Schwarz P, Withrow S, Curtis C, et al. Partial maxillary resection as a treatment for oral cancer in 61 dogs. J Am Anim Hosp Assoc 1991;27:617.
59. Salisbury S, Thacker H, Pantzer E, et al. Partial maxillectomy in the dog comparison of suture materials and closure techniques. Vet Surg 1985;14:265.
60. Matthiesen D, Manfra M. Results and complications associated with partial mandibulectomy and maxillectomy techniques. Probl Vet Med 1990;2:248.
61. Bryant K, Moore K, McAnulty J. Angularis oris axial pattern buccal flap for reconstruction of recurrent fistulae of the palate. Vet Surg 2003;32:113.
62. Sivacolundhu R. Use of local and axial pattern flaps for reconstruction of the hard and soft palate. Clin Techn Small Anim Pract 2007;22:61.
63. Smith M. Island palatal mucoperiosteal flap for repair of oronasal fistula in a dog. J Vet Dent 2001;18:127.
64. de Souza H, Amorim F, Corgozinho K, et al. Management of the traumatic oronasal fistula in the cat with a conical silastic prosthetic device. J Feline Med Surg 2005;7:129.
65. Smith M. Oronasal fistula repair. Clin Techn Small Anim Pract 2000;15:243.
66. Kramer A, Walsh P, Seguin B. Hemipelvectomy in dogs and cats: technique overview, variations, and description. Vet Surg 2008;37:413.
67. Karakousis C, Emrich L, Driscoll D. Variants of hemipelvectomy and their complications. Am J Surg 1989;158:404.
68. Straw R, Withrow S, Powers B. Partial or total hemipelvectomy in the management of sarcomas in nine dogs and two cats. Vet Surg 1992;21:183.
69. Kraybill W, Standiford S, Johnson F. Posthemipelvectomy hernia. J Surg Oncol 1992;51:38.

Complications of Minimally Invasive Surgery in Companion Animals

Philipp D. Mayhew, BVM&S, MRCVS

KEYWORDS
- Complications • Surgery • Laparoscopy • Thoracoscopy
- Minimally invasive

Minimally invasive surgery (MIS) has become increasingly popular in recent years for diagnosis and treatment of an ever expanding list of disease processes in small animal patients. Reports in the veterinary literature have documented a large number of MIS alternatives to traditional open surgery albeit mostly in small cohorts of patients. In human medicine, a paradigm change from open to MIS procedures occurred in the late 1980s and early 1990s when procedures such as laparoscopic cholecystectomy (LC) were first described and subsequently taught to general surgeons in practice. Significant advantages of MIS have been documented by many investigators and include significant decreases in postoperative pain, length of hospital stay, and analgesic requirements, as well as many other types of morbidity with some procedures now being performed on an outpatient basis.[1–3] Along with these advantages, however, has come a recognition that MIS procedures are not without surgical morbidity and in some cases may be associated with higher levels or different types of complications compared to open surgery. An example of this was the increased incidence of common bile duct lacerations, a rare complication of open cholecystectomy, which became more prevalent during the early learning curve for LC.[4]

In veterinary medicine, the field of MIS is still very much in its infancy and further evidence-based studies need to focus on larger patient cohorts evaluated prospectively to document in detail the complications that are associated with different procedures. Some evidence exists in veterinary patients to support the hypothesis that MIS may decrease the severity or incidence of certain morbidities compared to open surgery. Ovariohysterectomy and pericardectomy models have been used to demonstrate a decrease in postoperative pain after MIS compared to open surgery.[5,6] A more rapid return to normal postoperative activity has been documented using

Disclosure: The author has nothing to disclose.
School of Veterinary Medicine, Department of Surgical and Radiological Sciences, University of California-Davis, One Shields Avenue, Davis, CA 95616, USA
E-mail address: philmayhew@gmail.com

accelerometry in canine laparoscopy-assisted ovariectomy and gastropexy models.[7,8] In addition, there is some evidence that the incidence of postoperative surgical site infections may be decreased in veterinary patients undergoing MIS procedures.[9] These studies have begun to provide evidence to support the use of MIS in veterinary patients, but a great deal more work is required to evaluate the morbidity associated with the wide range of MIS procedures now being performed in the veterinary field.

ANESTHESIA-RELATED COMPLICATIONS IN MIS

Although both laparoscopic and thoracoscopic procedures are generally well tolerated in small animals there are several important physiological alterations unique to these interventions that should be taken into consideration when performing anesthesia for MIS.

Creation of a pneumoperitoneum is central to most laparoscopic procedures in order to create a working space in which to operate. Alternatives to pneumoperitoneum such as gasless laparoscopy or "lift" laparoscopy have been evaluated in both human and veterinary studies but have not gained widespread use to date.[10,11] Pneumoperitoneum is usually created by insufflation of the abdomen with CO_2. CO_2 has several favorable characteristics as an insufflating agent: it is inexpensive, noninflammable, colorless, and rapidly excreted. Nitrous oxide has been proposed as an alternative for abdominal insufflations, but N_2O is capable of supporting combustion and so its use in combination with any electrocautery device is dangerous. Helium has been shown to produce less peritoneal inflammation than CO_2 and may have a protective effect against port site metastasis compared to CO_2.[10] Thus, although CO_2 insufflation is considered the current standard of care, alternative gases such as helium may gain greater clinical use in the future.

Physiological changes induced by CO_2 pneumoperitoneum are largely the result of 2 mechanisms: the rapid absorption of CO_2 across the peritoneal membrane and the compressive effect of pneumoperitoneum on the diaphragm. Pressure on the diaphragm will decrease tidal volume and effective ventilation especially at higher pressure (>20 mm Hg).[12] Excessively high $PaCO_2$ stimulates catecholamine release, which increases heart rate, arterial blood pressure, and cardiac output, leading eventually to severe acidosis and possibly arrythmias.[13,14] Monitoring the adequacy of ventilation through end-tidal capnography and/or blood gas analysis, is therefore an essential component of anesthetic monitoring during laparoscopy. Positive-pressure ventilation with a mechanical ventilator is essential for control of ventilatory rate and maintenance of tidal volume in animals under general anesthesia. Other effects of increased intra-abdominal pressure (IAP) include depression of cardiac output, increases in systemic vascular resistance, and a decrease in hepatic blood flow.[15] These parameters were adversely affected at IAPs of 16 mm Hg but not 12 mm Hg in one canine study.[15] Gas embolism is a rare but potentially fatal consequence of high-pressure pneumoperitoneum or the direct inoculation of gases into vascular spaces during laparoscopic access and insufflation.[16] For these reasons, it is generally recommended that IAP be carefully monitored intraoperatively with the use of a mechanical insufflator and that IAP should not exceed 12 to 15 mm Hg.[12–15] In reality a very good working space can usually be obtained at IAPs of 8 to 12 mm Hg.

During thoracoscopy, trocar-cannula assemblies that lack a one-way valve are generally used so that upon entry of the first cannula into the chest a pneumothorax will form. Some thoracoscopic interventions can be performed using the working space that is created by a pneumothorax alone. This is generally true for simpler procedures such as diagnostic thoracoscopy procedures, creation of a pericardial windows (PW), or thoracic duct ligation (TDL).[17–19] For these types of procedure, complications of anesthesia are expected to be similar to those associated with "open" thoracotomy.

To increase the working space during more advanced thoracoscopic procedures, thoracic insufflation or one-lung ventilation (OLV) are generally used. Examples of procedures where OLV is considered either highly desirable or mandatory include lung lobectomy and cranial mediastinal mass resection. Thoracic insufflation even at low intrathoracic pressures (3 mm Hg), causes significant cardiopulmonary depression and is therefore not used frequently.[20] In comparison, OLV is generally well tolerated although its use can also be associated with several important physiological changes as well as complications. A significant ventilation-perfusion mismatch occurs during OLV as a result of nonventilated lung tissue remaining perfused. Significant decreases in PaO_2, arterial oxygen content, and oxygen saturation occur, although none of these changes were deemed to be clinically significant in one study in normal dogs.[21] Various techniques can be used to create OLV including the use of bronchial blockers, selective intubation, or double-lumen endobronchial intubation.[22] Reports in the veterinary literature have mainly documented the use of endobronchial blockers[5,23,24] and double-lumen endobronchial intubation.[25–27] Regardless of which technique is used to establish OLV, great care needs to be taken monitoring anesthesia as significant intraoperative complications can arise. These can broadly be divided into physiological consequences of OLV and complications associated with physical movement of the tube or blocker intraoperatively. The most common physiological effects of OLV have been discussed and are generally not clinically significant in normal animals, but may become so in patients with significant cardiopulmonary disease.[21,22] Intraoperative tube or blocker displacement most commonly results in loss of OLV intraoperatively, impairing the surgeon's ability to complete the procedure. Bronchoscopy-guided replacement of the tube or blocker into the correct position will usually be required to remedy this situation. Less commonly, if a bronchial blocker or DLT slips cranially out of the mainstem bronchus into the trachea, it is possible for an acute airway obstruction to occur, resulting in total cessation of ventilation. This must be noticed immediately and will necessitate tube repositioning. Placing the OLV tube in the operating room rather than in the anesthesia preparation area will minimize movement of the patient and minimize risk of initial displacement.[24] After placement, every effort should be made by both surgeon and anesthetist to minimize movement of the patient. A further complication associated with endobronchial blockers and DLTs is bronchial wall damage associated with excessive bronchial cuff pressures. Small-volume bronchial cuff injection has been shown to increase cuff pressures dramatically and substantial variation in cuff pressures across different tube types exists.[28] Using low-pressure/high-volume cuffs such as the Rusch double-lumen tube is likely to be preferable to other tubes that exert higher cuff pressures.[28] Although cuff injuries have not been reported to date in the veterinary literature, bronchial ischemia and necrosis, pneumothorax, and pneumomediastinum have been reported in humans after OLV. To decrease this risk, it is advised that appropriate sized tubes are used, that patients are not moved with the cuff in place without deflating it, and that prolonged intubation be avoided as much as possible.[29]

COMPLICATIONS ASSOCIATED WITH LAPAROSCOPIC AND THORACOSCOPIC ACCESS

The first step in any laparoscopic or thoracoscopic procedure is safe access into the peritoneal or pleural cavity. There are a number of different techniques available for achieving access, but intrinsic to any technique is the possibility of iatrogenic damage

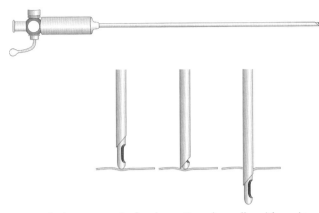

Fig. 1. A Veress needle is composed of a sharp-tipped needle with an inner spring-loaded blunt-tipped obturator. As the needle is inserted into the peritoneal cavity, the sharp needle penetrates the body wall. As soon as body wall resistance is lost, the blunt obturator springs forward to prevent iatrogenic penetration of viscera.

to intracavitary structures during initial port placement. In human laparoscopy it has been shown that initial access to the peritoneal cavity is the most dangerous step in any laparoscopic procedure. One large study of 103,852 cases showed that 82% of vascular injuries and 75% of visceral injuries occur at the time of first trocar insertion.[30]

In small animal laparoscopy, 2 main options exist for abdominal access; the open (Hasson) technique and the closed (Veress needle) technique. A third option called "optical entry" uses specialized disposable trocar-cannula assemblies that allow the telescope to be placed into the trocar during inserting thus allowing visualization of the tissue planes during passage through the body wall. Optical entry is gaining popularity in human surgery but is currently limited in veterinary applications by the high cost of the specialized single-use disposable trocar-cannula assemblies required.

Using the Hasson technique, a mini-laparotomy is created at a subumbilical location and a blunt trocar is used to insert the first cannula for introduction of the telescope. A Veress needle is a specialized instrument that uses a spring loaded, blunt-tipped obturator housed within a sharp-tipped needle component. The sharp component of the needle will penetrate the body wall whose resistance will force the blunt obturator to retract into the shaft (**Fig. 1**). Upon penetration of the body wall, however, resistance is lost, allowing the blunt-tipped obturator to spring forward thereby shielding the abdominal viscera from injury (see **Fig. 1**).

Several large studies have shown that iatrogenic injuries to abdominal structures occur with slightly greater frequency after use of closed techniques when compared to open.[30-32] However, the Veress needle is still used far more commonly due to its perceived speed, decreased incidence of air leakage, and smaller associated incision size. In one recent human study, only 2.5% of 500,179 laparoscopy cases were performed using an open Hasson technique.[30] In veterinary species different challenges exist with regard to laparoscopic access. Most small animals have substantially less fat deposits around the umbilical site than humans do, making an open Hasson technique simpler. However, use of the open and closed approaches has remained largely a personal choice among veterinary surgeons with studies of

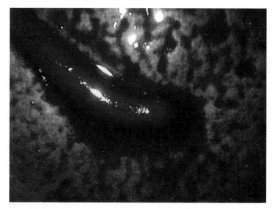

Fig. 2. A curvilinear laceration can be seen on the surface of the spleen. This type of injury is typical for trocar-associated lacerations that occur during placement of the first trocar-cannula assembly or from careless cannula manipulation during surgery.

laparoscopic procedures, being fairly evenly split between the 2 techniques. No large veterinary studies exist comparing the different access techniques in cats and dogs, although access-related complications have been reported.[7,16,33–35]

Splenic laceration is the most frequently reported access injury in cats and dogs with incidences of 3% to 18% being reported in several small studies.[7,33–35] In the majority of cases, splenic laceration occurs in association with initial Veress needle or trocar insertion (**Fig. 2**). Other mechanisms of iatrogenic splenic laceration include inadvertent pressure during instrument manipulation or the blind movement of deeply positioned cannulae, the tips of which may come into contact with the spleen during manipulation. It is rare for a splenic laceration to result in bleeding that is of hemodynamic significance to the patient, and conversion to open abdominal surgery or treatment with blood products is very rarely required after this complication. However, any form of hemorrhage within the peritoneal cavity adversely affects visualization and has been shown to extend surgical time in an ovariectomy model.[35] Generally, the splenic laceration should be located and observed until cessation of the bleeding has occurred. If necessary, a small piece of oxidized regenerated cellulose (Surgicel) can be placed over the area. In rare cases, if the hemorrhage is severe, conversion to an open approach is reasonable and partial or complete splenectomy may be indicated.

Injury to visceral organs is another important access-related injury in human laparoscopy and has been shown to occur in 0.06% to 0.083% of cases.[30–32] Veress needle entry was statistically more likely to result in visceral injury compared to the open approach in one human study.[31] These injuries result in conversion to an open approach in approximately 65% of cases.[30] In small animals, to the author's knowledge, no reports of visceral injury during access have been described, possibly due to the more frequent use of open techniques in small animal species.

Even less information is available with regard to the incidence of access injury during thoracoscopic interventions in small animals. In general, the first portal established is either a paraxiphoid or an intercostal portal. Injuries during paraxiphoid port placement have not been reported in small animals, possibly because of the lack of large vascular structures close to this entry site. When the initial portal is intercostal or indeed when further instrument ports are placed intercostally after placement of the telescope portal, incising in the middle of the intercostal space is imperative to avoid iatrogenic damage to the intercostal artery and vein that run parallel and caudal to each rib. Bleeding from intercostal vessels can be profuse and will generally not cease spontaneously.[23,24] In these cases placement of a circumcostal suture proximal and distal to the bleeding vessel is usually necessary. Direct injury to underlying lung parenchyma during first trocar placement is possible despite the lungs tending to fall away from the thoracic wall as soon as a pneumothorax forms. If a blunt trocar is used, contact with lung tissue is unlikely to cause iatrogenic damage. For intercostal trocar insertion, the use of blunt dissection through the thoracic wall prior to insertion of the trocar-cannula assembly may help to reduce iatrogenic damage to blood vessels and lung parenchyma during entry.

COMPLICATIONS SPECIFIC TO LAPAROSCOPIC TECHNIQUES

Diagnostic laparoscopy has been used for many years for the collection of samples from a variety of organs in the abdomen. Laparoscopic or laparoscopy-assisted biopsy of the liver, kidney, pancreas, gastrointestinal tract, spleen, and mesenteric lymph node are all techniques that are used frequently.[36–41] Laparoscopic liver biopsy can result in significant hemorrhage, although rarely is it severe enough to warrant intervention. It has been described using laparoscopic cup biopsy forceps or an Harmonic Scalpel, and both techniques have been shown to be associated with little hemorrhage in healthy dogs.[39,40] A vessel-sealing device was shown to decrease bleeding from a liver biopsy site in one study compared to cup biopsy forceps.[40] The possibility of more severe hemorrhage should not be discounted as one clinical study of diagnostic laparoscopic procedures reported that emergent conversion to an open approach was required in 6.3% of the cases due to bleeding complications.[42] Splenic biopsy was recently described using a 5-mm cup biopsy forceps in a cohort of 15 dogs and cats and was not associated with excessive hemorrhage or the need for conversion in any patient.[41] Segments of gelatin sponge were placed at the surgical site to aid in hemostasis.[41] Biopsy of the gastrointestinal tract has thus far only been described using a laparoscopy-assisted technique.[36] Laparoscopy-assisted intestinal resection and anastomosis for removal of mass lesions from the small or large intestines have been reported in 2 dogs and 2 cats and were not associated with any complications.[43] Since that time the author has performed several more laparoscopy-assisted intestinal mass resections and found that conversion to open laparotomy can become necessary when the mass has adhesions to surrounding organs or the margins of the mass cannot be clearly visualized.

Laparoscopic sterilization was first described by Wildt in 1985.[44] Since then, a large number of laparoscopic ovariohysterectomy (OVH) and ovariectomy (OVE) techniques have been described in the literature,[6,8,33–35,45–48] using a variety of port configurations and hemostatic techniques for pedicle ligation. Postoperative pain has been shown to be reduced when fewer ports are used,[49] and several reports have shown an apparent improvement in pain scores and postoperative activity in animals after laparoscopic sterilization compared to those undergoing an open surgical technique.[6,8] The most commonly reported complication of laparoscopic sterilization procedures is hemorrhage associated with pedicle ligation. The use of a vessel-sealing device has been shown to reduce hemorrhage in comparison to extracorporeal ligation or clip application, although in all cases bleeding was judged to be clinically inconsequential.[34] Bipolar electrocoagulation has also been shown to be superior to either monopolar electrocoagulation or the use of an Nd:Yag laser in prevention of mesovarial bleeding during laparoscopic OVE.[47,48]

Gastropexy has been used for many years to prevent the occurrence or recurrence of gastric-dilation volvulus (GDV) syndrome in dogs. Recently, several minimally invasive gastropexy techniques have been described and evaluated. The laparoscopy-assisted gastropexy described by Rawlings and others has been evaluated most rigorously and is associated with a very low incidence of complications.[50,51] Initial occurrence of abscessation at the site of the body wall incision occurred in a small number of dogs but was judged to be associated with a technical error where full-thickness stay sutures in the stomach were retained in the final wound closure.[50] Once these stay sutures were no longer used and the partial-thickness gastric seromuscular incision was sutured without gastric penetration, this complication appears to have been alleviated.[50] Seroma formation is probably the most common complication of laparoscopy-assisted gastopexy but is usually self-limiting. Risk of seroma formation can be minimized by careful apposition of all body wall layers, thus eliminating dead space. Long-term evaluation of laparoscopy-assisted gastropexy has been performed in 20 dogs, and in all cases the gastropexy was intact on ultrasonographic evaluation at 1 year postoperatively.[51] In one study comparing the laparoscopy-assisted technique to an intracorporeally sutured totally laparoscopic technique, the laparoscopy-assisted gastropexy was shown to be a faster technique but was associated with a somewhat slower return to normal activity postoperatively.[7] A variety of other minimally invasive gastropexy techniques have been evaluated, but no studies have directly compared the surgical morbidity of one technique to that of another.

A technique for laparoscopy-assisted cystotomy was first described in 2003 and has since undergone a number of modifications.[52] There are few reported technique-specific complications associated with laparoscopy-assisted cystotomy, although no studies have compared the technique to traditional cystotomy with regard to completeness of urolith removal or long-term recurrence of urolithiasis post-treatment.

As more advanced laparoscopic techniques are developed in veterinary medicine and greater case numbers are evaluated, more information concerning the surgical morbidity of these techniques will emerge. Advanced techniques that are already in use include laparoscopic cholecystectomy, adrenalectomy, and ureteronephrectomy. Although early experience has been encouraging, very small numbers of cases have been reported in dogs so limited conclusions can be drawn from these studies with regard to morbidity.[53,54]

COMPLICATIONS SPECIFIC TO THORACOSCOPIC PROCEDURES

A number of thoracoscopic techniques have now been described in small animals including pericardial window formation,[5,25] subphrenic pericardectomy,[17,27] lung lobectomy,[24,55,56] thoracic duct ligation,[19,23] ligation of patent ductus arteriosus,[57] resection of vascular ring anomalies,[58] and cranial mediastinal mass resection.[26] Anesthetic complications have been discussed above but constitute an important source of potential morbidity and can be associated with any thoracoscopic procedure.

PW formation was one of the first described thoracoscopic techniques used in veterinary medicine and can easily be performed in most breeds without OLV. In some breeds with very low thoracic depth-to-width ratios (eg, brachycephalic breeds), lack of working space can provide a significant challenge and care must be taken not to cause iatrogenic damage to lung parenchyma during the procedure. In brachycephalic breeds, the author has found that OLV may still be helpful even for PW creation. PW is used to treat neoplasia-associated as well as idiopathic pericardial effusion.

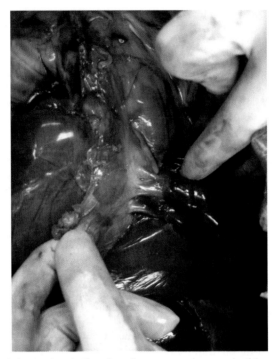

Fig. 3. An iatrogenic laceration to the phrenic nerve can be seen in this necropsy image. This occurred during a subphrenic pericardectomy procedure. Visualization of the phrenic nerve must be maintained at all times to avoid this complication.

Complications of this technique can include lung laceration, phrenic nerve transsection, and hemorrhage, although all are uncommon.[25] Iatrogenic damage to the underlying epicardium or coronary vessels during dissection is a possibility, and care needs to be taken, especially if a vessel-sealing device is used for tissue transsection. These devices are very helpful to minimize hemorrhage but all have some degree of lateral thermal spread, so elevation of the device above the level of the epicardium is important to avoid thermal damage to underlying structures. Recurrence of pericardial effusion due to stenosis of the window or adhesion of the pericardium back onto the epicardium appears to be uncommon after this procedure.[17,25] Thoracoscopic subphrenic pericardectomy has now also been described in dogs both with and without one-lung ventilation.[17,27] This technique is similar to the PW although an effort is made to remove all pericardial tissue ventral to the phrenic nerve. This may increase the likelihood of iatrogenic damage to the phrenic nerve (**Fig. 3**), a complication that has been described in one experimental study in dogs.[27] Iatrogenic damage to the atrial appendages must also be avoided during this procedure. A thoracoscopic technique for right atrial mass resection after pericardectomy was recently documented using the EndoGIA stapler in a dog.[59] Small well-circumscribed masses involving the right atrial appendage may be resected in this fashion, but just as in open surgery, it may be challenging to achieve a complete margin of resection.[59]

Thoracoscopic lung lobectomy (TLL) has been described for management of primary and metastatic lung masses as well as resection of pulmonary blebs/bullae associated with spontaneous pneumothorax.[24,56] This exciting new technique has the potential to significantly reduce morbidity in comparison with open thoracotomy for lung lobectomy. In humans advantages of TLL include a reduced volume of thoracic drainage, decreased postoperative pain, shorter hospital stays, and a more rapid return to normal function.[1,60] One experimental report of lung biopsy and complete lobectomy using OLV did not report any surgical complications in 8 healthy dogs.[55] In a subsequent clinical study, TLL was used for lung tumor removal in 9 dogs.[24] Successful thoracoscopic resection was achieved in 5/9 dogs, while conversion to an open technique was required in 4 dogs.[24] Conversion was required in these dogs was due to loss of visibility secondary to bleeding from an intercostal artery in 1 dog, loss of intraoperative OLV in 2 dogs, and difficulty accessing the right middle lung lobe in 1 dog.[24] No significant complications were seen in the dogs in which a TLL was completed without conversion. With such little data to evaluate it is unclear whether TLL will have a significant effect on morbidity and mortality levels compared to open surgical resection in veterinary patients. Case selection for TLL, as for most other MIS techniques, is the key to success. Smaller and more peripherally located masses are most likely to be resectable using thoracoscopy, especially in the early part of a surgeon's learning curve.[24] With greater experience of the surgical technique as well as OLV, it is likely that a greater proportion of cases will become amenable to TLL.

A minimally invasive thoracic duct ligation technique was first evaluated in dogs by Radlinsky,[23] and the results of the technique have since been reported in small numbers of clinical cases.[19,61] A significant complication of this technique may be the failure to ligate all branches of the thoracic duct, although this problem can equally occur after open thoracic duct ligation.[23,62] No studies have directly compared the efficacy of thoracic duct ligation after thoracoscopic surgery to that obtained using open techniques. Early data suggest that success, as defined by resolution of pleural effusion and clinical signs, may be similar between techniques, although a controlled prospective clinical study will be required to confirm this.[19,61]

Several other thoracoscopic techniques have been described in very small numbers of animals including ligation of persistent ductus arteriosus and vascular ring anomalies as well as thymoma resection.[26,57,58] All of these advanced techniques require careful case selection and experience in MIS. Further studies are required to evaluate the level of morbidity and mortality involved to be able to accurately assess whether they offer a significant advantage over traditional "open" techniques.

CONVERSION FROM MIS TO OPEN TECHNIQUES

Conversion from a minimally invasive to an open approach may be necessary for a variety of different reasons, and conversion rates are often reported in studies describing various MIS procedures. Two types of conversion exist: "emergent conversions" in which an intraoperative complication occurs that cannot be remedied without open access and "elective conversions" where a complication has not occurred but an MIS approach will not allow the procedure to be completed.[63] In humans, the conversion rates and risk factors for conversion have been reported for many different laparoscopic and thoracoscopic procedures. General factors that may predispose patients to conversion of MIS procedures include a diagnosis of malignancy, increasing patient body weight or body condition score, and surgeon experience.[63]

The conversion rate in a cohort of diagnostic laparoscopic procedures performed at a single institution in 94 dogs and cats was 21% with 65% of these being judged to be elective conversions and 35% judged to be emergent conversions.[42] The most common reasons for elective conversions were poor visibility due to adhesions and the presence of solitary tumors that were presumably not judged to be resectable by laparoscopy. Emergent conversions were due to hemorrhage from organ biopsy or trocar insertion along with a single case of iatrogenic biliary tract rupture.[42]

Reports of conversion rates for therapeutic laparoscopic procedures in the veterinary literature mostly involve small numbers of cases of simpler laparoscopy-assisted interventions and are generally low. As practitioners gradually take on more complex techniques, we may find that both complication and conversion rates gradually start to increase.

Conversion is also necessary in a subset of individuals undergoing thoracoscopic surgery. In humans, thoracoscopic procedures were associated with a 17% overall complication rate in one large study of 1066 procedures.[64] The conversion rate to open surgery was 1.7%.[65] It is well recognized that in human medicine a learning curve exists with thoracoscopic procedures and that, generally, operative experience in 30 to 60 cases is required before factors such as perioperative blood loss and operative time start to decrease.[65,66] In veterinary patients, thoracoscopic pericardectomy, lung lobectomy, and thoracic duct ligation are the only procedures in which case series with significant numbers of clinical cases have been reported. One report of thoracoscopic lung lobectomy in dogs was associated with a significant early conversion rate, although 2 of 4 conversions were directly related to loss of OLV intraoperatively.[24]

In all MIS cases, appropriate criteria for conversion to an open surgical approach should be established by the surgical team. These might include a time limit set on adequate progress being made intraoperatively. If timely completion is not achieved, then conversion is performed. Anesthetic complications or equipment malfunction should also be seen as a reason to convert. Finally, emergent conversion should always be performed if life-threatening complications occur. In all cases where an MIS procedure is being performed, the possibility of conversion should be considered and discussed with the owners prior to surgery. Surgeons should have prior experience with the open version of the procedure and the patient should be prepared as for open surgery, so that if conversion becomes necessary, it can be performed immediately. Equipment necessary for an open surgical approach should also be available on the sterile equipment table.

POSTOPERATIVE COMPLICATIONS

Port-site complications after MIS procedures are generally associated either with seroma formation, surgical site infection (SSI), or, rarely, herniation. Seroma formation is possible at any surgical site if dead space is not adequately eliminated and has been reported in dogs after laparoscopic sterilization.[33,45] In humans, numerous studies have compared SSI rates after MIS to those seen after open procedures and most have concluded that use of an MIS is associated with a reduction in the rate of SSI.[67–69] In veterinary patients, less data are available, but one study has reported that MIS procedures may have a lower SSI rate compared to open surgery in dogs and cats.[9] Of 558 patients in this study, the open surgery group had a 5.5% SSI rate compared to a 1.7% SSI rate in the MIS group.[9] Care should be taken in interpretation of this data, however, as an MIS approach was significantly associated with SSI rate only on univariate analysis of the data. Herniation of thoracic or abdominal contents through port incisions is rare but has been reported with the use of port sites as small as 5 mm (**Fig. 4**).[45] For this reason, it is advised to close the fascial sheath of the body wall in all port closures that involve incisions of 5 mm or greater.

Port-site metastasis is a potential complication when neoplastic lesions are resected and withdrawn through small portal incisions. Metastasis of a pericardial

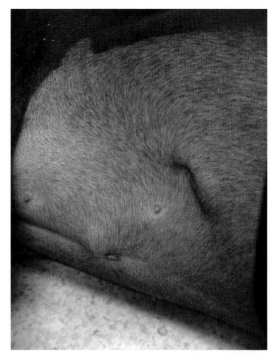

Fig. 4 Herniation of tissue can be seen at the subumbilical site of a 5-mm laparoscopic portal after a laparoscopy-assisted gastropexy procedure had been performed (the gastropexy site can also be seen in a paramedian location). Closure of the fascial layer of the body wall is recommended at all portal sites that are 5 mm or greater to avoid this complication.

mesothelioma to a port site after thoracoscopic PW has been described in the veterinary literature.[70] This process was initially considered to be a result of direct inoculation of neoplastic cells during traumatic extirpation of tissue through small port incisions. However, it was found that the use of specimen retrieval bags to remove neoplastic or infected tissue, although highly recommended, does not completely prevent port-site metastasis. There is now general recognition that a more complex interplay of factors such as the local immune response, pneumo-peritoneum, and surgical technique may all play a role in the etiopathogenesis of port site metastasis.[71]

SUMMARY

MIS is an exciting new field in veterinary medicine, which in time will transform the standard of care for a substantial subset of surgical patients. At this time, the process of establishing which procedures lend themselves well to an MIS approach is ongoing. Surgical morbidity is always a major concern and all MIS procedures can be associated with access, anesthesia, and procedure-specific morbidity, especially when surgeons are at an early stage in their learning curve. Veterinary surgeons must continue to be diligent in reporting the success and complication rates of MIS procedures to allow more evidence-based analysis of surgical morbidity and mortality as this field continues to develop.

REFERENCES

1. Lee J, El-Tamer M, Schifftner T, et al. Open and laparoscopic adrenalectomy: Analysis of the national surgical improvement program. J Am Coll Surg 2008;206: 953–61.
2. Villamizar NR, Darrabie MD, Burfeind WR, et al. Thoracoscopic lobectomy is associated with lower morbidity compared with thoracotomy. J Thorac Cardiovasc Surg 2009;138:419–25.
3. Calland JF, Tanaka K, Foley E, et al. Outpatient laparoscopic cholecystectomy: Patient outcomes after implementation of a clinical pathway. Ann Surg 2001;233: 704–15.
4. Deziel DJ, Millikan KW, Economou SG, et al. Complications of laparoscopic cholecystectomy: A national survey of 4292 hospitals and an analysis of 77,604 cases. Am J Surg 1993;165:9–14.
5. Walsh PJ, Remedios AM, Ferguson JF, et al. Thoracoscopic versus open partial pericardectomy in dogs: comparison of post-operative pain and morbidity. Vet Surg 1999;28:472–9.
6. Devitt CM, Cox RE, Hailey JJ. Duration, complications, stress, and pain of open ovariohysterectomy versus a simple method of laparoscopic-assisted ovariohysterectomy in dogs. J Am Vet Med Assoc 2005;227:921–7.
7. Mayhew PD, Brown DC. Prospective evaluation of two intra-corporeally sutured prophylactic laparoscopic gastropexy techniques compared to laparoscopic-assisted gastropexy in dogs. Vet Surg 2009;38:738–46.
8. Culp WTN, Mayhew PD, Brown DC. The effect of laparoscopic versus open ovariectomy on postsurgical activity in small dogs. Vet Surg 2009;38:811–7.
9. Mayhew PD, Freeman LJ, Kwan T, Brown DC. Prospective comparison of postoperative wound infection rates after minimally invasive versus open surgery. In: Proceedings of the Veterinary Endoscopy Society Annual Meeting. Cancun, Mexico; 2009. p. 35.
10. Neuhaus SJ, Gupta A, Watson DI. Helium and other alternative insufflation gases for laparoscopy. Surg Endosc 2001;15:553–60.
11. Fransson BA. Lift laparoscopy in small animals. In: Proceedings of the American College of Veterinary Surgeons Annual Symposium. Seattle (WA); 2010. p. 368–9.
12. Gross ME, Jones BD, Berstresser DR, et al. Effects of abdominal insufflation with nitrous oxide on cardiorespiratory measurements in spontaneously breathing isoflurane anesthetized dogs. Am J Vet Res 1993;54:1352–8.
13. Quandt JE. Anesthetic considerations for laser, laparoscopy and thoracoscopy procedures. Clin Tech Small Anim Pract 1999;14:50–5.
14. Weil AB. Anesthesia for Endoscopy in Small Animals. Vet Clin Small Anim 2009;39; 839–48.
15. Ishizaki Y, Bandai Y, Shimomura K, et al. Safe intraabdominal pressure of carbon dioxide pneumoperitoneum during laparoscopic surgery. Surgery 1993;114:549–54.
16. Gilroy BA, Anson LW. Fatal air embolism during anesthesia for laparoscopy in a dog. J Am Vet Med Assoc 1987;190:552–4.
17. Dupre GP, Corlouer JP, Bouvy B. Thoracoscopic pericardectomy performed without pulmonary exclusion in 9 dogs. Vet Surg 2001;30:21–7.
18. Kovak JR, Ludwig LL, Bergman PJ, et al. Use of thoracoscopy to determine the etiology of pleural effusion in dogs and cats: 18 cases (1998-2001). J Am Vet Med Assoc 2002;221:990–4.

19. Allman DA, Radlinsky MG, Ralph AG, et al. Thoracoscopic thoracic duct ligation and pericardectomy for treatment of chylothorax in dogs. Vet Surg 2010;39:21–7.
20. Daly CM, Swalec-Tobias K, Tobias AH, et al. Cardiopulmonary effects of intrathoracic insufflation in dogs. J Am Anim Hosp Assoc 2002;38:515–20.
21. Kudnig ST, Monnet E, Riquelme M, et al. Effect of one-lung ventilation on oxygen delivery in anesthetized dogs with an open thoracic cavity. Am J Vet Res 2003;64: 443–8.
22. Bailey JE, Pablo LS. Anesthetic and physiologic considerations for veterinary endo-surgery. In: Freeman LJ, editor. Veterinary endosurgery. 1st edition. St. Louis (MO): Mosby Inc; 1999. P. 85.
23. Radlinsky MG, Mason DE, Biller DS, et al. Thoracoscopic visualization and ligation of the thoracic duct in dogs. Vet Surg 2002;31:138–46.
24. Lansdowne JL, Monnet E, Twedt DC, et al. Thoracoscopic lung lobectomy for treatment of ling tumors in dogs. Vet Surg 2005;34:530–5.
25. Jackson J, Richter KP, Launer DP. Thoracoscopic partial pericardectomy in 13 dogs. J Vet Intern Med 1999;13:529–33.
26. Mayhew PD, Friedberg JS. Video-assisted thoracoscopic resection of non-invasive thymomas using single-lung ventilation in two dogs. Vet Surg 2008;37:756–62.
27. Mayhew KN, Mayhew PD, Sorrell-Raschi L, et al. Thoracoscopic sub-phrenic peri-cardectomy using double-lumen endobronchial intubation for alternating one-lung ventilation.Vet Surg 2009;38:961–6.
28. Brodsky JB, Adkins MO, Gaba DM. Bronchial cuff pressure of double-lumen tubes. Anesth Analg 1989;69:608–10.
29. Anantham D, Jagadesan R, Tiew PEC. Clinical review: Independent lung ventilation in critical care. Critical Care 2005;9:594–600.
30. Champault G, Cazacu F, Taffinder N. Serious trocar accidents in laparoscopic surgery: a French survey of 103,852 operations. Surg Laparosc Endosc 1996;6: 367–70.
31. Bonjer HJ, Hazebroeck EJ, Kazemier G, et al. Open versus closed establishment of pneumoperitoneum in laparoscopic surgery. Br J Surg 1997;84:599–602.
32. Catarci M, Carlini P, Gentileschi P, et al. Major and minor injuries during the creation of pneumoperitoneum. A multicenter study of 12,919 cases. Surg Endosc 2001;15: 566–9.
33. Davidson EB, Moll HD, Payton ME. Comparison of laparoscopic ovariohysterectomy and ovariohysterectomy in dogs. Vet Surg 2004;33:62–9.
34. Mayhew PD, Brown DC. Comparison of three techniques for ovarian pedicle hemo-stasis during laparoscopic-assisted ovariohysterectomy. Vet Surg 2007;36:541–7.
35. Dupre G, Fiorbianco V, Skalicky M, et al. Laparoscopic ovariectomy in dogs: Com-parison between single portal and two-portal access. Vet Surg 2009;38:818–24.
36. Rawlings CA, Howerth EW, Bement S, et al. Laparoscopic-assisted enterosotomy tube placement and full-thickness biopsy of the jejunum with serosal patching in dogs. Am J Vet Res 2002;63:1313–9.
37. Harmoinen J, Saari S, Rinkinen M, et al. Evaluation of pancreatic forceps biopsy by laparoscopy in healthy beagles. Vet Therapeutics 2002;3:31–6.
38. Rawlings CA, Diamond H, Howerth EW, et al. Diagnostic quality of percutaneous kidney biopsy specimens obtained with laparoscopy versus ultrasound guidance in dogs. J Am Vet Med Assoc 2003;223:317–21.
39. Rawlings CA, Howerth EW. Obtaining quality biopsies of the liver and kidney. J Am Anim Hosp Assoc 2004;40:352–8.
40. Barnes RF, Greenfield CL, Schaeffer DJ, et al. Comparison of biopsy samples obtained using standard endoscopic instruments and the harmonic scalpel during

laparoscopic and laparoscopic-assisted surgery in normal dogs. Vet Surg 2006;35:243–51.

41. Radhakrishnan A. Laparoscopic splenic biopsy in dogs and cats: 15 cases. In: Proceedings of the American College of Veterinary Surgeons Symposium. Seattle (WA); 2009. p. E48.

42. Buote NJ, Kovak-McClaran JR, Schold JD. Conversion from diagnostic laparoscopy to laparotomy: Risk factors and occurrence. Vet Surg 2011;40:106–14.

43. Gower S, Mayhew PD. Laparoscopic-assisted intestinal resection and anastomosis using a novel wound retraction device. In: Proceedings of the American College of Veterinary Surgeons Symposium. San Diego (CA); 2008. p. E14.

44. Wildt DE, Lawler DF. Laparoscopic sterilization of the bitch and queen by uterine horn occlusion. Am J Vet Res 1985;46:864–9.

45. Austin B, Lanz OI, Hamilton SM, et al. Laparoscopic ovariohysterectomy in nine dogs. J Am Anim Hosp Assoc 2003;39:391–6.

46. Hancock RB, Lanz OI, Waldron DR, et al. Comparison of postoperative pain after ovariohysterectomy by harmonic scalpel-assisted laparoscopy compared with median celiotomy and ligation in dogs. Vet Surg 2005;34:273–82.

47. Van Goethem B, Rosenvelt KW, Kirpensteijn J. Monopolar versus bipolar electrocoagulation in canine laparoscopic ovariectomy: a nonrandomized, prospective clinical trial. Vet Surg 2003;32:464–70.

48. Van Nimwegen SA, Van Swol CFP, Kirpensteijn J. Neodymium:yttrium aluminium garnet surgical laser versus bipolar electrocoagulation for laparoscopic ovariectomy in dogs. Vet Surg 2005;34:353–7.

49. Case JB, Marvel SJ, Boscan P, et al. Comparison of surgical time and post-operative pain among dogs fellowing laparoscopic ovariectomy with one, two or three instrument cannulas. In: Proceedings of the Veterinary Endoscopy Society Annual Meeting. Breckenridge (CO); 2010. p. 10.

50. Rawlings CA, Foutz TL, Mahaffey MB, et al. A rapid and strong laparoscopic-assisted gastropexy. Am J Vet Res 2001;62:871–5.

51. Rawlings CA, Mahaffey MB, Bement S. Prospective of laparoscopic-assisted gastropexy in dogs susceptible to gastric dilatation. J Am Vet Med Assoc 2002;221: 1576–81.

52. Rawlings CA, Mahaffey MB, Barsanti JA, et al. Use of laparoscopic-assisted cystoscopy for removal of urinary calculi in dogs. J Am Vet Med Assoc 2003;222:759–62.

53. Pelaez MJ, Bouvy BM, Dupre GP. Laparoscopic adrenalectomy for treatment of unilateral adrenocortical carcinomas: techniques, complications and results in seven dogs. Vet Surg 2008;37:444.

54. 54)Mayhew PD, Mehler SJ, Radhakrishnan A. Laparoscopic cholecystectomy of uncomplicated gall bladder mucocele in six dogs. Vet Surg 2008;37:555.

55. Garcia F, Prandi D, Pena T, et al. Examination of the thoracic cavity and lung lobectomy by means of thoracoscopy in dogs. Can Vet J 1998;39:285–91.

56. Brissot HN, Dupre GP, Bouvy BM, et al. Thoracoscopic treatment of bullous emphysema in 3 dogs. Vet Surg 2003;32:524–9.

57. Borenstein N, Behr L, Chetboul V, et al. Minimally invasive patent ductus arteriosus occlusion in 5 dogs. Vet Surg 2004;33:309–11.

58. MacPhail CM, Monnet E, Twedt DC. Thoracoscopic correction of a persistent right aortic arch in a dog. J Am Anim Hosp Assoc 2001;37:577–81.

59. Crumbaker DM, Rooney MB, Case JB. Thoracoscopic subtotal pericardectomy and right atrial mass resection in a dog. J Am Vet Med Assoc. 2010;237:551–4.

60. Stammberger U, Steinacher C, Hillinger S, et al. Early and long-term complaints following video-assisted thoracoscopic surgery: evaluation in 173 patients. Eur J Cardio-thorac Surg 2000;18:7–11.

61. Mayhew PD, Mayhew KN, Culp WTN, et al. Minimally invasive treatment of idiopathic chylothorax in four dogs. In: Proceedings of the Veterinary Endoscopy Society Annual Meeting. Cancun, Mexico; 2009. p. 31.

62. Birchard SJ, Cantwell HD, Bright RM. Lymphangiography and ligation of the canine thoracic duct: a study in normal dogs and three dogs with chylothorax. J Am Anim Hosp Assoc 1982;18:769–77.

63. Halpin VJ, Soper NJ. Decision to convert to open methods. In: Whelan RL, Fleashman JW, Fowler DL, editors. The SAGES manual of perioperative care in minimally invasive surgery. New York: Springer; 2006. p. 296–303.

64. Winter H, Meimarakis G, Pirker M, et al. Predictors of general complications after video-assisted thoracoscopic surgical procedures. Surg Endosc 2008;22:640–5.

65. Toker A, Tanju S, Ziyade S, et al. Learning curve in videothoracoscopic thymectomy: how many operations and in which situations? Eur J Cardiothoracic Surg 2008;34:155–8.

66. Zhao H, Bu L, Yang F, et al. Video-assisted thoracoscopic surgery lobectomy for lung cancer: The learning curve. World J Surg 2010;34:2368–72.

67. Biscione FM, Couto RC, Pedrosa TM, et al. Comparison of the risk of surgical site infection after laparoscopic cholecystectomy and open cholecystectomy. Infect Control Hosp Epidemiol 2007;28:1103–6.

68. Imai E, Ueda M, Kanao K, et al. Surgical site infection risk factors identified by multivariate analysis for patient undergoing laparoscopic, open colon and gastric surgery. Am J Infect Control 2008;36:727–31.

69. Sekhar N, Torquati A, Youssef T, et al. A comparison of 399 open and 568 laparoscopic gastric bypasses performed during a 4-year period. Surg Endosc 2007;21:665–8.

70. Brisson BA, Reggeti F, Bienzle D. Portal site metastasis of invasive mesothelioma after diagnostic thoracoscopy in a dog. J Am Vet Med Assoc 2006;229:980–3.

71. Castillo OA, Vitagliano G. Port site metastasis and tumor seeding in oncologic laparoscopic urology. Urology 2008;71:372–78.

Complications of Ovariohysterectomy and Orchiectomy in Companion Animals

Christopher A. Adin, DVM

KEYWORDS
- Spay • Neuter • Ovariohysterectomy • Orchiectomy
- Castration • Complications

Ovariohysterectomy (OVH) and orchiectomy are two of the most commonly performed surgeries in companion animal practice. Techniques for accomplishing surgical sterilization vary widely between geographic areas. While a ventral midline OVH is the standard technique in the United States, veterinarians in continental Europe commonly use a ventral midline ovariectomy, and practitioners in the United Kingdom perform flank OVH.[1] Interestingly, retrospective analyses have shown no significant differences in the rate of stump pyometra, urinary incontinence, or other complications when these techniques are compared, so there is no strong rationale to prefer one technique over another.[2–5] In fact, a recent prospective study showed that there were no significant differences in operative time or pain scores when ovariectomy was compared to OVH, calling into question the previous assertions that ovariectomy is faster and carries less morbidity.[6] Given the audience of the current publication, the author will refer to the OVH as the standard procedure in this text but will refer other techniques as indicated.

Given the frequency with which sterilization procedures are performed, it is not surprising that a number of complications have been described, including hemorrhage, wound healing complications, ovarian remnant syndrome,[7] stump pyometra, uterine stump abscess/granuloma formation,[8,9] obstipation,[10] ureteral trauma,[8,11–13] inadvertent prostatectomy,[14,15] vaginoperitoneal fistula formation,[16] enterocutaneous fistula formation,[17] gossypyboma,[17,18] and urinary incontinence.[19,20] Interestingly, the overall incidence of complications is high (around 20% in one representative study),[21] and when the incidence of common complications is compared between retrospective studies performed over time, it does not appear that any major

The author has nothing to disclose.
Department of Veterinary Clinical Sciences, College of Veterinary Medicine, The Ohio State University, 601 Vernon Tharp Street, Columbus, OH 43210, USA
E-mail address: adin.1@osu.edu

Vet Clin Small Anim 41 (2011) 1023–1039
doi:10.1016/j.cvsm.2011.05.004
0195-5616/11/$ – see front matter © 2011 Elsevier Inc. All rights reserved.

improvements have been made in the incidence of common postoperative complications over the past 30 years.[21–25]

COMPLICATIONS OF OVARIOHYSTERECTOMY
Hemorrhage

Hemorrhage has been described by some authors as the most common complication associated with OVH,[23,24] with a 79% incidence of intraoperative hemorrhage being reported in 1 group of 87 dogs greater than 50-lb body undergoing OVH at a teaching hospital.[24] In this same study, the rate of hemorrhage was only 2% in 290 dogs that were under 50-lb body weight, suggesting that large body size and intra-abdominal fat cause a significant increase in the risk of this complication. Other retrospective analyses of OVH reported a much lower rate of intraoperative hemorrhage, ranging from 4%[25] to 9%.[21] Specific criteria for characterizing hemorrhage are not described in any of these retrospective studies, and it is likely that some authors reported only clinically significant or major hemorrhage (dropped pedicle), while others reported any hemorrhage that was identified in the medical record. Despite these discrepancies in the prevalence of intraoperative bleeding, postoperative mortality due to ongoing hemorrhage is extremely rare. Not 1 of the 968 animals described in three retrospective studies of canine OVH was reported to have died due to postoperative hemorrhage and all but one were successfully addressed prior to abdominal closure.[21,24,25] Another study suggested that postoperative death due to hemorrhage occurred in 1 of 1016 dogs and in 1 of 1459 cats undergoing elective sterilization or declaw surgeries.[22] Given the low mortality reported in these and other published reports, it appears that intraoperative hemorrhage during OVH rarely translates into life-threatening postoperative hemorrhage.

Diagnosis/Therapy

Detection of intra-abdominal hemorrhage can be difficult, and clinical signs of intrahemorrhage after OVH involve nonspecific findings such as a slow recovery from anesthesia, pale mucous membranes, and tachycardia. A clinical observation is that many dogs with acute postoperative hemoperitoneum will leak large volumes of nonclotting, bloody fluid from the incision, a sign that may be mistakenly attributed to hemorrhage from subcutaneous vessels. Animals with the aforementioned signs should be examined for the presence of significant hemoperitoneum using ultrasound imaging and abdominocentesis. In the absence of an ultrasound machine, abdominocentesis can be performed blindly using 20-gauge needles placed in paramedian locations along the ventral abdomen, using appropriate aseptic technique. Insertion of the needles 3 to 4 cm from midline avoids the falciform ligament, which can clog the needle and prevent successful detection of fluid. Nonclotting abdominal fluid with a packed cell volume (PCV) that approximates or exceeds the animal's peripheral blood PCV is diagnostic for intra-abdominal hemorrhage. Prior to considering surgical intervention, coagulation testing should be considered. Depending upon the breed and history, evaluation of prothrombin time, activated partial thromboplastin time, buccal mucosal bleeding time, and platelet count should be performed, ruling out preexisting inherited or acquired defects in hemostasis, before considering surgical exploration. It is important to realize that elective sterilization surgery is often the first invasive procedure that is performed on an animal and would therefore be the most likely time for discovery of a congenital disorder in hemostasis. Using data obtained on physical examination, ultrasound examination, and hematologic testing, the clinician must decide whether intra-abdominal hemorrhage should be treated in a conservative manner (abdominal pressure bandage, intravenous fluid therapy) or by surgical exploration and religation of the pedicles. One recent report suggested that therapy with abdominal pressure bandages was successful in 3 of 4 dogs with postoperative bleeding, while surgery was required on 1 dog that failed conservative therapy.[21]

Avoidance

Intraoperative hemorrhage during ovariohysterectomy is most commonly associated with rupture of the right ovarian pedicle during attempted release of the suspensory ligament.[21] Occurrence of this complication has been attributed largely to rough tissue handling by novice surgeons, with many of the reports arising from teaching institutions where surgery is performed by fourth-year veterinary students.[21,24,25] One early study suggested no difference in complication rate when surgeries were performed by veterinary surgeons, although students tended to perform elective surgeries while veterinary surgeons performed some OVHs in dogs with underlying diseases (eg, pyometra).[25] Another common cause of ovarian pedicle hemorrhage is insufficient knot-tying technique, a problem that is most often revealed when a surgeon-in-training attempts to ligate a large, fat-filled pedicle in a mature female dog. In a training institution, avoidance of ovarian pedicle rupture is facilitated by encouraging ample abdominal exposure through incisions that extend from the umbilicus to the last mammary teat, allowing access to the right ovarian pedicle, which is located in the craniodorsal abdomen. Rather than strumming the suspensory ligament, the author recommends grasping the cranial edge of the suspensory ligament between the thumb and index finger, sliding the thumb and finger down into the incision, and breaking the supensory ligament with a twisting motion of the finger and thumb right at the point of attachment on the body wall. This technique allows for controlled rupture of the cranial edge of the suspensory ligament at a location that is distant from the origin of the vascular pedicle. Ligation is performed using 3-clamp technique, with each ovarian pedicle being double-ligated and transfixed. When rupture of a pedicle does occur, hemorrhage from the small ovarian and uterine vessels in prepubertal bitches is typically slow, giving the surgeon ample time to lengthen the incision and retract the duodenum to the left, using the mesoduodenum to hold back the viscera before attempting to grasp the dropped pedicle. The pedicle should be grasped with the tip of a mosquito hemostat, being careful to avoid inadvertent trauma to the ureter, aorta, vena cava, and renal artery and vein that lie in the adipose tissue of the retroperitoneal space. A similar maneuver is used to expose the left ovarian pedicle, placing the small intestines and spleen medial to the mesocolon and retracting the descending colon to the right. Hemorrhage from the uterine pedicle is identified by retroflexing the bladder (pulling the apex of the bladder in a ventrocaudal direction) and exposing the uterine stump, which lies between the urinary bladder and the descending colon. It should be noted that it is often difficult to identify active bleeding during reexploration of the abdomen, even in an animal that has experienced significant intra-abdominal hemorrhage. Presumably, decreases in perfusion pressure associated with general anesthesia and positioning in dorsal recumbency may temporarily decrease hemorrhage from ovarian or uterine pedicles. For this reason, the author recommends re-ligation of all pedicles at the time of surgery, regardless of intraoperative findings.

Wound Healing Complications

Although understated in most textbook descriptions of elective sterilization surgery, problems associated with incisional healing are some of the most frequently reported complications following OVH surgery, far exceeding the incidence of intraoperative

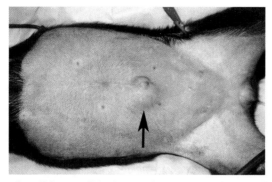

Fig. 1. An abdominal wall hernia (*black arrow*) was noted 7 days after ventral midline ovariohysterectom in a domestic short-haired cat. The etiology of the swelling was diagnosed based on palpation of an associated abdominal wall defect.

hemorrhage in some studies.[21] It is interesting to note that the incidence of incisional swelling, wound infection, and abdominal dehiscence has not decreased over the past 40 years, although original reports of OVH used surgical gut for closure of the linea alba and subcutaneous tissues—a technique that would now be considered below the standard of care that is achieved in modern teaching hospitals.[1,21,25] In a related manner, the use of preoperative or postoperative analgesia was not described in early reports of ovariohysterectomy,[24] with anesthetic protocols consisting of only a tranquilizer (acetylpromazine), anticholinergic, short-acting barbiturate induction (thiamylal), and inhaled halothane as a general anesthetic agent. Following this protocol, the authors described a 74% rate of self-inflicted incisional trauma in a group of 87 large dogs, with a 43% incidence in 476 cats, a complication that may have been related to postoperative pain. Development of wound complications has also been related to duration of surgery, with an increased incidence of postoperative swelling and wound infections occurring after surgeries that lasted longer than 90 minutes and in anesthetic episodes lasting longer than 120 minutes.[21] Wound infection occurs with a similar rate after elective OVH as in the general population undergoing elective surgery and ranges from 2.2% to 5.7%.[21,22] Seroma formation along the ventral midline is also a quite common complication due to the dependent location of the wound, which facilitates collection of fluid. This complication must be distinguished from the subcutaneous swelling that is associated with more serious abdominal wall dehiscence and herniation of the falciform fat or small intestine (**Fig. 1**). Fortunately, ventral midline incisional dehiscence is extremely rare, occurring in less than 1% of over 2000 cases of elective sterilization surgery.[22] Diagnosis of abdominal wall herniation is usually made by palpation of a defect in the abdominal closure in association with the appearance of a subcutaneous soft tissue mass effect. Unless self-induced trauma has occurred, the skin closure is typically intact and hernia repair can be performed on a semielective basis. Confirmation of the diagnosis can be made with plain radiography, which may show a defect in the ventral abdominal wall on lateral projections or by using abdominal ultrasound examination.

Avoidance

Abdominal wall dehiscence that occurs during the first 7 days after surgery is most commonly due to technical errors, including failure to incorporate the external rectus fascia, inappropriate suture size, or knot failure. Many of these technique errors can be avoided by use of proper surgical technique. The author recommends clearing of subcutaneous tissues from the external rectus fascia for approximately 1 cm on either side of the linea alba to facilitate proper incorporation of the external rectus fascia during closure. The linea may be closed in either a continuous or an interrupted appositional suture pattern, using monofilament, absorbable suture material. Due to the slow healing rate of abdominal wall fascial incisions, a suture with prolonged retention of tensile strength is recommended, such as polydioxanone or polyglyconate. Perioperative antibiotics are not commonly recommended during OVH procedures, although the surgery classifies as a clean contaminated procedure.[21] Based on the high rate of postoperative wound infection that was reported when surgical time exceeded 90 minutes,[21] the prophylactic use of cephalosporin antibiotics should be considered in training institutions when procedure time is expected to be prolonged.

Ovarian Remnant Syndrome

Ovarian remnant syndrome is a rare complication of OVH in dogs and cats.[26–28] Residual ovarian tissue most commonly results from incomplete resection of the ovary during the initial surgery,[26,27] although 1 experimental study showed that fragments of ovarian tissue can become revascularized through the mesentery or omentum, maintaining functional status indefinitely.[26,27,29] Although this complication is attributable to surgical error, retrospective studies have shown that the vast majority of animals that develop this complication had their original surgery performed by an experienced veterinarian, not by a veterinary student or recent graduate.[26,27] Diagnosis is typically suspected in dogs with a history of OVH that later develop clinical signs of proestrus or estrus, with most commonly reported signs including vaginal discharge, vulvar swelling, and behavioral changes (**Fig. 2**).[26,27] Confirmation of the diagnosis can be made using vaginal cytology, hormonal testing, abdominal ultrasound, and exploratory laparotomy. A recent retrospective study by Ball et al reported that vaginal cytology and hormone assays (serum estrogen >20 pg/mol, progesterone >2 or luteinizing hormone concentrations >1 ng/mL) do not serve as reliable predictors of ovarian remnant syndrome.[27] In that same study, abdominal ultrasound was a useful diagnostic aid in dogs with ovarian remnant syndrome, correctly identifying the ovarian tissue location in 6 of 9 dogs showing signs of proestrus or estrus and in 3 of 3 dogs with no clinical signs. Ultrasonographic appearance of the ovarian tissue was described as being a soft tissue or cystic (hypoechoic) mass, with variable acoustic enhancement, echogenic fluid, or anechoic follicles.[27] Retained ovarian tissue can nearly always be visually identified at the site of original ovariectomy at the time of abdominal exploration (see **Fig. 2**).

Therapy

Surgical exploration and resection of retained ovarian tissue have led to resolution of clinical signs in all reported cases of ovarian remnant syndrome.[26,27] It has been suggested that performing the exploratory surgery during a time of active proestrus, estrus, or diestrus can facilitate identification of ovarian tissue due to the presence of follicles, corpora leutea, and increased size of the ovarian vascular pedicle.[27,28] Retained ovarian tissue is typically noted to be located in close association with the fibrous tissue that marks the location of the original ovarian pedicle ligation and can be distinguished from surrounding adipose tissue by the darker coloration and firm character of ovarian tissue (see **Fig. 2**).[27] Ovarian pedicle remnants are located caudal to the kidneys and are often in close association with the ureters. Thus, the surgeon must take great care in identifying the ureter prior to resecting the ovarian remnant, to

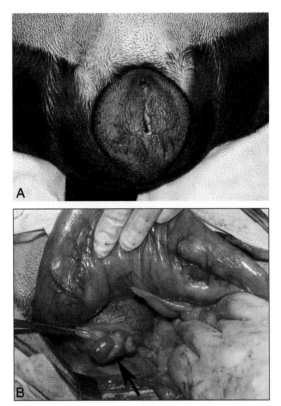

Fig. 2. Marked vulvar enlargement and serosanguinaous vaginal discharge are noted in a dog with ovarian remnant ovarian syndrome (*A*). An ovarian remnant (*B*) is easily distinguished as a multilobulated mass of tissue (*black arrow*) caudal to the left kidney.

avoid causing inadvertent ureteral trauma. If there is any doubt in identifying the ovarian tissue, fibrous tissues associated with both ovarian ligature sites are resected and submitted for histopathology.

Avoidance

The ovary can be very difficult to visualize, especially in dogs, due to the large amount of adipose tissue associated with the mesosalpinx in this species. As a result, a variety of strategies have been used to ensure complete removal of the ovary during OVH. First, adequate exposure is obtained in the initial midline abdominal incision so that the ovary can be completely exteriorized during clamp placement. The suspensory ligament is ruptured or stretched to a degree that allows mobilization of the ovary so that there is adequate space to place two hemostatic clamps on the ovarian pedicle without encroaching on the ovary. Because visualization of the ovary is often obscured by fat in the mesosalpinx, digital palpation of the ovary is performed while placing the hemostatic clamps on the ovarian pedicle, making sure to place the clamps at least 1 cm proximal (or deep) to the ovary on the ovarian pedicle. Ligatures are then placed proximal to the clamp, ensuring that the ovary will be completely resected when the pedicle is severed distal to the ligatures. As a final precaution, the ovary is examined directly before releasing the ovarian pedicle. The ovary can then be examined for completeness of resection by inserting a Metzenbaum scissor blade into the opening of the ovarian bursa, incising the bursa until the mesosalpinx is reflected.

Stump Pyometra

A common misconception is that stump pyometra occurs as a result of incomplete resection of the uterine body. In fact, numerous large studies performed in Europe have demonstrated that ovariectomy alone (without removal of the uterus) prevents the later occurrence of pyometra with equal efficacy as complete OVH.[5] It is important to remember that the pathophysiology of stump pyometra is identical to that of classic canine pyometra, involving repeated exposure of the uterus to progesterone from either an ovarian remnant or, much more rarely, the therapeutic administration of exogenous progestogens. Thus, stump pyometra is not caused by retained uterine tissue; it is actually a rarely reported complication of ovarian remnant syndrome. Interestingly, a recent report of ovarian remnant syndrome in dogs described that 11 of 12 uterine stumps that were submitted for histopathology had evidence of cystic endometrial hyperplasia.[27] Stump pyometra can occur with an open cervix, causing obvious clinical signs of purulent vaginal discharge in a dog with a previous history of OVH. In dogs with a closed cervix, signs are of pyometra are nonspecific (eg, lethargy, fever, decreased appetite),[30] and diagnosis of closed stump pyometra can be extremely difficult when clinical signs are not directly referable to the urogenital tract. A key diagnostic finding is the presence of a fluid-filled uterine stump on abdominal ultrasound in a dog that has a history of previous OVH. Further examination by a skilled operator may allow detection of the retained ovarian tissue that is invariably the cause of this complication. Ultrasound-guided fine needle aspiration of the uterine fluid can be performed to allow cytologic interpretation and confirm diagnosis, but results are unlikely to alter the plan for surgical intervention and aspirates have a risk of seeding the abdomen with bacteria.

Therapy

Resolution of stump pyometra is achieved by resection of the uterine stump at the level of the cervix. A caudal midline celiotomy is performed and the uterine stump is located by retroflexing the urinary bladder and identifying the uterus between dorsal to the urinary bladder and ventral to the colon. The uterine stump is double-ligated and transfixed with absorbable monofilament suture, just cranial to the cervix. Inverting the uterine stump with a Parker Kerr oversew is now considered unnecessary and may even contribute to walling off bacteria in the remaining uterine lumen. Instead, the uterine stump is flushed copiously with sterile 0.9% NaCl. If there is remaining concern about ongoing contamination, the omentum may be sutured to the end of the uterine stump to form a fibrin seal while providing physiologic drainage of the area.

Avoidance

Uterine stump pyometra is one manifestation of ovarian remnant syndrome. As a result, avoidance strategies are identical to those described above and are directed at ensuring complete removal of the ovaries at the time of sterilization surgery.

Ureteral Injury

The ureters travel through the retroperitoneal space caudal to the kidney and are crossed by the gonadal arteries, where they can be inadvertently traumatized or ligated during OVH (**Fig. 3**). At their distal insertion into the bladder, the feline ureters

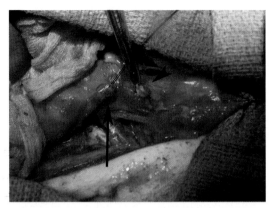

Fig. 3. Abdominal exploration was performed in a dog that was suffering from uroabdomen 1 week after ventral midline ovariohysterectom. The right ureter (*black arrow*) had been traumatized during ligation of the uterine pedicle (*black arrowhead*). A right ureterone-phrectomy was performed. (*Courtesy of* Andrew Mercurio, DVM, The Ohio State University.)

are also rather closely associated with the uterine body where they are in danger of being ligated with the uterine pedicle, particularly when the bladder is full and in a more cranial position. Despite this anatomic proximity with the urogenital tract, there are only 3 individual case reports of ureteral injury secondary to OVH in dogs.[11–13] although it is likely that this complication is far more common and goes undetected, as unilateral ureteral obstruction would not cause azotemia in a previously healthy animal. Clinical signs in the reported cases were highly varied. In 1 dog, ureteral injury was detected due to severe clinical signs associated with uroabdomen 5 days after unilateral ureteral transaction.[11] In the other 2 case reports, ureteral obstruction occurred as a late complication, with suture reactions adjacent to the ureter causing extramural ureteral compression at 1 and 9 years after OVH.[12,13] Diagnosis of ureteral injury is typically obtained using a combination of imaging modalities since no single modality is ideal for all situations. Intravenous urography is most useful in detecting the location of upper urinary tract rupture in animals with normal renal function, but abdominal ultrasound is more adept at imaging the urinary tract in cases of chronic obstruction, when deteriorated renal function can limit the detectable contrast that reaches the collecting system.

Therapy
Ureteral repair is technically demanding and, in smaller animals, requires the use of microsurgical instruments and an operating microscope. As such, animals with suspected ureteral injury after OVH should be referred to a surgeon with the equipment and experience required to successfully perform these surgeries. Repair of acute ureteral laceration is typically accomplished by end-to-end or end-to-side ureteral anastomosis.[11] Swelling of the tissues at the anastomotic site is common in the immediate postoperative period, while stricture can occur in a more delayed fashion at 3 to 4 weeks after surgery. To maximize the ureteral diameter at the site of anastomosis, each end of the ureter is spatulated by inserting a scissor into the cut end and incising longitudinally to expose the ureteral lumen. Anastomosis is then performed using 6-0 to 10-0 suture in a simple interrupted pattern. Stenting of the ureter by bridging the anastomotic site with a red rubber catheter or ureteral stent can

minimize the risk of anastomotic leakage and preserve the lumen diameter. Ureteral lacerations or obstructions that are located near the urinary bladder are treated by resection of the distal segment and neoureterocystostomy (ureteral implantation into the bladder apex). Anastomosis with the urinary bladder has a lower complication rate than ureteroureterostomy and is technically simpler to perform.[31,32] In cases where ureteral injury is irreparable or where no residual renal function is present, unilateral ureteronephrectomy can be performed.

Avoidance

Ureteral injury is avoided by constantly being aware of the anatomic location and proximity of the ureter to the operative site. Inadvertent injury to the ureter can occur if a surgeon grasps to retrieve a dropped ovarian pedicle that has retracted into the retroperitoneal fat caudal to the kidney. Due to the slow rate of blood loss from an ovarian pedicle, it is recommended that a surgeon take the time to increase exposure by lengthening the abdominal incision cranial to the umbilicus and using suction or laparotomy sponges to improve vision of the dropped pedicle. The pedicle is then grasped carefully with noncrushing Debakey forceps and elevated away from the ureter before clamping the vessel with a hemostat. Inadvertent incorporation of the ureters in the uterine stump ligation is facilitated by complete preoperative emptying of the urinary bladder during preparation of the skin. The empty bladder moves caudally in the abdomen, pulling the ureters away from the region of uterine stump ligation and improving visualization during ligation.

Bowel Obstruction

Numerous early studies and case reports described the development of bowel obstruction following uncomplicated ovariohysterectomy.[10,23,33–35] In each of these early studies, bowel obstruction occurred as a result of granuloma or abscess formation around a pedicle that had been ligated using multifilament nonabsorbable suture material.[9,10,23,33–36] Although the use of multifilament nonabsorbable suture has been largely replaced by the use of monofilament absorbable suture, uterine stump abscessation is still reported.[9] In addition, a new phenomenon of colonic obstruction due to the formation of fibrous adhesions of the broad ligament, uterine stump, and colon has been described.[10] Presenting signs are nonspecific (ie, lethargy, vomiting, dysuria, and constipation) and are often attributable to compression of the adjacent colon and urinary bladder neck in affected animals. Granulomas and abscesses may be detected between the urinary bladder and colon during abdominal palpation or imaging studies[9,36] (**Fig. 4**), while fibrous adhesions appear as an extraluminal compression of the colonic lumen.[10] The detection of leukocytosis, pyrexia, or hypoechoic fluid in association with a uterine stump mass is consistent with abscess formation.[9,36] Colonic obstruction after OVH has been described in both cats and dogs, with insufficient information to discern a species predisposition.[10,34,35]

Treatment

Conservative therapy with stool softeners, highly digestible diet, and anti-inflammatory medications may be attempted in animals with partial colonic obstruction due to granuloma formation. Animals with fibrous adhesions or abscesses would not be expected to respond well to medical management and surgical intervention is recommended. A ventral midline exploratory surgery is performed and the cause of obstruction is assessed. In animals with uterine stump granulomas or abscesses, complete resection is performed if possible. In animals with inflammation involving the ureters or the neurovascular supply of the urinary bladder, partial resection and

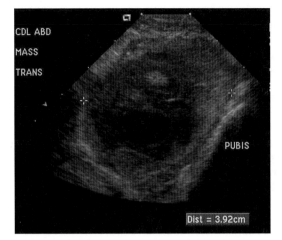

Fig. 4. Ultrasonographic image of a uterine stump abscess in a 3-year-old whippet that underwent ventral midline OVH 1 week prior to presenting for pollakiuria.

omentalization are indicated to avoid iatrogenic injury.[9] Fibrous adhesions are disrupted using blunt and sharp dissection to free the colon and relieve obstruction.[10] The prognosis is good in animals that undergo surgical therapy and whose clinical signs resolve without need for further interventions.[9,10]

Avoidance

Historical information would suggest that the use of multifilament nonabsorbable suture for ligations is contraindicated during elective OVH.[36] Prevention of adhesions is never completely ensured, although strategies to minimize serosal irritation would include avoidance of bowel dessication, eliminating powder from surgical gloves prior to surgery, and using gentle tissue handling during surgery.

Acquired Urinary Incontinence

Urethral sphincter mechanism incompetence (USMI) is a form of acquired urinary incontinence that can develop after OVH in dogs. Estrogen increases the number of alpha receptors and the affinity of those receptors to adrenergic binding, increasing urethral smooth muscle tone. Removal of the positive influence of estrogen on urethral tone is the major mechanism involved in acquired USMI, although estrogen replacement therapy is only successful in restoring continence in 60% of affected dogs, suggesting that other factors contribute to this condition. While USMI is an indirect result of surgery, it is arguable that this problem should be listed as the most common complication after OVH. The relative risk of USMI is increased 7.8-fold by OVH,[37] and most retrospective studies estimate that nearly 1 in 5 dogs develop incontinence after OVH.[38] Signs of urinary incontinence can begin any time between 2 weeks and 10 years after OVH, with an average of 2.9 years.[38-40] Incontinence is most commonly noted during sleep and recumbency but may also manifest during times of excitement or nervousness.[39,40] Large breed dogs appear to be at increased risk, with incidence approaching 30% in dogs greater than 20-kg body weight.[38] Diagnosis is largely based on a history of acquired incontinence that developed after OVH, although complete blood count, serum biochemistry panel, urinalysis, abdominal ultrasound, and cystoscopy are often recommended to rule out other metabolic, infectious or anatomic conditions that may be contributing to incontinence. Definitive diagnosis requires urodynamic studies to document the changes in the urethral pressure profile associated with USMI.[41] In clinical practice, many veterinarians use a therapeutic trial as an initial method of both treatment and diagnosis of the condition.

Therapy

The vast majority of dogs with USMI will respond to treatment with the sympathomimetic drug phenylpropanolamine (PPA). A prospective placebo-controlled study reported an 85% success rate in resolving incontinence when PPA was dosed at 1 mg/kg 3 times daily.[42] Side effects of this alpha agonist drug are predictable and include restlessness, anorexia, and hypertension. Dosing is titrated until incontinence is controlled or side effects are noted. Estrogen-related drugs such as diethylstilbesterone (DES) are synergistic with PPA and can be added to the treatment regimen in dogs that are refractory to PPA alone.[43] Bone marrow suppression is a rare complication of DES administration, and complete blood counts should be monitored serially in dogs that are receiving the drug.[43] Several procedures are available for dogs that fail to respond to medical therapy or develop drug-related side effects, including submucosal collagen injection, colposuspension, and placement of an artificial urethal sphincter.[44–47]

Avoidance

Historically, authors asserted that the rate of incontinence was increased when dogs were spayed before the first estrus cycle or when the cervix was removed during OVH; however, subsequent studies in larger groups of animals have disproved these theories[20,37] and there are no known methods to avoid this problem, aside from avoiding OVH entirely. Based on the incidence of USMI after OVH and on the significance of urinary incontinence in a pet dog, this is an area that deserves great attention by the veterinary community. In particular, research into alternative methods for sterilization would seem appropriate, given the high incidence of incontinence after traditional OVH.

Complications of Orchiectomy

Hemorrhage

Orchiectomy is performed through a prescrotal incision in mature dogs. The vascular pedicle can be double-ligated and transfixed through a closed technique, or an incision is made in the parietal vaginal tunic to expose the vascular pedicle, allowing direct ligation of the pampiniform plexus. In contrast to OVH, overt hemorrhage following orchiectomy is most often related to bleeding from the tunic and is therefore self-limiting, causing incisional hemorrhage, subcutaneous bruising, and scrotal hematoma. Scrotal hematoma was reported to occur in 7 dogs and 2 cats in a series of 218 animals undergoing elective sterilization surgery, although the data were not presented in a manner that allowed calculation of overall incidence.[22] Serious hemorrhage from the vascular pedicle is actually harder to detect, as vessels can retract into the abdomen and cause hemoperitoneum with few external signs of hemorrhage. Animals with significant intracavitary hemorrhage will present with more subtle signs, such as pale mucous membranes, tachycardia, and slow recovery from anesthesia. Diagnosis should be carried out with evaluation of blood coagulation, platelet function, and abdominal ultrasound examination as described for hemorrhage following OVH.

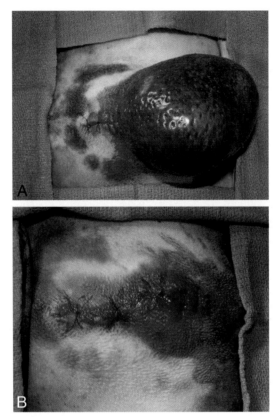

Fig. 5. This large scrotal hematoma (*A*) was diagnosed 48 hours after closed orchiectomy in an adult male mixed breed dog. The dog was treated by scrotal ablation (*B*).

Treatment

Initial treatment of mild scrotal hematoma formation involves cryotherapy (ice packing for 10 minutes every 4 hours) and sedation to minimize activity in the immediate postoperative period. Dogs with severe scrotal hematoma often go on to suffer from necrosis of the scrotal skin, and scrotal ablation is recommended in the early postoperative period to minimize morbidity to the animal (**Fig. 5**). In animals with significant abdominal hemorrhage secondary to failed ligation of the testicular pedicle, abdominal exploration is performed via a parapreprutial skin incision and caudal midline abdominal approach through the linea alba.

Avoidance

Prophylactic scrotal ablation should be considered in older intact dogs to avoid the risk of scrotal edema, hematoma formation, and poor cosmetic outcome after orchiectomy. It has been suggested that performance of a closed castration (without incising the parietal tunic) decreases the incidence of scrotal hematoma following orchiectomy.[48] Nonetheless, open castration provides a more secure ligation of the large pampiniform plexus and is recommended in dogs greater than 20-kg body weight.[49,50]

Inadvertent Prostatectomy

Cryptorchidism is a common congenital anomaly in dogs, with 9% of 466 animals undergoing castration surgery at a veterinary teaching hospital having been diagnosed as unilaterally or bilaterally cryptorchid.[22] Intra-abdominal testicles are removed through a parapreputial caudal abdominal approach to avoid the development of testicular neoplasia in the retained testis. Unintended removal of the prostate is a rare but devastating complication of cryptorchid castration.[14,15,51,52] Due to inadequate exposure and improper identification of anatomic structures, the surgeon grasps an ovoid object in the caudoventral abdomen and removes it, mistakenly identifying the prostate instead of the retained intra-abdominal testicle. Unfortunately, the prostatic urethra is resected with the prostate, leading to uroabdomen, or, if the urethra and bladder neck are ligated, to complete urinary obstruction and rapidly progressive uremia.[14] Diagnosis of this problem is largely based on detection of azotemia and anuria in association with a recent history of cryptorchid castration. Confirmation of urethral trauma or ligation can be performed by positive contrast urethrography (**Fig. 6**).

Treatment

Surgical exploration through a caudal abdominal approach is performed as soon as the patient is stabilized. The urethral transection is repaired by reanastomosis with the urinary bladder neck using interrupted sutures in an appositional pattern. The author recommends the use of magnification ($\times 3.5$) and availability of microsurgical instrumentation to facilitate direct apposition of urethral mucosa with a fine (5-0 to 6-0) monofilament absorbable suture material, minimizing the likelihood of urine leakage or postoperative stricture. Anastomosis is performed over a urinary catheter to prevent inadvertent incorporation of the back wall during suture placement (see **Fig. 6**). A Foley urinary catheter is maintained for 5 to 7 days to facilitate bridging of the repair with urothelium. Although complete prostatectomy is associated with a high rate of incontinence when performed in dogs with malignant neoplasia, a functional outcome is often achieved in previously healthy dogs that have undergone inadvertent prostatectomy.[14,51]

Avoidance

Prevention of inadvertent prostatectomy can be achieved by obtaining definitive identification of anatomy during cryptorchid castration. A paramedian caudal abdominal incision is made extending along the entire length of the prepuce and terminating at the cranial aspect of the pubic bone. The prepuce is retracted and a ventral midline abdominal incision is carried out in similar fashion. The urinary bladder is retroflexed so that the dorsal bladder neck and trigone can be examined. The paired, white deferent ducts are identified near the trigone as they course over the ureters and insert on the dorsal surface of the prostate. The ductus deferens are used to locate the retained testicle(s) by tracing each duct to its origin from the epididymis of the abdominal testicle or, for a descended testis, until it exits through the inguinal ring. Although the intra-abdominal testicle may be atrophied or affected by a neoplastic process, the characteristic appearances of the epididymis and the vascular pampiniform plexus are helpful in confirming the origin of the tissue before resection. Keep in mind that an undescended testicle lacks the parietal vaginal tunic, exposing the vascular pedicle, ductus deferens, and gubernaculum to direct examination. Exposure of the vascular anatomy facilitates both identification of the testicle and subsequent ligation of the vascular pedicle. Resected tissue is submitted for histopathologic examination to confirm removal of the testicle and to investigate for

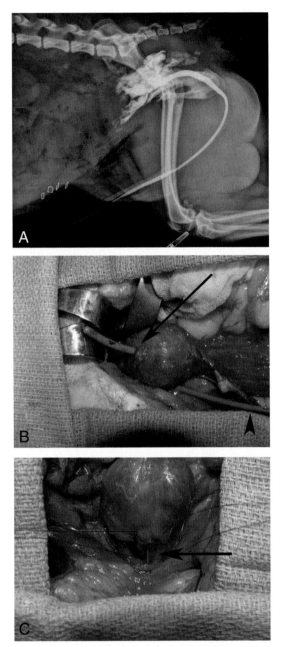

Fig. 6. Positive contrast urethrography (*A*) showing extravasation of contrast from the post prostatic urethra in a dog that underwent abdominal cryptorchidectomy 24 hours earlier. Urethral transection had occurred, due to confusion of the prostate with the abdominal testicle. Antegrade passage of a urinary catheter from the urinary bladder shows the site of urethral transection caudal to the prostate (*B, black arrow*). A second catheter was placed retrograde from the penis (*B, arrowhead*), allowing identification of the pelvic urethra. The prostatic urethra was anastomosed to the pelvic urethra over a urinary catheter (*C, black arrow*). (*Courtesy of* Dr Stephen Birchard, The Ohio State University.)

the development of testicular neoplasia, which occurs at a higher rate in retained testes.[49]

REFERENCES

1. Howe LM. Surgical methods of contraception and sterilization. Theriogenology 2006; 66(3):500–9.
2. Coe RJ, Grint NJ, Tivers MS, et al. Comparison of flank and midline approaches to the ovariohysterectomy of cats. Vet Rec 2006;159(10):309–13.
3. Whitehead M. Ovariohysterectomy versus ovariectomy. Vet Rec 2006;159(21): 723–4.
4. Veenis M. Ovariectomy vs. ovariohysterectomy. J Am Anim Hosp Assoc 2004;40(3): 170.
5. van Goethem B, Schaefers-Okkens A, Kirpensteijn J. Making a rational choice between ovariectomy and ovariohysterectomy in the dog: a discussion of the benefits of either technique. Vet Surg 2006;35(2):136–43.
6. Peeters ME, Kirpensteijn J. Comparison of surgical variables and short-term postoperative complications in healthy dogs undergoing ovariohysterectomy or ovariectomy. J Am Vet Med Assoc 2011;238(2):189–94.
7. Heffelfinger DJ. Ovarian remnant in a 2-year-old queen. Can Vet J 2006;47(2):165–7.
8. Kanazono S, Aikawa T, Yoshigae Y. Unilateral hydronephrosis and partial ureteral obstruction by entrapment in a granuloma in a spayed dog. J Am Anim Hosp Assoc 2009;45(6):301–4.
9. Campbell BG. Omentalization of a nonresectable uterine stump abscess in a dog. J Am Vet Med Assoc 2004;224(11):1788, 1799–803.
10. Coolman BR, Marretta SM, Dudley MB, et al. Partial colonic obstruction following ovariohysterectomy: a report of three cases. J Am Anim Hosp Assoc 1999;35(2): 169–72.
11. Mehl ML, Kyles AE. Ureteroureterostomy after proximal ureteric injury during an ovariohysterectomy in a dog. Vet Rec 2003;153(15):469–70.
12. Kyles AE, Douglass JP, Rottman JB. Pyelonephritis following inadvertent excision of the ureter during ovariohysterectomy in a bitch. Vet Rec 1996;139(19):471–2.
13. Ruiz de Gopegui R, Espada Y, Majo N. Bilateral hydroureter and hydronephrosis in a nine-year-old female german shepherd dog. J Small Anim Pract 1999;40(5):224–6.
14. Schulz KS, Waldron DR, Smith MM, et al. Inadvertent prostatectomy as a complication of cryptorchidectomy in four dogs. J Am Anim Hosp Assoc 1996;32(3):211–4.
15. Sereda C, Fowler D, Shmon C. Iatrogenic proximal urethral obstruction after inadvertent prostatectomy during bilateral perineal herniorrhaphy in a dog. Can Vet J 2002;43(4):288–90.
16. Holt PE, Bohannon J, Day MJ. Vaginoperitoneal fistula after ovariohysterectomy in three bitches. J Small Anim Pract 2006;47(12):744–6.
17. Frank JD, Stanley BJ. Enterocutaneous fistula in a dog secondary to an intraperitoneal gauze foreign body. J Am Anim Hosp Assoc 2009;45(2):84–8.
18. Merlo M, Lamb CR. Radiographic and ultrasonographic features of retained surgical sponge in eight dogs. Vet Radiol Ultrasound 2000;41(3):279–83.
19. Arnold S, Arnold P, Hubler M, et al. Urinary incontinence in spayed female dogs: frequency and breed disposition]. Schweiz Arch Tierheilkd 1989;131(5):259–63.
20. Stocklin-Gautschi NM, Hassig M, Reichler IM, et al. The relationship of urinary incontinence to early spaying in bitches. J Reprod Fertil Suppl 2001;57:233–6.
21. Burrow R, Batchelor D, Cripps P. Complications observed during and after ovariohysterectomy of 142 bitches at a veterinary teaching hospital. Vet Rec 2005;157(26): 829–33.

22. Pollari FL, Bonnett BN, Bamsey SC, et al. Postoperative complications of elective surgeries in dogs and cats determined by examining electronic and paper medical records. J Am Vet Med Assoc 1996;208(11):1882–6.

23. Pearson H. The complications of ovariohysterectomy in the bitch. J Small Anim Pract 1973;14(5):257–66.

24. Berzon JL. Complications of elective ovariohysterectomies in the dog and cat at a teaching institution: Clinical review of 853 cases. Vet Surg 1979;8:89–91.

25. Dorn AS, Swist RA. Complications of canine ovariohysterectomy. J Am Anim Hosp Assoc 1977;13:720–4.

26. Miller DM. Ovarian remnant syndrome in dogs and cats: 46 cases (1988-1992). J Vet Diagn Invest 1995;7(4):572–4.

27. Ball RL, Birchard SJ, May LR, et al. Ovarian remnant syndrome in dogs and cats: 21 cases (2000-2007). J Am Vet Med Assoc 2010;236(5):548–53.

28. Wallace MS. The ovarian remnant syndrome in the bitch and queen. Vet Clin North Am Small Anim Pract 1991;21(3):501–7.

29. DeNardo GA, Becker K, Brown NO, et al. Ovarian remnant syndrome: revascularization of free-floating ovarian tissue in the feline abdominal cavity. J Am Anim Hosp Assoc 2001;37(3):290–6.

30. Pretzer SD. Clinical presentation of canine pyometra and mucometra: a review. Theriogenology 2008;70(3):359–63.

31. Mehl ML, Kyles AE, Pollard R, et al. Comparison of 3 techniques for ureteroneocystostomy in cats. Vet Surg 2005;34(2):114–9.

32. Hardie RJ, Schmiedt C, Phillips L, et al. Ureteral papilla implantation as a technique for neoureterocystostomy in cats. Vet Surg 2005;34(4):393–8.

33. Joshua JO. The spaying of bitches. Vet Rec 1965;77:642–6.

34. Muir P, Goldsmid SE, Bellenger CR. Megacolon in a cat following ovariohysterectomy. Vet Rec 1991;129(23):512–3.

35. Smith MC, Davies NL. Obstipation following ovariohysterectomy in a cat. Vet Rec 1996;138(7):163.

36. Boza S, Lucas X, Zarelli M, et al. Late abscess formation caused by silk suture following hysterectomy in a female dog. Reprod Domest Anim 2009.

37. Thrusfield MV, Holt PE, Muirhead RH. Acquired urinary incontinence in bitches: its incidence and relationship to neutering practices. J Small Anim Pract 1998;39(12):559–66.

38. Arnold S, Arnold P, Hubler M, et al. Urinary incontinence in spayed female dogs: frequency and breed disposition. Schweiz Arch Tierheilkd 1989;131(5):259–63.

39. Holt PE. Urinary incontinence in dogs and cats. Vet Rec 1990;127(14):347–50.

40. Thrusfield MV. Association between urinary incontinence and spaying in bitches. Vet Rec 1985;116(26):695.

41. Holt PE. Urethral pressure profilometry in the anaesthetised bitch: a comparison between double and single sensor recording. Res Vet Sci 1989;47(3):346–9.

42. Scott L, Leddy M, Bernay F, et al. Evaluation of phenylpropanolamine in the treatment of urethral sphincter mechanism incompetence in the bitch. J Small Anim Pract 2002;43(11):493–6.

43. Page SW. Diethylstilboestrol — clinical pharmacology and alternatives in small animal practice. Aust Vet J 1991;68(7):226–30.

44. Rawlings C, Barsanti JA, Mahaffey MB, et al. Evaluation of colposuspension for treatment of incontinence in spayed female dogs. J Am Vet Med Assoc 2001;219(6):770–5.

45. Holt PE, Gregory SP. Can urethral pressure profilometry predict the response to colposuspension in bitches? Vet Rec 1991;128(12):281–2.

46. Adin CA, Farese JP, Cross AR, et al. Urodynamic effects of a percutaneously controlled static hydraulic urethral sphincter in canine cadavers. Am J Vet Res 2004;65(3):283–8.
47. Arnold S, Hubler M, Lott-Stolz G, et al. Treatment of urinary incontinence in bitches by endoscopic injection of glutaraldehyde cross-linked collagen. J Small Anim Pract 1996;37(4):163–8.
48. Fossum TW. Surgery of the kidney and ureter. In: Fossum TW, editor. Small animal surgery. 3rd edition. St Louis: Mosby; 2007. p. 635–62.
49. Boothe HW. Testes and epididymides. In: Slatter DH, editor. Textbook of small animal surgery, vol 2. 3rd edition. Philadelphia: Saunders; 2003. p. 1521–30.
50. Fingland RB. Ovariohysterectomy. In: Bojrab MJ, editor. Current techniques in small animal surgery. 4th edition. Baltimore (MD): Williams & Wilkins; 1998. p. 489–96.
51. Yarrow TG. Inadvertent prostatectomy as a complication of cryptorchidectomy. J Am Anim Hosp Assoc 1996;32(5):376–7.
52. Powers MY, Campbell BG, Weisse C. Porcine small intestinal submucosa augmentation urethroplasty and balloon dilatation of a urethral stricture secondary to inadvertent prostatectomy in a dog. J Am Anim Hosp Assoc 2010;46(5):358–65.

Surgical Site Infections in Small Animal Surgery

Laura L. Nelson, DVM, MS

KEYWORDS

• Surgery • Infection • Antimicrobial resistance • Nosocomial
• Veterinary • Prevention

Surgical site infections (SSIs) are among the most common nosocomial infections in human patient populations, accounting for 16% of such infections in all patients and 38% of nosocomial infections among surgical patients in the United States.[1] Although similar reporting of nosocomial infections does not exist in the veterinary field, SSI has been described as a complication of 0.8% to 18.1% of small animal surgical procedures, with significant variation associated with surgery type.[2–8]

The development of SSI can result in a variety of consequences including poor cosmesis, increased medication costs, revision surgery, prolonged wound management, tissue destruction, risk of drug side effects, increased client cost, and patient death. In a 1992 analysis of SSI in human surgical patients, each infection resulted in 7.3 additional hospital days and an additional $3152 in charges.[1] In both human and veterinary medicine, surgical site and other nosocomial infections are increasingly complicated by the emergence of multidrug-resistant (MDR) pathogens that, without attention to isolation and barrier protocols, may be spread through the hospital environment to affect other patients.[9–15] Although the morbidity and mortality associated with MDR pathogens have not been thoroughly investigated in small animal practice, MDR infections are associated with poorer outcomes in humans.[15]

SSIs cannot be completely eliminated, but preventive strategies represent the most economical and effective means of reducing their impact. These strategies include adherence to aseptic principles during surgery, the judicious use of antimicrobial prophylaxis (AMP), identification of at-risk patient populations, and protection of the surgical wound in the postoperative period. When SSI does occur, accurate and timely identification of infection, appropriate assessment of the extent of infection, culture-based antibiotic therapy, appropriate wound management, and attention to infection control protocols are important to ensure the best outcome. Finally, surveillance protocols are critical to identify systematic breaks in surgical asepsis, inadequate perioperative care protocols, and patterns of antimicrobial resistance. This article will review the

The author has nothing to disclose. This work was not supported by any funding agencies.
Department of Small Animal Clinical Sciences, Michigan State University College of Veterinary Medicine, A162 Veterinary Medical Center, East Lansing, MI 48824, USA
E-mail address: Michae19@cvm.msu.edu

classification and definitions of SSI, evaluate patient and environmental risk factors for infection, and explore prevention and treatment strategies.

STANDARD DEFINITIONS AND CLASSIFICATION

The diagnosis of SSI requires interpretation of both clinical and laboratory information and is subject to a certain degree of subjectivity. Standard definitions for SSI have been developed to improve consistency in diagnosis and reporting, without which surveillance data are difficult or impossible to interpret. The Centers for Disease Control and Prevention National Nosocomial Infections Surveillance (NNIS) system, established in 1970 to monitor reported trends in nosocomial infections in US hospitals, has developed standardized surveillance criteria for defining SSIs (**Table 1**).[1] This classification system can be applied to veterinary patients. Though a subjective diagnosis of SSI by the attending clinician or surgeon is sufficient based on this classification scheme, bacterial culture and antimicrobial sensitivity testing should be performed in all cases to confirm the presence of bacterial infection and, more important, to guide antimicrobial interventions in an era of antimicrobial resistance. The lack of consistent diagnostic criteria has made studies of SSI in veterinary patients difficult to compare.[2–7]

EPIDEMIOLOGY

The risk of SSI for a given surgery is a dynamic relationship between the size of the bacterial inoculum, the virulence of the bacteria, and the resistance of the host as represented in the following formula[16]:

$$\text{Infection Risk} = \frac{\text{Contamination} \times \text{Virulence}}{\text{Host Resistance}}$$

Each of these factors merits consideration in the assessment of risk and the development of prevention protocols for SSI.

The expected degree of wound contamination is usefully defined by surgical wound classification, which uses descriptive case features to grade the degree of intraoperative microbial contamination predicted during surgery (**Table 2**).[1,17] This classification is limited by its inability to account for broad variations between surgical procedures within a category (eg, forequarter amputation and stifle arthrotomy) and its use *preoperatively* to predict *intraoperative* contamination.[1] As a predictor of SSI risk, wound classification is clinically useful to define the appropriate use of antibiotics (prophylactic vs therapeutic), and wound closure strategy (primary closure vs open wound management). The incidence of SSI by wound classification is listed in **Table 3**. Wound classification is also useful in the definition of SSI risk (see **Table 3**).[2,4] Veterinary SSI rates have also been described for specific clean surgical procedures, often in the context of antimicrobial prophylaxis (AMP).[5–7] Published infection rates for specific procedures in human surgery have been also been used to identify specific risk factors and prevention strategies for SSI.[1,18,19]

Despite the logical association of wound contamination with SSI incidence, patient factors are also critically important in SSI development. The NNIS describes three categories of variables that have been shown to be reliable predictors of SSI risk: (1) estimations of the intrinsic degree of microbial contamination of the surgical site, (2) measurements of surgical duration, and (3) markers for host susceptibility.[1] The American Society of Anesthesiology (ASA) classifies patients according to physical status score (**Table 4**), which has served as a useful indicator of host susceptibility.[1,20] Patient ASA status at the time of surgery is a significant predictor of SSI risk in humans.[1,17]

Table 1	
Criteria for SSI definition	
Superficial Incisional	Infection occurs within 30 days after operation and involves only skin or subcutaneous tissue of the incision.[a]
	and at least one of the following:
	1. Purulent drainage, with or without laboratory conformation, from the superficial incision
	2. Organisms isolated from an aseptically obtained culture of fluid or tissue from the superficial incision
	3. At least one of the following signs or symptoms of infection: pain or tenderness, localized swelling, redness, or heat *and* superficial incision is deliberately opened by surgeon, *unless* incision is culture-negative
	4. Diagnosis of superficial incisional SSI by the surgeon or attending clinician
	[a]*Does not include suture abscess.*
Deep Incisional	Infection occurs within 30 days after operation (within 1 year if implant is left in place) and appears to be related to the deep soft tissues (eg, fascial and muscle layers) of the incision.[a]
	and at least one of the following:
	1. Purulent drainage from the deep incision but not from the organ/space component of the surgical site
	2. A deep incision spontaneously dehisces or is deliberately left open by a surgeon when the patient has at least one of the following signs or symptoms: fever, localized pain, or tenderness, unless site is culture-negative
	3. An abscess or other evidence of infection involving the deep incision is found on direct examination, during reoperation, or by histopathologic or radiographic examination
	4. Diagnosis of a deep incisional SSI by a surgeon or attending clinician
	[a]*Infections that involve both superficial and deep incision sites and organ/space infections that drain through the incision are reported as deep incisional SSI.*
Organ/Space	Infection occurs within 30 days after operation (within 1 year if implant is left in place) and involves any part of the anatomy (eg, organs or spaces), other than the incision, which was opened or manipulated during an operation *and*
	at least one of the following:
	1. Purulent drainage from a drain that is placed through a stab wound into the organ/space
	2. Organisms isolated from an aseptically obtained culture of fluid or tissue in the organ/space
	3. An abscess or other evidence of infection involving the organ/space that is found on direct examination, during reoperation, or by histopathologic or radiologic examination
	4. Diagnosis of an organ/space SSI by a surgeon or attending clinician

Adapted from Mangram AJ, Horan TC, Pearson ML, et al. Guideline for prevention of surgical site infection, 1999. Hospital Infection Control Practices Advisory Committee. Infect Control Hosp Epidemiol 1999;20(4):250–78, with permission.

Stratification of SSI risk according to patient status or comorbidity has not been well evaluated in veterinarian medicine but is likely to be similarly important. A list of risk factors for SSI development in humans is depicted in **Box 1**.[17] The influence of specific comorbidities on SSI in veterinary patients is uncertain.

Table 2 Wound classification	
Clean	Nontraumatic, uninfected operative wounds that involve only integumentary and musculoskeletal soft tissues
Clean-contaminated	Operative wounds in which a hollow viscus (including the gastrointestinal, genitourinary, and respiratory tracts) is opened under controlled circumstances (eg, routine enterotomy, cystotomy)
Contaminated	Bacteria have been extensively introduced into a normally sterile body cavity, but for a period of time too brief to allow infection to become established during surgery (e.g. acute penetrating abdominal injury, major breach in asepsis during bowel surgery)
Dirty	Surgery is performed to control established infection (eg, peritonitis due to enterotomy dehiscence, total ear canal ablation)

Data from Barie PS, Eachempati SR. Surgical site infections. Surg Clin North Am 2005;85(6):1115–35, viii–ix.

Finally, environmental and procedural factors play an important role in SSI risk (see **Box 1**). In veterinary medicine, procedural factors associated with SSI include prolonged anesthetic and surgical time, student surgeon, lack of appropriate AMP, clipping hair prior to induction, numbers of people in the operating room, duration of hospitalization, drain placement, and early suture removal.[2,4,5] These factors increase SSI risk through increasing wound contamination, reducing host resistance to infection, or both.

STRATEGIES FOR SSI PREVENTION

Due to the morbidity and expense associated with SSI development, preventive strategies are strongly emphasized. Few of the preventive measures discussed later have been validated in veterinary surgery but are adapted from best practice recommendations in the human medical field based on variable levels of evidence.[1] A scoring system can be used to categorize the strength of each recommendation, with category IA representing the strongest recommendation and less substantiated risks being assigned a category of "unresolved issue" (**Box 2**). In the discussion below, this scoring system will be used to identify the strength of the recommendation for several risk factors of SSI, allowing the reader to understand the relative contribution of each recommendation.

Table 3 SSI rates by wound classification	
Classification	**Infection Rates**
Clean	2.5%[a]; 2.0%–4.9%[b]
Clean-contaminated	4.5%[a]; 3.5%–4.5%[b]
Contaminated	5.8%[a]; 4.6%–9.1%[b]
Dirty	18.1%[a]; 6.7%–17.8%[b]

[a] Vasseur and colleagues 1988.[4]
[b] Eugster and colleagues 2004.[2]

Table 4	
American Society of Anesthesiology (ASA) physical status classification system	
ASA 1	A normal, healthy patient
ASA 2	A patient with mild systemic disease
ASA 3	A patient with severe systemic disease
ASA 4	A patient with severe systemic disease that is a constant threat to life
ASA 5	A moribund patient who is not expected to survive without the operation
ASA 6	A declared brain-dead patient whose organs are being removed for donor purposes

Data from American Society of Anesthesiologists. ASA Physical Status Classification. Available at: http://www.asahq.org/. Accessed January 25, 2011.

Preoperative Measures

Patient preparation

Before surgery, the patient should be examined for evidence of bacterial infection, including evaluation of the skin and urinary tract, and surgery postponed pending resolution of infection if possible (IA).[1] Uncontrolled disease states such as diabetes mellitus (IB) or hyperadrenocorticism, obesity, malnutrition, anemia (IB), parasitism, and hypovolemia should be addressed to the extent feasible prior to surgery.[1] The enhancement of nutritional support or discontinuation of systemic corticosteroids solely as a means of preventing SSI is controversial.[1] Bathing of human surgical patients with an antiseptic agent 24 hours prior to surgery has been recommended (IB), but the effects of presurgical bathing are uncertain in veterinary patients. If significant soiling of the coat or evidence of ectoparasitism is present, preoperative bathing and/or treatment with an appropriate insecticide is advisable. Care should be taken to ensure complete drying of densely haired patients to prevent skin irritation.

Hair removal should be performed with clean, appropriately serviced clippers after anesthetic induction and immediately before the surgical procedure (IA).[1,5,21] Clipping prior to anesthetic induction has been associated with higher rates of SSI in dogs.[5] Following hair removal, the incision site should be thoroughly washed to remove gross contamination prior to antiseptic skin preparation (IB).[1] After removing gross contamination, an appropriate antiseptic should be used for final aseptic skin preparation (IB), with the antiseptic applied in concentric circles moving toward the periphery of the prepared area (II).[1]

Preparation of surgical team

Members of the surgical team should keep nails short and avoid the use of artificial nails (IB).[1] Nail polish and jewelry should also be removed (unresolved issue and category II, respectively).[1] Prior to aseptic preparation, hands and arms should be washed with a nonmedicated soap and water to remove gross debris. Subungual areas should be cleaned with a nail file.[1] Hands and forearms up to the elbows should be treated with an appropriate aqueous scrub for 2 to 5 minutes, with care taken to keep hands away from the body and above the elbows before gown and gloves are donned (IB).[1] The use of brushes is discouraged, as aqueous scrubbing with the sponge only is equally effective and potentially less damaging to the skin.[22] Recontamination of the hands during rinsing if taps are contaminated with bacteria (*Pseudomonas* spp, in particular) has been raised as a potential limitation of aqueous scrub use.[22] Though the antiseptic used for surgical hand preparation remains an

---

Box 1
Risk factors for SSI development

Patient factors:

Ascites

Chronic inflammation

Corticosteroid therapy (controversial)

Obesity

Diabetes

Extremes of age

Hypocholesterolemia

Hypoxemia

Peripheral vascular disease

Postoperative anemia

Prior site irradiation

Recent operation

Remote infection

Skin carriage of staphylococci

Skin disease in the area of incision

Undernutrition

Environmental factors:

Contaminated medications

Inadequate disinfection/sterilization

Inadequate skin antisepsis

Inadequate ventilation

Treatment factors:

Drains

Emergency procedure

Hypothermia

Inadequate antibiotic prophylaxis

Oxygenation (controversial)

Prolonged preoperative hospitalization

Prolonged operative time

Adapted from Barie PS, Eachempati SR. Surgical site infections. Surg Clin North Am 2005;85(6): 1115-35; with permission.

---

area of surgeon preference, chlorhexidine gluconate has been shown to be superior to povidone-iodine in the prevention of SSI associated with clean-contaminated surgery.[23]

Alcohol-based surgical hand rubs have been introduced as an antiseptic alternative to traditional aqueous scrubs. Compared to alcohol-based scrubs, aqueous scrubs

---

Box 2
Strength of recommendation

Category IA: Strongly recommended for implementation and supported by well-designed experimental, clinical, or epidemiological studies

Category IB: Strongly recommended for implementation and supported by some experimental, clinical, or epidemiological studies and strong theoretical rationale

Category II: Suggested for implementation and supported by suggestive clinical or epidemiological studies or theoretical rationale

No recommendation; unresolved issue: Practices for which insufficient evidence or no consensus regarding efficacy exists

Data from Mangram AJ, Horan TC, Pearson ML, et al. Guideline for prevention of surgical site infection, 1999. Hospital Infection Control Practices Advisory Committee. Infect Control Hosp Epidemiol 1999;20(4):250–78.

---

are associated with more skin irritation and dermatitis, which may result in greater bacterial carriage on the skin.[22] In addition, alcohol-based rubs have overall *greater* antimicrobial efficacy than currently available aqueous scrubs.[22] The combination of alcohols with long-acting compounds such as chlorhexidine gluconate or hexachlorophene limit bacterial regrowth on gloved hands, though the degree of initial reduction of skin flora after alcohol application is sufficient to prevent bacterial regrowth to baseline for over 6 hours.[22] Hands should be free of gross debris and dry prior to application of an approved hand rub that is labeled for operative use.[22]

The goal of surgical hand preparation is to reduce the release of skin bacteria from the hands of the surgical team in case of glove puncture. Surgical gloves become punctured in up to 35% of cases after 2 hours of surgery and 80% of glove punctures are not noted by the surgeon.[22,24] Perforation of surgical gloves increases the risk of SSI, particularly in patients not receiving AMP.[25] The high prevalence of MDR bacteria on the hands of medical professionals, including veterinary surgeons, makes prevention of transmission of skin bacteria to the surgical wound particularly important.[26] Methicillin-resistant *Staphylococcus aureus* (MRSA) outbreaks in veterinary patients have been associated with colonized surgeons and staff.[27,28] The management of surgical personnel who are carriers of MDR bacteria remains controversial, but current recommendations do *not* support their exclusion unless they have been linked epidemiologically to dissemination of the organism in a clinical setting (IB).[1] Surgical team members with draining skin lesions should be cultured and excluded from duty until the infection has been resolved (IB).[1]

Antimicrobial use

The NNIS recommends that a prophylactic antimicrobial agent be administered only when indicated and selected based on efficacy against the most common pathogens causing SSI for a specific operation and in light of published recommendations (IA)."[1] AMP should be administered intravenously such that bactericidal concentrations are achieved in serum and tissues when the incision is made and maintained at therapeutic levels throughout surgery until at most a few hours after wound closure in the operating theater (IA).[1] Antimicrobial drug protocols for AMP in veterinary patients have been described.[29]

The appropriate use of AMP in clean veterinary orthopedic surgery has been researched more thoroughly than for other surgery types, though conclusions of such studies are occasionally conflicting.[3,6,8] Vasseur et al did not identify a difference in SSI rates among clean, largely orthopedic procedures with and without perioperative ampicillin administration.[3] This prospective study included only procedures completed within 90 minutes with no breaks in aseptic technique and performed by two experienced surgeons.[3] A later retrospective study by Vasseur et al found a significantly lower SSI rate in patients receiving AMP for clean procedures, but the benefits of AMP were not observed in procedures less than 90 minutes in duration or performed by a surgeon or resident.[4] In a second prospective study comparing the efficacy of two AMP protocols vs. placebo on reducing SSI rates in clean orthopedic surgery, Whittem et al found a significantly higher SSI rate in dogs receiving placebo (15.6%) when compared with dogs receiving penicillin G (2.6%) and cefazolin (4.9%).[6] Indications for AMP have not been significantly evaluated for clean soft tissue procedures.

The use of postoperative antibiotics for clean procedures is not supported by the human medical literature, though its use in veterinary surgery, particularly following orthopedic procedures, is commonplace.[1,30,31] Two recent retrospective studies evaluating SSI rates after tibial plateau-leveling osteotomy (TPLO) have described relatively high overall SSI rates (6.1% and 6.6%),with postoperative antibiotic administration associated with significant reductions in SSI occurrence.[30,31] Because of the retrospective nature of these studies, it is uncertain whether postoperative antibiotic administration truly prevented infection or reduced the identification of SSI in the postoperative period. Concerns with postoperative antimicrobial administration are its limited benefit in the prevention of SSI paired with increased risk of the development of MDR pathogens.[17,32] Careful study of the risks vs true benefits of postoperative antibiotic administration are indicated before the prophylactic use of postoperative antibiotics in clean and clean-contaminated procedures is recommended.

Because of a lack of clear guidelines for AMP in veterinary surgery, the following recommendations based on current practice and the human medical literature are proposed: (1) Clean procedures: AMP should be considered where bone is incised, a prosthesis inserted, where infection would be considered catastrophic, for high-risk patients (a poorly defined category in veterinary medicine), or when surgery is expected to be more than 90 minutes in duration.[29] Such therapy should be instituted within 60 minutes of the onset of surgery, with re-dosing intraoperatively as indicated by the antibiotic used.[17,29,33] Antibiotic therapy should be discontinued no more than 12 to 24 hours postoperatively. (2) Clean-contaminated procedures: AMP is indicated, with the drug administered selected based on the expected flora of the site of contamination (gastrointestinal tract, urogenital tract, etc).[29] The same guidelines for dosing onset and treatment duration for clean surgery apply. (3) Contaminated procedures: same general guidelines as for clean-contaminated procedures apply. If existing infection or purulent exudate is suspected at the time of surgery, the procedure should be considered dirty and therapeutic rather than prophylactic antimicrobial therapy used. (4) Dirty procedures: broad-spectrum antibiotic therapy appropriate for likely pathogens should be administered before surgery and continued into the postoperative period until culture and sensitivity results allow narrowing of the antimicrobial spectrum.[29] The acquisition of samples for culture and sensitivity ideally occurs before antibiotic therapy is commenced, but such therapy should not be empirically withheld from patients prior to surgery, particularly if they are exhibiting signs of sepsis or systemic inflammatory response syndrome. The author recognizes that these recommendations are both derivative and dogmatic, and strongly promotes the further study of AMP in veterinary surgery.

Intraoperative Measures

Asepsis in the operating room

Issues related to hospital design (including surgical suites and isolation) and cleaning and disinfection protocols have been recently reviewed and will not be extensively discussed in this chapter.[1,34,35] The importance of proper operating room design and management and of effective equipment sterilization protocols in limiting SSI is emphasized (IB).[1] Proper surgical attire, including a surgical mask, cap, or hood to fully cover hair on the head and face, and a clean scrub suit should be worn by all persons in the operating room (IB).[1] Shoe covers are not recommended for the prevention of SSI.[1] The risk of SSI has been reported to increase by 1.3 times with each additional person in the operating room.[2] Relatively large numbers of observers are common during surgical procedures at veterinary teaching hospitals. To facilitate operative instruction while maintaining optimal patient safety, consideration should be given to the installation of audiovisual recording equipment.[36]

All surgical team members should wear sterile gloves put on after donning a surgery gown (IB).[1] The type of surgical glove used is at the surgeon's preference. Due to the prevalence of surgical glove perforation during surgery and the association of glove perforation with SSI in some circumstances, consideration should be given to regular glove changes, particularly during long procedures.[24,25] Double-gloving has also been shown to reduce the incidence of SSI in joint replacement surgery and holes in the inner glove.[24]

Surgical gowns and drapes should be used routinely and should serve as an effective barrier when wet (IB).[1] Considerable controversy exists regarding the appropriateness of reusable cloth gowns and drapes vs. their single-use counterparts. In general, reusable cloth gowns and drapes are less effective barriers against fluid and bacterial translocation than single-use non-woven drapes.[37,38] In addition, there is significant variability between the barrier properties of reusable gowns and the effects of repeated laundering on the maintenance of those properties.[39] Despite clear differences in experimental permeability, the association of reusable cloth gown and drape use with increased SSI rates is not well-established.[40] The author recommends that any reusable gowns and drapes be well-maintained and that launderings be tracked to allow identification and retirement of gowns and drapes when recommended by the manufacturer. The use of an impermeable barrier (appropriate single-use, nonwoven material) should be incorporated into the patient's drapes for all major procedures due to the inadequacy of woven drapes to resist bacterial translocation when damp. The use of single-use gowns, if not routine, should be considered for surgeries that demand exceptional levels of asepsis, such as total joint arthroplasty, and in procedures expected to involve a significant amount of fluid (e.g. celiotomy for septic abdomen). Distal limb wraps for extremity surgery should include a sterile, impermeable barrier to prevent bacterial strike-through.[41]

The use of adhesive incise drapes has been promoted in human and veterinary surgery as a means of reducing incisional contamination from skin microflora.[42,43] Such drapes create a semi-occlusive barrier that allows passage of gases and moisture while preventing bacterial translocation. Some incise drapes have been impregnated with iodophors to decrease bacterial populations beneath the drape.[42,43] Veterinary and human studies of incise drapes have failed to demonstrate a significant reduction in SSI rates over conventional draping techniques, with some human studies suggesting that they may increase infection rates.[42,44] In addition, adherence of incise drapes to the edges of the incision was inconsistent in one veterinary report.[42] Cyanoacrylate-based microbial sealants have been introduced as an alternative means of blocking transfer of skin bacteria to the surgical wound.[43,45] Though use of these preparations has not been evaluated in veterinary patients, human reports suggest that they are more effective than traditional skin antisepsis/ draping or incise drapes at reducing wound contamination.[43,45] These preparations merit further investigation in veterinary patients.

Surgical technique

Surgeons are able to make the surgical site less favorable to bacterial colonization by adhering to careful technique. Tissue should be handled gently, effective hemostasis maintained, devitalized tissue removed, and dead space closed (IB).[1,46] Foreign bodies, including implants, synthetic mesh, suture, and charred tissue, should be minimized in the surgical wound, as they significantly decrease the wound's resistance to infection (IB).[46] Closed suction drains are preferred when drainage is necessary, with the drain tube placed through a separate incision distant from the operative incision (IB).[1] Drains should be removed as soon as possible (IB).[1] The use of drains has been associated with increased SSI incidence in veterinary patients.[2]

Suture is the most common synthetic material left behind in surgical wounds. Pathogenic bacteria, including *S aureus,* have been demonstrated to form biofilms, defined as extracellular polymeric substances composed of proteins, lipids, polysaccharides, and extracellular DNA that enclose bacteria and make their elimination very difficult.[47] Such biofilms have been shown to form on suture, with bacterial growth favored on braided *vs.* monofilament suture.[47] Reduction of the susceptibility of a surgical wound to bacterial infection can be facilitated by avoiding nonabsorbable and multifilament sutures.[47] Inappropriately large suture and excessively large or numerous knots should be avoided. The use of triclosan-coated sutures may be another means of decreasing suture-associated infection.[48]

Clean and clean-contaminated wounds can be closed primarily. The optimal closure strategy for contaminated wounds is controversial in human surgery and is likely dependent on factors other than wound classification alone.[17] If the incision is significantly contaminated, the surgeon should consider a delayed primary closure to ensure optimal drainage in the immediate postoperative period.[17] Infected or "dirty" wounds should be managed open and allowed to heal by second intention or until the establishment of a healthy wound bed that can be secondarily closed. In veterinary medicine, septic peritonitis can be successfully managed through open abdominal drainage or primary fascial closure with or without the placement of closed-suction drains.[49–51] Incisional closure with skin staples has been associated with higher incidence of SSI in one small animal report.[31]

Patient care

Maintenance of normal core body temperature is an important factor in decreasing SSI incidence in humans, though hypothermia has not been identified as a risk factor in veterinary patients.[5,17] The effects of perioperative hypothermia on surgical patients have been reviewed.[52] Maintenance of normothermia can be accomplished through the use of active surface rewarming, including circulating water blankets and forced air warming blankets.[52] The use of forced air warming blankets was not associated with increased wound contamination in one study.[53] Active core rewarming through pleural or peritoneal lavage should be considered when significant hypothermia is present. Because of the efficiency of pleural and peritoneal lavage in altering core body temperature, any lavage fluids used intraoperatively should be warmed to 104° to 109°F (40–43°C) to allow rewarming.[52] The use of cool or room-temperature lavage on pleural and peritoneal surfaces is avoided.

Prolonged anesthesia alone (independent of surgery length) has been associated with increased SSI risk in veterinary patients.[2,5] The significance of this finding is uncertain, but may relate to impairment of the host immune response by prolonged exposure to anesthetic drugs.[5] The risk associated with prolonged anesthesia should be considered in patients undergoing extensive preoperative diagnostics and efforts made to minimize overall anesthesia time. Other factors in operative patient care that may improve host defenses include appropriate volume replacement, the administration of supplemental oxygen, and administration of appropriate analgesia.[54]

Postoperative care

The incision should be protected by a sterile dressing for 24 to 48 hours if it has been closed primarily (IB).[1] Wound coverage beyond this period is not of demonstrated benefit, and may make monitoring of the incision for signs of inflammation more difficult.[8] Caretakers should wash hands before and after dressing changes and any contact with the surgical site (IB).[1] The use of disposable, nonsterile examination gloves is recommended when handling surgical wounds and patients known or suspected to have an SSI. Because the duration of hospitalization is associated with increased risk of MDR infection, preoperative and postoperative hospitalization should be minimized.[11]

Surveillance

The development and implementation of a hospital infection control program is important to establish policies regarding antimicrobial use, monitor the incidence and resistance patterns of nosocomial pathogens, promote and enforce hand-washing/hygiene protocols, and establish protocols for isolation of patients with nosocomial and MDR infections.[8,55] A comprehensive discussion of such a protocol is beyond the scope of this chapter. As a more targeted policy intervention, the use of surgical safety checklists to minimize surgical complications has been recently advocated in the human field.[56] The use of checklists decreased the overall complication rate in patients undergoing noncardiac surgery in a multi-institutional, international study from 18.4% to 11.7% in one study.[56]

MANAGEMENT OF SSIs

Clear guidelines for SSI management are lacking (in marked contrast to the plethora of data regarding preventive strategies), but general principles of management are described in **Box 3**.[17,57] Infections limited to mild incisional cellulitis without evidence of a wound abscess or deeper extension of infection may be amenable to oral antibiotic therapy alone.[18]

MULTIDRUG-RESISTANT PATHOGENS IN SURGICAL SITE INFECTIONS

Mechanisms of antimicrobial resistance in small animal veterinary patients and considerations related to MDR SSI have been recently reviewed.[32,58,59] Information regarding antimicrobial selection for some commonly identified MDR pathogens is reviewed below.

MRSA

MRSA is an important human pathogen that is becoming increasingly recognized in veterinary patients. MRSA strains possess an altered penicillin-binding protein that

---

Box 3
Principles of SSI management

1. Open the incision and débride necrotic fat, skin, and fascia as needed. Determine if the incision extends into any body cavities involved in the original surgery.

2. Address the source of contamination, if ongoing (eg, dehiscence of enterotomy incision).

3. Obtain samples of tissue or aseptically collected fluid (exudate) for aerobic and anaerobic culture.

4. Manage the wound with an appropriate dressing (wet-to-dry gauze, negative-pressure wound therapy, or other), with regular dressing changes to monitor wound progress.

5. Antimicrobial therapy may not be indicated in all instances, but should be guided by culture and sensitivity results and instituted when there is evidence of cellulitis, fever, or leukocytosis. Initial therapy should be broad-spectrum and accommodate pathogens likely to be associated with the original procedure.

6. Implant removal should be considered if involved in the SSI, particularly if not functionally important (eg, bone plate on healed fracture).

7. Close or reconstruct the incision after a healthy wound bed has been re-established and culture results known *or* allow to heal by second intention.

---

confers resistance to all β-lactam antibiotics, including all penicillins, carbapenems, and cephalosporins.[59] Treatment should be based on the results of culture and sensitivity, with some caveats. Fluoroquinolones should be avoided due to poor prediction of in vivo response from in vitro susceptibility and rapid development of resistance.[58] Chloramphenicol is often an option, though side effects and consequences of human exposure should be considered. Trimethoprim-sulfas and aminoglycosides (amikacin) may also be useful, provided diligent monitoring for side effects and renal damage is performed.[58] Vancomycin is commonly used to treat MRSA infections in humans, which has led to the development of vancomycin-resistant forms (VRSA).[32] The use of vancomycin in veterinary patients is voluntarily restricted at many institutions to help preserve its effectiveness. When MRSA infection is identified, infection control precautions and client counseling are important to limit its spread to humans and other animals.[28] MRSA infection has not been found to be more likely to result in significant morbidity and mortality than methicillin-susceptible *S. aureus* infections in dogs.[12]

Other Methicillin-Resistant Staphylococci

Methicillin resistance has also been reported in *Staphylococcus pseudintermedius*, *Staphylococcus schleiferi coagulans*, and coagulase-negative staphylococci. Treatment strategies are similar for these isolates as for MRSA, with less concern about zoonotic transmission.[58]

Enterococci

These gram-positive bacteria are common opportunistic pathogens in which antimicrobial resistance is very common. Enterococci are inherently resistant to all cephalosporins, some penicillins, clindamycin, and trimethoprim.[58] Vancomycin-resistant enterococci (VRE) are an emerging concern. Treatment with ampicillin alone or with aminoglycosides (provided that high aminoglycoside minimum inhibitory concentrations are not needed) can be successful in many cases.[58] Chloramphenicol may also be considered.[58] Because enterococci tend to persist in the environment, attention to adequate environmental disinfection protocols and barrier precautions is important.

Pseudomonas

Pseudomonas spp are common opportunistic pathogens, due in part to their ability to persist in the environment and their resistance to many antiseptics. *Pseudomonas,* like *Staphylococcus*, produces biofilms that can make elimination of infection from an implant difficult. There is good agreement between in vivo and in vitro susceptibility results for *Pseudomonas*. Resistance to fluoroquinolones is relatively common, but susceptibility to aminoglycosides is often present.[58]

SUMMARY

SSIs represent a significant source of morbidity, mortality, and cost associated with small animal surgery. The most well-established and effective strategies to reduce the impact of SSIs are preventive and focus on bolstering host immunity to infection and decreasing the degree of wound contamination during surgery. When SSI is identified, the use of consistent definitions and culture-based therapy help to facilitate surveillance efforts. For SSIs more severe than mild cellulitis of the immediate incisional area, débridement and open wound management are important keys to successful treatment. The selection of antibiotics to treat SSIs should be based on bacterial culture, particularly due to the increasing incidence of MDR-resistant pathogens in veterinary patients.

REFERENCES

1. Mangram AJ, Horan TC, Pearson ML, et al. Guideline for prevention of surgical site infection, 1999. Hospital Infection Control Practices Advisory Committee. Infect Control Hosp Epidemiol 1999;20(4):250–78 [quiz: 279–80].
2. Eugster S, Schawalder P, Gaschen F, et al. A prospective study of postoperative surgical site infections in dogs and cats. Vet Surg 2004;33(5):542–50.
3. Vasseur PB, Paul HA, Enos LR, et al. Infection rates in clean surgical procedures: a comparison of ampicillin prophylaxis vs a placebo. J Am Vet Med Assoc 1985;187(8): 825–7.
4. Vasseur PB, Levy J, Dowd E, et al. Surgical wound infection rates in dogs and cats. Data from a teaching hospital. Vet Surg 1988;17(2):60–4.
5. Beal MW, Brown DC, Shofer FS. The effects of perioperative hypothermia and the duration of anesthesia on postoperative wound infection rate in clean wounds: a retrospective study. Vet Surg 2000;29(2):123–7.
6. Whittem TL, Johnson AL, Smith CW, et al. Effect of perioperative prophylactic antimicrobial treatment in dogs undergoing elective orthopedic surgery. J Am Vet Med Assoc 1999;215(2):212–6.
7. Weese JS, Halling KB. Perioperative administration of antimicrobials associated with elective surgery for cranial cruciate ligament rupture in dogs: 83 cases (2003-2005). J Am Vet Med Assoc 2006;229(1):92–5.
8. Weese JS. A review of post-operative infections in veterinary orthopaedic surgery. Vet Comp Orthop Traumatol 2008;21(2):99–105.
9. Gibson JS, Morton JM, Cobbold RN, et al. Multidrug-resistant E. coli and enterobacter extraintestinal infection in 37 dogs. J Vet Intern Med 2008;22(4):844–50.
10. Weese JS, Faires M, Rousseau J, et al. Cluster of methicillin-resistant Staphylococcus aureus colonization in a small animal intensive care unit. J Am Vet Med Assoc 2007;231(9):1361–4.

11. Ogeer-Gyles J, Mathews KA, Sears W, et al. Development of antimicrobial drug resistance in rectal Escherichia coli isolates from dogs hospitalized in an intensive care unit. J Am Vet Med Assoc 2006;229(5):694–9.

12. Faires MC, Traverse M, Tater KC, et al. Methicillin-resistant and -susceptible Staphylococcus aureus infections in dogs. Emerg Infect Dis 2010;16(1):69–75.

13. Jones RD, Kania SA, Rohrbach BW, et al. Prevalence of oxacillin- and multidrug-resistant staphylococci in clinical samples from dogs: 1,772 samples (2001–2005). J Am Vet Med Assoc 2007;230(2):221–7.

14. Tomlin J, Pead MJ, Lloyd DH, et al. Methicillin-resistant Staphylococcus aureus infections in 11 dogs. Vet Rec 1999;144(3):60–4.

15. Wilson MA. Skin and soft-tissue infections: impact of resistant gram-positive bacteria. Am J Surg 2003;186(5A):35S–41S; discussion 42S–3S, 61S–4S.

16. Cheadle WG. Risk factors for surgical site infection. Surg Infect (Larchmt) 2006; 7(Suppl 1):S7–11.

17. Barie PS, Eachempati SR. Surgical site infections. Surg Clin North Am 2005;85(6): 1115–35, viii–ix.

18. Lazenby GB, Soper DE. Prevention, diagnosis, and treatment of gynecologic surgical site infections. Obstet Gynecol Clin North Am 2010;37(3):379–86.

19. Hedrick TL, Heckman JA, Smith RL, et al. Efficacy of protocol implementation on incidence of wound infection in colorectal operations. J Am Coll Surg 2007;205(3): 432–8.

20. American Society of Anesthesiologists. ASA Physical Status Classification. Available at: http://www.asahq.org/. Accessed January 25, 2011.

21. Brown DC, Conzemius MG, Shofer F, et al. Epidemiologic evaluation of postoperative wound infections in dogs and cats. J Am Vet Med Assoc 1997;210(9):1302–6.

22. Widmer AF, Rotter M, Voss A, et al. Surgical hand preparation: state-of-the-art. J Hosp Infect 2010;74(2):112–22.

23. Noorani A, Rabey N, Walsh SR, et al. Systematic review and meta-analysis of preoperative antisepsis with chlorhexidine versus povidone–iodine in clean-contaminated surgery. Br J Surg 2010;97(11):1614–20.

24. Character BJ, McLaughlin RM, Hedlund CS, et al. Postoperative integrity of veterinary surgical gloves. J Am Anim Hosp Assoc 2003;39(3):311–20.

25. Misteli H, Weber WP, Reck S, et al. Surgical glove perforation and the risk of surgical site infection. Arch Surg 2009;144(6):553–8 [discussion: 558].

26. Burstiner LC, Faires M, Weese JS. Methicillin-resistant Staphylococcus aureus colonization in personnel attending a veterinary surgery conference. Vet Surg 2010;39(2): 150–7.

27. McLean CL, Ness MG. Methicillin-resistant Staphylococcus aureus in a veterinary orthopaedic referral hospital: staff nasal colonisation and incidence of clinical cases. J Small Anim Pract 2008;49(4):170–7.

28. Leonard FC, Abbott Y, Rossney A, et al. Methicillin-resistant Staphylococcus aureus isolated from a veterinary surgeon and five dogs in one practice. Vet Rec 2006;158(5): 155–9.

29. Greene CE. Infectious diseases of the dog and cat. 3rd edition. St. Louis (MO)/ London: Saunders Elsevier; 2006.

30. Fitzpatrick N, Solano MA. Predictive variables for complications after TPLO with stifle inspection by arthrotomy in 1000 consecutive dogs. Vet Surg 2010;39(4):460–74.

31. Frey TN, Hoelzler MG, Scavelli TD, et al. Risk factors for surgical site infection-inflammation in dogs undergoing surgery for rupture of the cranial cruciate ligament: 902 cases (2005–2006). J Am Vet Med Assoc 2010;236(1):88–94.

32. Tenover FC. Mechanisms of antimicrobial resistance in bacteria. Am J Med 2006; 119(6 Suppl 1):S3–10 [discussion S62–70].

33. Marcellin-Little DJ, Papich MG, Richardson DC, et al. Pharmacokinetic model for cefazolin distribution during total hip arthroplasty in dogs. Am J Vet Res 1996;57(5): 720–3.

34. Portner J, Johnson J. Guidelines for reducing pathogens in veterinary hospitals: disinfectant selection, cleaning protocols, and hand hygiene. Compend Contin Educ Vet 2010;32(5):E1–12.

35. Portner J, Johnson J. Guidelines for reducing pathogens in veterinary hospitals: hospital design and special considerations. Compend Contin Educ Vet 2010;32(5): E1–8.

36. Cosman PH, Shearer CJ, Hugh TJ, et al. A novel approach to high definition, high-contrast video capture in abdominal surgery. Ann Surg 2007;245(4):533–5.

37. Blom A, Estela C, Bowker K, et al. The passage of bacteria through surgical drapes. Ann R Coll Surg Engl 2000;82(6):405–7.

38. Blom AW, Gozzard C, Heal J, et al. Bacterial strike-through of re-usable surgical drapes: the effect of different wetting agents. J Hosp Infect 2002;52(1):52–5.

39. Leonas KK. Effect of laundering on the barrier properties of reusable surgical gown fabrics. Am J Infect Control 1998;26(5):495–501.

40. Rutala WA, Weber DJ. A review of single-use and reusable gowns and drapes in health care. Infect Control Hosp Epidemiol 2001;22(4):248–57.

41. Vince KJ, Lascelles BD, Mathews KG, et al. Evaluation of wraps covering the distal aspect of pelvic limbs for prevention of bacterial strike-through in an ex vivo canine model. Vet Surg 2008;37(4):406–11.

42. Owen LJ, Gines JA, Knowles TG, et al. Efficacy of adhesive incise drapes in preventing bacterial contamination of clean canine surgical wounds. Vet Surg 2009;38(6):732–7.

43. Bady S, Wongworawat MD. Effectiveness of antimicrobial incise drapes versus cyanoacrylate barrier preparations for surgical sites. Clin Orthop Relat Res 2009; 467(7):1674–7.

44. Webster J, Alghamdi AA. Use of plastic adhesive drapes during surgery for preventing surgical site infection. Cochrane Database Syst Rev 2007;4:CD006353.

45. Wilson SE. Microbial sealing: a new approach to reducing contamination. J Hosp Infect 2008;70(Suppl 2):11–4.

46. Heinzelmann M, Scott M, Lam T. Factors predisposing to bacterial invasion and infection. Am J Surg 2002;183(2):179–90.

47. Henry-Stanley MJ, Hess DJ, Barnes AM, et al. Bacterial contamination of surgical suture resembles a biofilm. Surg Infect (Larchmt) 2010;11(5):433–9.

48. Edmiston CE, Seabrook GR, Goheen MP, et al. Bacterial adherence to surgical sutures: can antibacterial-coated sutures reduce the risk of microbial contamination? J Am Coll Surg 2006;203(4):481–9.

49. Mueller MG, Ludwig LL, Barton LJ. Use of closed-suction drains to treat generalized peritonitis in dogs and cats: 40 cases (1997–1999). J Am Vet Med Assoc 2001; 219(6):789–94.

50. Lanz OI, Ellison GW, Bellah JR, et al. Surgical treatment of septic peritonitis without abdominal drainage in 28 dogs. J Am Anim Hosp Assoc 2001;37(1):87–92.

51. Staatz AJ, Monnet E, Seim HB 3rd. Open peritoneal drainage versus primary closure for the treatment of septic peritonitis in dogs and cats: 42 cases (1993–1999). Vet Surg 2002;31(2):174–80.

52. Armstrong SR, Roberts BK, Aronsohn M. Perioperative hypothermia. J Vet Emerg Crit Care 2005;15(1):32–5.

53. Huang JK, Shah EF, Vinodkumar N, et al. The Bair Hugger patient warming system in prolonged vascular surgery: an infection risk? Crit Care 2003;7(3):R13–6.
54. Sessler DI. Non-pharmacologic prevention of surgical wound infection. Anesthesiol Clin 2006;24(2):279–97.
55. Weese JS. Investigation of antimicrobial use and the impact of antimicrobial use guidelines in a small animal veterinary teaching hospital: 1995–2004. J Am Vet Med Assoc 2006;228(4):553–8.
56. Weiser TG, Haynes AB, Dziekan G, et al. Effect of a 19-item surgical safety checklist during urgent operations in a global patient population. Ann Surg 2010;251(5):976–80.
57. Stevens DL. Treatments for skin and soft-tissue and surgical site infections due to MDR Gram-positive bacteria. J Infect 2009;59(Suppl 1):S32–9.
58. Weese JS. A review of multidrug resistant surgical site infections. Vet Comp Orthop Traumatol 2008;21(1):1–7.
59. Umber JK, Bender JB. Pets and antimicrobial resistance. Vet Clin North Am Small Anim Pract 2009;39(2):279–92.

Index

Note: Page numbers of article titles are in **boldface** type.

Vet Clin Small Anim 41 (2011) 1057–1068
doi:10.1016/S0195-5616(11)00130-6
0195-5616/11/$ – see front matter © 2011 Elsevier Inc. All rights reserved.

vetsmall.theclinics.com

Moving?

Make sure your subscription moves with you!

To notify us of your new address, find your **Clinics Account Number** (located on your mailing label above your name), and contact customer service at:

Email: journalscustomerservice-usa@elsevier.com

800-654-2452 (subscribers in the U.S. & Canada)
314-447-8871 (subscribers outside of the U.S. & Canada)

Fax number: 314-447-8029

Elsevier Health Sciences Division
Subscription Customer Service
3251 Riverport Lane
Maryland Heights, MO 63043

*To ensure uninterrupted delivery of your subscription, please notify us at least 4 weeks in advance of move.